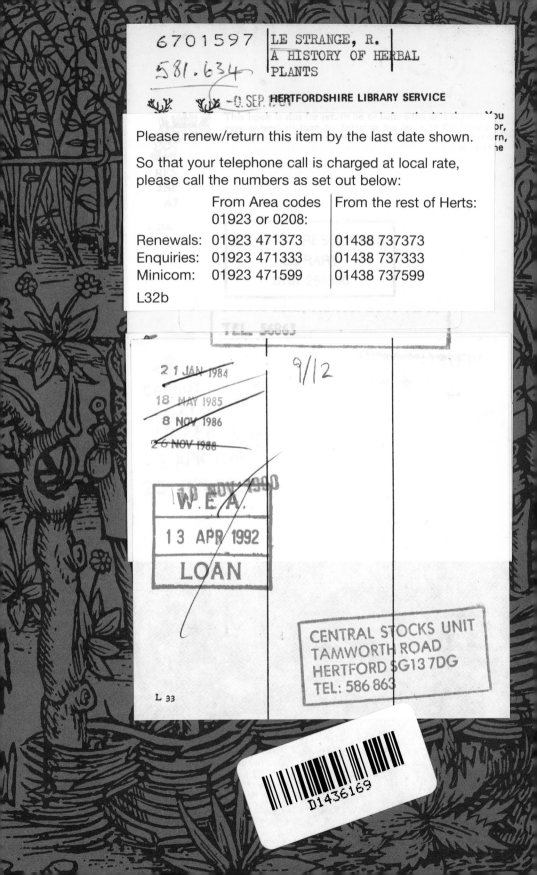

A History of
Herbal Plants

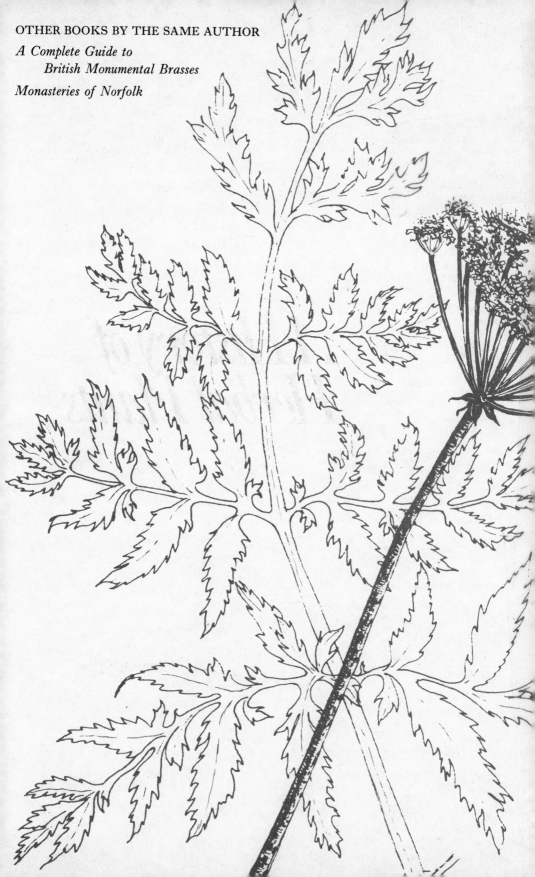

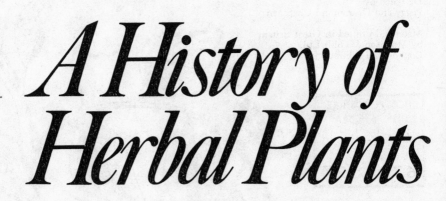

A History of
Herbal Plants

Richard le Strange
Illustrated by Derek Cork

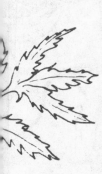

Foreword by Anthony Huxley

ANGUS AND ROBERTSON·PUBLISHERS

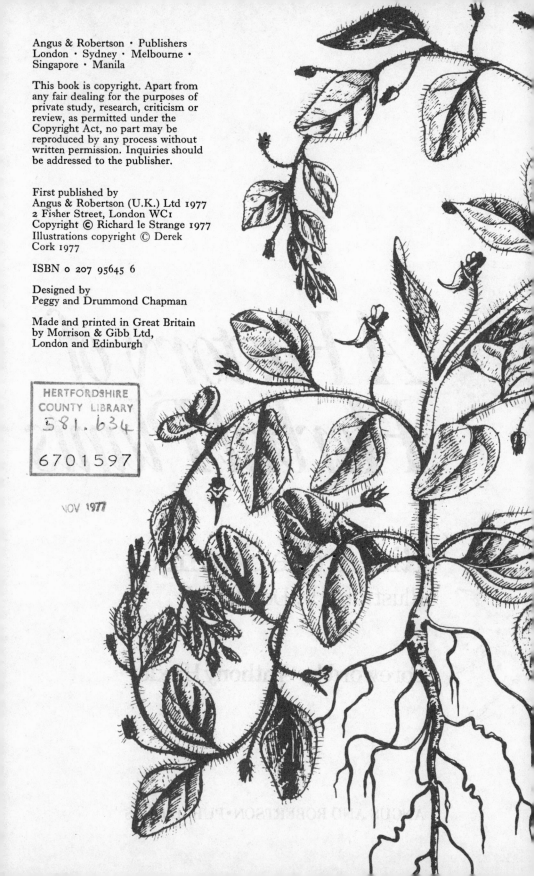

Angus & Robertson · Publishers
London · Sydney · Melbourne ·
Singapore · Manila

First published by
Angus & Robertson (U.K.) Ltd 1977
2 Fisher Street, London WC1
Copyright © Richard le Strange 1977
Illustrations copyright © Derek
Cork 1977

ISBN 0 207 95645 6

Designed by
Peggy and Drummond Chapman

Made and printed in Great Britain
by Morrison & Gibb Ltd,
London and Edinburgh

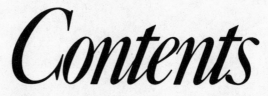

Contents

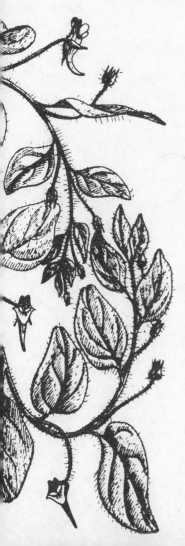

Acknowledgements

I should like to thank the library and other staff of the University of East Anglia and the John Innes Institute, Norwich, and the Librarian of Kew Gardens for help in the course of research for this book. I would especially like to thank Mrs Elizabeth Atchison, the Librarian of the John Innes Institute, for allowing me to make use of their library, and for access to the numerous herbals and medicinal books housed in the 'special collection' there.

To Liz, for typing the manuscript

Foreword

The world of plants has been vital to mankind since intelligence began to glimmer. Branches and leaves sheltered early man, burning wood warmed him, fruits, seeds and roots fed him. Gradually, by a process of trial and error which must have caused many a fatality, he sorted out plants he could eat and those he could not, and gradually also discovered certain qualities beyond mere edibility – pain-killing, soothing, relief of fevers, help with sleep.

The earliest records of such beneficial plants appear to be nearly 5000 years old, in a Chinese Pharmacopoeia. The ancient Sumerians recorded around a thousand medicinal plants over 4000 years ago, and succeeding civilisations all had their herbal experts, or doctors, who could help their fellows in adversity.

There are, of course, innumerable other uses of plants, but the possibilities for healing or harm with which 'herbs' were endowed most touched man's essentially superstitious nature, and it was the collection and study of these diverse plants which formed the basis of botanical knowledge for many centuries.

At the same time another facet of man's nature, that of desiring power over his fellows, endowed some plants with special mythical powers. Priests of early religions began a link between plants and ritual, magic and witchcraft which has not ceased today.

As that famous herbalist Mrs Hilda Leyel once observed, 'botany and medicine came down the ages hand in hand until the seventeenth century; then both arts became scientific, their ways parted . . . The botanical books ignored the medicinal properties of plants and the medical books contained no plant lore.' Mrs M. Grieve's massive *A Modern Herbal*, which Mrs Leyel put into book form, was the only real twentieth century attempt to collect together all the viable information on the subject, and this present volume is a worthy successor, in a somewhat different style. Where, in my view,

it improves on Mrs Grieve – and indeed on most books written by out and out herbalists – is in the sorting out of real medicinal values from imagined ones which have accrued over centuries of witchcraft, folk use, and through the 'doctrine of signatures', whereby the resemblance of a plant to a part of the body decreed its medical potential, often with no real basis.

In this study, Richard le Strange brings in botany, history and folk lore, and makes good and entertaining use of quotations from herbal writers from Dioscorides onwards. Man's ingenuity, credulity, and above all, perhaps, his insatiable curiosity, are all displayed in this massive, deeply researched volume which provides anyone interested in plants with a vast mine of unfamiliar material, pleasantly augmented by Derek Cork's numerous line drawings. Where plants have uses beyond herbalism these are mentioned, including flavouring of food, but it is not by any means a culinary handbook. It is rather that marriage of botany and plant-based medicine whose demise Mrs Leyel bemoaned, placed in an up-to-date context.

The 1970s have seen an increasing awareness of the vital part plants have to play in mankind's continued existence on this planet – not just much-manipulated crop plants, but true wild ones, in a few cases still only known through the practices of 'primitive' peoples. At the same time we are pulling the natural vegetation off the skin of the earth in an alarming fashion. At the time of writing, it is estimated that at least 40 per cent of primeval tropical forest has been irremediably destroyed, and with it an unknown host of species potentially valuable to mankind.

It is books like *A History of Herbal Plants* which, I believe, will continue to strengthen awareness of the world of plants, so much taken for granted, yet potentially so beneficial to us all.

Anthony Huxley, 1977.

Introduction

Today it is more for enjoyment than for any practical use that most of us care for the flowers, shrubs and trees growing wild about us. Our ancestors enjoyed them, too, but were also carefully taught from early childhood of their numerous other values, not only as medicinal plants, but as dyes, spices, grains and strewing herbs to mention only a few. Many of these simple uses are now in danger of becoming completely lost. Some indeed have already been long forgotten, as have the plants' common and descriptive names, and the legendary tales, poetry and magical rhymes spun around them.

The employment of plant life by man dates far back in history to the most ancient of times, when, having found that certain plants could be eaten as food, it was discovered the stem fibres of some kinds, such as the Nettle, could be woven into garments, while their juices could be turned into dyes for applying to the hair and body. One of the more familiar species belonging to the latter group is the Woad, which yielded the bluish dye worn by Britain's native warriors when Julius Caesar first invaded their shores in 55 B.C. The dye was probably applied, not only to frighten the Roman soldiers, but to protect against wounds, for Woad certainly helps to stay bleeding by acting as a simple but reliable styptic.

The more attractive and aromatic flowers were also worn on festive occasions and were added, together with a selection of fermented fruits, leaves, seeds and barks, to a variety of intoxicating wines and beers, as man gradually became aware that some of these concoctions brought relief in sickness and eased pain. Evidence that the Poppy was used in this way has been found in some early cave dwellings, where its seed was probably administered for its soporific effects.

Another point that constantly impresses me is that over the centuries every single plant mentioned in the following text, whether poisonous or not, has been sampled for food, or patiently experimented with in an effort to find out about its medicinal use. How many people succumbed to the more virulent sorts before the proper dose was found will never be known – but it was surely many thousands. Nevertheless, these simple cures have continuously and slowly evolved over the centuries from nearly every country in the world. Who, for example, discovered that a Tincture of Opium from the Poppy would stop children's crying, or that the oil from the beans of the Castor Tree, in small amounts, made a reliable purgative, while two or three of the beans themselves if eaten would prove fatal within a few hours; or alternatively that the extracted oil would bring relief when applied to burns and septic wounds, besides making a useful fuel for lamps? Yet both these plants must have been regularly used for these purposes in Egypt around 1500 B.C. since their seed has been excavated from some of the ancient tombs there. Who, even further back in recorded history, discovered that Chaulmoogra Oil from the Hydnocarpus genus of trees was efficacious in the treatment of leprosy? This cure is mentioned in the *Pharmacopoeia* of the Emperor Shen Nung of China, a document dating from between 2730 and 3000 B.C. Who decided that the dose of this bitter-tasting liquid should be 10 to 20 drops after meals, and that it should be applied also to the part affected? The same herbal describes such medicinal plants as the Indian Hemp, Aconite, Opium Poppy, Croton and Rhubarb – plants still commonly prescribed today, besides mentioning many inorganic remedies such as arsenic, sulphur and iron. The Indian Hemp appears to have been commonly administered throughout all periods of Chinese history, and was employed as an anaesthetic or narcotic draught by Hua Tu (A.D. 115–205), one of the most famous of their ancient surgeons, before he began an operation. Nor were the Indian physicians lagging far behind, although one of their earlier Sanskrit writings of about 1500 B.C. suggests the 'cure' of many diseases was effected by incantations and spells. A series of later works, dating from approximately 700 B.C. reveals much more medicinal information. Part of this work is now attributed to Susruta, the famous Hindu physician who probably lived in the fifth century A.D., and who prescribed over 750 medicinal herbs alone. These were mostly used as external applications, as in ointments and baths, or were inhaled or added to snuffs and sneezing powders. A further 1,000 medicinal plants were recorded on tablets *c.* 2200 B.C., in a sort of Sumerian herbal found in Isin, a district of Babylon.

Hippocrates was the first of the Greeks to regard medicine as a science. He was born in 460 B.C. on the little island of Kos off the coast of Asia Minor. As a distinguished physician, he travelled regularly in foreign countries, researching into and practising medicine. Most of his *Materia medica* was derived from the vegetable kingdom – he used purgatives, sudorifics, diuretics and injections as internal remedies, and ointments, plasters and linaments as applications, leaving a list of some 400 simple remedies to the world at his death. Some of the plants he prescribed are in common use today, including the Mint, Poppy, Mugwort, Sage, Rosemary, Rue and Verbena. Another famous Greek was Theoprastus of Athens, a biologist-botanist, born at Eresus in Lesbos in 370 B.C. He produced a number of manuscripts, including *Historia Plantarum*, which became the standard botanical textbook for

Ricinus communis

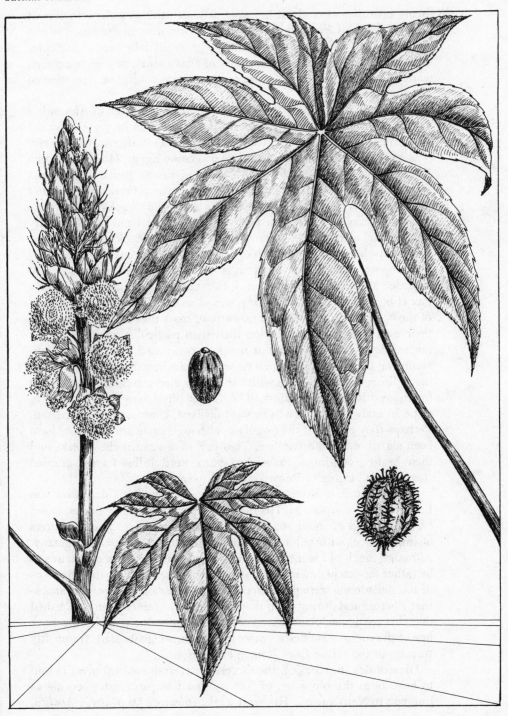

many centuries after. In it he explained such things as how to extract gum Myrrh and Frankincense by making incisions in the stems of the plants. These early Greek doctors were generally followers of Asclepias the god of Medicine (see the genus of that name), and administered various preparations of aromatic roots and flowers in the treatment of internal complaints.

Although no record of it remains, the Medical School of Alexandria in Egypt should be mentioned here. It was founded in 332 B.C. by the Ptolemies, a year before the death of the conqueror after whom the city was named. Alexander the Great had overcome Egypt, Greece and Asia Minor before sweeping through Persia as far as India. His armies included not only soldiers, but scientists too, who set down the learning of the conquered countries in the 700,000 or more books of the Alexandrian School. All were destroyed when the School and the University – which had attracted the foremost contemporary Greek scholars – were burned to the ground by a mob of Christian fanatics in A.D. 391.

It appears that in the early days of Rome, when Greece was still regarded as the centre of the world, the state of medicine was at a fairly low ebb, while the art of healing was considered beneath the dignity of the ordinary Roman. In the majority of cases the sick simply became their own physicians, employing their own particular remedies, at the same time invoking the help of the gods concerned. One plant which, according to Horace, was much resorted to medicinally at this time was the ordinary Cabbage, eaten with wine or applied externally – a panacea for many ills and complaints. The Greek physicians who decided to settle in early Rome were in general disliked, if not openly distrusted. Perhaps they exploited the populace, although some are known to have been slaves of Roman families. This prejudice against the Greeks and their healing continued for several years until Julius Caesar granted them the full rights of Roman citizenship in 46 B.C.

One of the first Roman naturalists was Pliny the Elder, who was born in Verona in A.D. 23. His life's work amounted to 37 books, based on the writings of about 100 selected authors, covering 20,000 matters of importance, with volumes 20 and 27 dealing with medical botany. Although much of his information is fairly accurate, some of it tends to be rather far-fetched, with superstition creeping in. In his day the roots of the Belladonna were given to patients to chew on as a form of anaesthetic before and during painful operations. It has since been established that this particular plant, now known as Deadly Nightshade, was once one of the commonest herbs grown in Britain, where its seeds frequently turn up in the refuse from Roman excavations.

Dioscorides (fl. A.D. 60), the Greek writer and medical man, is said to have been the physician of Antony and Cleopatra, later serving as Surgeon to Nero's army. His great work, known as *De Materia Medica*, identified and described about 600 medicinal plants. The standard work for some 1500 years, it was much referred to throughout Europe during the medieval period.

It was in the Middle Ages that the writings of Galen became popular. Galen was born in Pergamos in Asia Minor in about A.D. 131, later becoming physician to the Emperor Marcus Aurelius. He had travelled extensively, studying philosophy at Pergamos and Smyrna, and medicine at Alexandria, returning to Pergamos at the age of 28 to become surgeon at the school of gladiators there. He is believed to have produced over 500 books and manuscripts, but unfortunately many of these were destroyed in a fire at his house in Rome. About 80 survived to be copied and repeatedly re-copied, especially during the Middle Ages. Many authorities today consider Galen to be the most distinguished physician of antiquity after Hippocrates. Galen's treatment of disease lay mainly in herbal remedies and from those who followed his methods developed the sect known as Eclectics, who employed both herbal and mineral substances. The Allopathic and Homoeopathic systems of medicine of the present day are based on his doctrines.

Besides making good use of plants and trees in their herbal medicine, both the Greeks and Romans employed the more aromatic species as cosmetics and perfumes. They burned the boughs as incense, or as fumigants in time of illness or plague, and used in salads many of the wild sorts now classed as weeds. The Romans became highly skilled in both horticulture and agriculture and introduced many culinary herbs to other countries within their empire, where some of them have since become naturalized. Other plants and numerous fruits, including Figs, Grapes, Plums, Pears, Cherries and Medlars, were cultivated in enormous orchards.

After the fall of the Roman Empire, the progress of medicine in the west was seriously affected and before long the use of these herbal preparations and remedies became obscured in myth and superstition, while very little appears to have been added by means of original research. Indeed the early Christians certainly retarded any progress that could have been made – medicinal cures had to take second place to the holy power of the church. Not only that, since the majority of diseases were thought of as heaven-sent punishment for sins committed it was believed that only prayer and repentance would alleviate them. Christian hospitals certainly existed. One of the earliest was founded by St Basil of Caesarea in A.D. 372, but even he is recorded as denying that illness and disease were of natural origin. His most frequent prescription was prayer and repentance.

It was left to the Arabian physicians to continue the research into medicine. They began by translating the original works of the Greeks into Arabic, adding their own observations and bringing into general use new drugs and plants such as Camphor, Saffron, Senna and Spinach. One of their most famous doctors was Avicenna, a Persian born near Bokhara in A.D. 980 who later became known as 'the Prince of Physicians'. His greatest work, the *Canon of Medicine*, frequently refers to the teachings of Galen and Aristotle and is still studied in the East. This very lengthy treatise was regularly used as a textbook in the European medical schools, including Montpellier, until the mid-seventeenth century. One of the commonest plants Avicenna administered 'to evacuate bile', was the Taraxacum or common Dandelion, which is still universally prescribed for the same purpose.

By the time that the invasion of the Mongols brought the flowering of Arabian culture to an end in the thirteenth century, the medical school of Salerno had been established for almost 500 years. This, the first organized medical school in Europe, was about 35 miles to the south of Naples and was originally a health resort for the Romans. Although little is known of its medical history it appears to have thrived chiefly in the time of the Crusades, from about 1090 to 1275. According to legend it was founded by four 'Masters' known as Adale the Arab, Salernus the Latin, Pontus the Greek and Elinus the Jew – its doors were open to all, irrespective of creed or nationality. One of the better known pupils of this famous school was Michael Scott (*c.* 1175). He prescribed equal parts of Opium, Mandragora and Henbane, pounded and mixed with water and used when it became necessary to saw or cut a man, by dipping a rag in the mixture and applying it to his nostrils. As a result, he claimed, the man would soon sleep so deep, that one could do what one wished with him.

Returning to the early Christian church, we find two saints, the twin brothers Cosmos and Damian, associated with the healing art and patron saints of surgery. They were actually Arab physicians who travelled extensively, preaching Christianity and healing the sick. Sadly both were beheaded in A.D. 303. By this time the monastic way of life was spreading to other countries – St Columba established his house, together with its herbarium and hospice, on the Scottish Isle of Iona in A.D. 563, while St Gall travelled to Switzerland to set up near Lake Constance his monastery with gardens containing such healing herbs as Pennyroyal, Mint, Rosemary, Cumin, Lily, Sage and Fennel. During the eighth century, the Emperor Charlemagne started to take an active interest in medicinal plants and about two years prior to his death issued a list of herbs that were to be cultivated within his domains, including Roses and Lilies, besides ordering the Houseleek to be planted on the roof-tops (a custom that still survives) to give added protection from lightning.

Very few original manuscripts of the Saxon period remain, but perhaps the most famous of these is the *Leech Book of Bald*, possibly a

Cinnamonum camphora

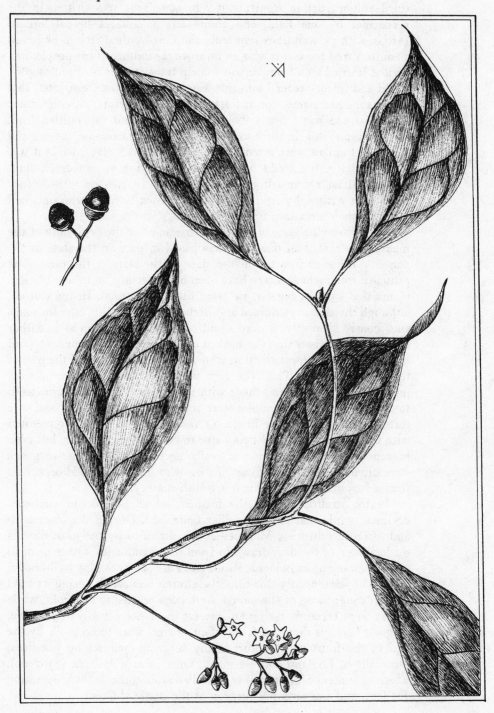

third edition, dating from about A.D. 900. This was written in the vernacular by one Bald, and combined the ancient herbal lore of Britain with prescriptions sent from the East by the Patriach of Jerusalem to Alfred the Great who, to improve the culture of his people, had invited learned men from abroad to help translate books of philosophy, travel and history from Latin into English. It has been estimated that the Saxons had names for at least 500 different plants, although their medicinal use was much entwined with myth and superstition from earlier pagan rites. In the *Leech Book of Bald*, for example, disease and illness in humans were often linked with malicious elves, while it was thought that cattle could be infected with flying venom or elf-shot. Saxon and later translations also exist of a fourth- or fifth-century *Herbarium* written by Apuleius, a little known Roman, who obtained much of his information from Dioscorides's writings.

So low was the state of European medicine at the beginning of the medieval period, that diagnosis was based in part on the state of the patient's urine and partly on the state of the stars at the time. The principal treatment seems to have been blood-letting, and the medicinal plants that were in regular use were little understood. In the church, although the sick were nursed and herbs prescribed, the 'cure for one's sins' consisted mostly of prayer and repentance, as much as in earlier times. In most cases this was backed up by the offering of prayers (and money) to the appropriate saint, who was believed to control the part of the body afflicted. Thus the sick with chest and lung complaints prayed to St Bernardine; those with infections of the gums and teeth to St Apollonia; back troubles were referred to St Lawrence, and sore throats and quinsy to St Blaise. Other saints were certainly credited with the power of not only being able to cure certain illnesses, but even to cause them. If surgery was really necessary the barber-surgeons were often brought in, a group of men who in England had organized themselves into guilds by the fourteenth century.

In the twelfth century the medical school of Salerno gradually declined, while that at Montpellier flourished. During the fourteenth and fifteenth centuries, Montpellier was attended by the most famous medical men of the day, drawn in from many countries. Other medical schools sprang up at Bologna, Padua and Paris, all becoming well-known centres of learning. By this time the church was slowly losing its hold on medicine: some of the monks were even practising for profit, while others were certainly taking an interest in, if not actually performing, surgery. Perhaps they had found their prayers were to no avail. By the end of the fourteenth century many surgeons had set up practices, especially in England and Germany. One, John of Arderne (1307–90), a former student of Montpellier, travelled around the country operating for fees, and was an army surgeon at the Battle of Crecy.

Value of
Medicinal
plants p XVII

Plants with one
Shaped leaves

Although the Christian church had stopped the scientific progress of medicine, it was also the duty of the Church to care for the sick, with the result that during the medieval period many hospitals were built throughout Europe and in the Holy Land where they were used by the Crusaders and pilgrims. In many cases, however, their administration had passed from the Church to lay institutions by the end of the fourteenth century, while in England Henry VIII later dissolved those that remained. Hundreds of leper and lazar houses also existed throughout Britain and Europe, but as the numbers of lepers decreased, so they were used to house the sick and poor instead.

The value of many medicinal plants administered in Europe at this time became based on what is known as the 'Doctrine of Signatures' or 'Similars', which taught that the healing herbs were signposted by God in some way for man's guidance – so as to show what disease or what part of the body the plant could be used for. This idea was developed by Paracelsus (1490–1541), the Swiss alchemist and physician, becoming very popular with the Puritans and such writers as William Coles, as in his book *The Art of Simpling* (see Lungwort and Walnut). For instance, plants with liver-shaped leaves were regarded as 'efficacious in bilious diseases', while plants containing a milky juice, such as the Lettuce, the fruit of the Almond and the juice of the Fig 'propagate milk in nursing mothers'. Numerous examples are listed, but in some the resemblances are rather far-fetched.

Gradually, herbalism and medicine were drifting apart. Nor were matters much helped by Culpeper in the seventeenth century, for he believed all disease and illness was governed by a planet, as were the hundreds of herbs he prescribed. Culpeper himself had, after a short apprenticeship to an apothecary in St Helen's, Bishopsgate, London, established in 1640 his own practice in Red Lion Street, Spitalfields, devoting himself to the study of astrology-medicine, publishing numerous but unorthodox medical tracts. They were much condemned by contemporary medical practioners, but even so enjoyed very large sales. In 1649 he incurred the wrath of the College of Physicians with his publication the *Physicall Directory*, having translated this from their Latin *Pharmacopoeia*. In the subsequent quarrels his views on astrology were held to be preposterous. Nevertheless as a physician Culpeper was greatly loved by the people, often treating his poorer patients without charge. His book *The English Physitian*, published in 1652, is now generally known in its enlarged form as Culpeper's Herbal and I make no apologies for quoting extensively from it in the following text. Such was Culpeper's popularity that his writings were taken to North America by the early settlers and widely consulted there not only in the treatment of the sick, but to ensure by use of astrological botany that the correct time was selected for the planting and harvesting of crops.

The books of other author-herbalists from which I have quoted include those of Turner, Gerard and Parkinson.

As many of the plants described in these works were not found in America, the settlers had to import them. The demand for seeds and roots and any new cures continued unabated for many years. The end result was that much of the European flora taken to America escaped from cultivation and became naturalized. Other plants simply naturalized themselves. The seeds of the Common Plantain, for example, probably reached that and other countries in sacks of grain.

As the housewife of this period was expected to have a good knowledge of medicinal herbs, besides employing them as flavourings, perfumes and dyes, she soon started to experiment with the native American plants, especially those known to have been used by the various Indian tribes. In turn, when these plants proved valuable medicinally or otherwise, so they were shipped to Europe, where they were enthusiastically received by botanist, herbalist and gardener alike, some later escaping from cultivation to become naturalized.

On their arrival in Virginia and New England, these early colonists also found the Indians growing several different varieties of Beans, Corns, Pumpkins and Gourds as food, besides Tobacco for smoking. Many other plants were collected as dyes, or for their fibre, which was employed in the making of cloth and clothing. One of the most widely prescribed of the Indians' herbs was the Ginseng or Five Finger Root (*Panax quinquefolium*). Its root was eaten as a medicinal 'cure-all', although it was some time before the colonists realized its potential value, or could even find the growing plant. In 1718, the Canadian Jesuits on discovering its true identity started to export the root to China, where a different species was held in high esteem. It had been prescribed there from about 3000 B.C., as a remedy for fatigue and as a means of invigorating the body, especially in old age.

The South American countries have provided the rest of the world with some wonderful medicinal cures. When the Spaniards conquered Mexico and Peru between 1531 and 1536, they were most impressed by the gardens of the native Indians and the plants and flowers cultivated for food, including the Sunflower and the Potato, and the herbs administered in medicine, such as the Coca and Tobacco.

Pedro de Cieza de Leon's book *Chronica del Peru*, published in Seville in 1553, mentions both the Potato and the Coca, or Cuco as it was known. It was this small shrubby tree, now botanically listed as *Erythrocylon coca*, that later provided the painkiller Cocaine. Although it has since been replaced by a synthetic substitute, Cocaine itself was formerly used by dentists as a local anaesthetic, and in hospitals as a spinal anaesthetic. The use of this plant goes back to pre-Inca times, to at least A.D. 500, for its leaves were found in a Peruvian burial urn dated

Panax quinquefolium

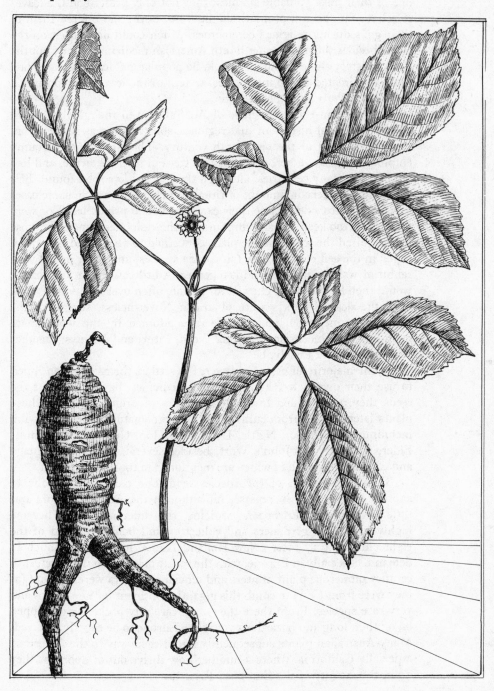

to the Nazca period. Medicinally the Inca priests regarded the Coca as one of their most valuable simples: they not only prescribed the leaves to relieve fatigue and promote stamina, but burnt and offered them to their gods during religious ceremonies. Much could be written on the Coca, besides the many other South American medicinal plants, but the Coca's history alone would fill a book. So popular is Coca chewing today, that an estimated 25–30 million lbs. weight of the leaves are consumed annually in Peru and Bolivia alone.

Mention must also be made of Australia, even though the known herbal-medicinal history of that region is short, dating as it does from towards the end of the eighteenth century. The Aborigines certainly employed the native herbs, shrubs and trees in their medicine, and had done so for many centuries, although the first settlers soon found their use involved a certain amount of ritual and chanting, and in some cases it was difficult to determine their exact medicinal principles. Nor were the settlers too keen on sampling some of these simples, especially those that required the leaves of the plant concerned to be chewed into quid, rolled in the ash of Red Gum (an Acacia species) and to be mixed with rabbit or wallaby hair to hold it together. A little of this tacky mixture would then be sucked or chewed for a time, often over a period of days, until the desired effects were obtained. Nevertheless, several of the Aborigines' medicinal plants were later adopted by the white man, including the Queensland Asthma Weed, Pituri and Drimys, together with some of the Eucalypts.

In the majority of cases, however, the settlers themselves continued to use their own better known herbal medicines, having brought the seeds they most valued from their country of origin. Many of these plants later escaped from cultivation to become naturalized in the wild, including the common Nettle, Dandelion, Hop, German Chamomile, Elder, Fumitory, St John's Wort, besides several species of Plantago and Chenopodium, all of which are mentioned in the following text.

This immigration of the species from one part of the globe to another also worked in reverse, for although the Australian flora was little employed in European medicine, the different species became highly valued by gardeners and collectors and before the end of the eighteenth century these 'New Holland Plants' had become much in demand, especially in Europe, with the result that during the nineteenth century numerous plant hunters and official collectors were sent out (as they were from Kew) to comb this gigantic continent for new forms and very rare species. From there they were carefully packed and shipped off on their long and hazardous voyage to Europe to be eagerly received. Many Australian plants subsequently found their way to the Americas, especially California, where a number now thrive out of doors, as they do in the vicinity of the European Riviera.

Erythrocylon coca

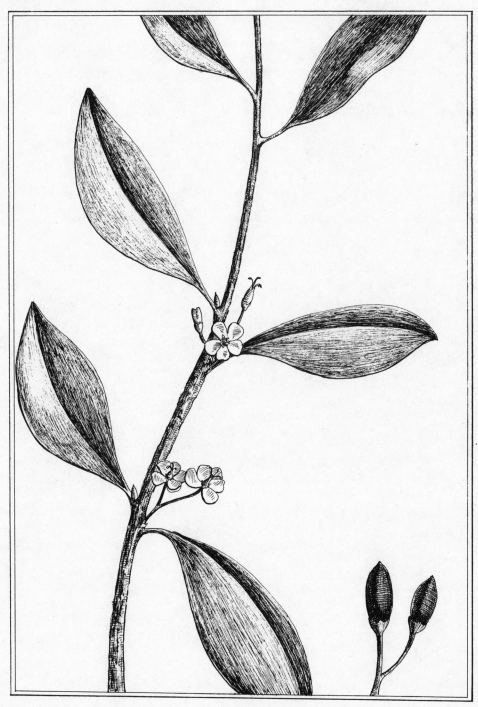

Botanical Notes

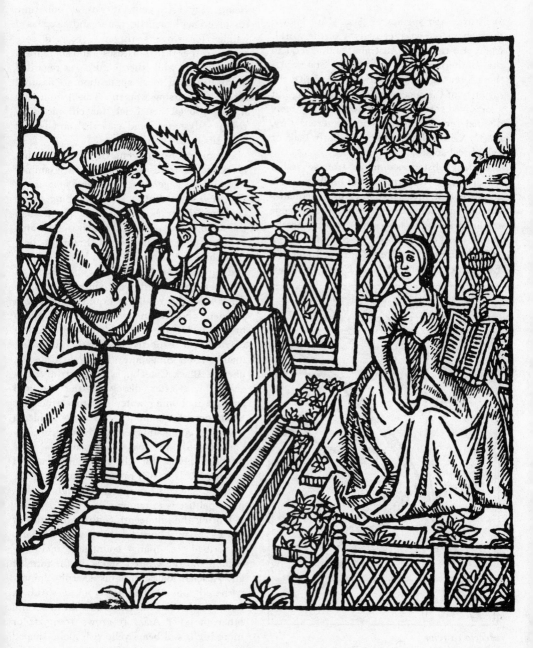

ACACIA

Leguminosae, the Pea family

Black Catechu, Pale Catechu,
Egyptian Thorn, Gum Acacia,
Babul Bark, Popinac

Well over 400 species of Acacia are known throughout the warmer regions of the world. Many are native to Australia, and several to the southern part of the United States. Although one or two are herbaceous plants, the majority of the species are quick-growing but short-lived shrubs or small trees, having finely divided fern-like leaves and numerous tiny, mostly yellow flowers borne in fluffy balls or cylindrical spikes.

Certain substances obtained from several of the species were formerly, and still are to a certain extent, prescribed in various medicines throughout the world. One such substance is obtained from the leaves, the shoots and the young wood of the Black Catechu (*A. catechu*, syn. *A. nigrum*). Native to Burma, India, the East Indies and the Malabar Coast, the Black

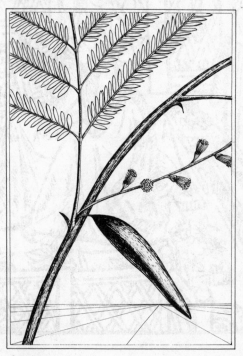

Acacia catechu

Catechu grows into a small, thickly barked tree, with spreading branches and bipinate leaves, and bears numerous whitish or yellowish flowers, followed by pea-like fruits. In the world markets this black, odourless and irregular-shaped cake-like mixture is known and sold as Cutch, or occasionally as Gambir. Being very astringent, it was at one time dissolved with a little water and used as a gargle 'for singer's throat – relaxed sore throat – other throat diseases – and sponginess of the gums', while the tincture was regarded as 'useful as a local application to fissured nipples of nursing women'. Taken internally it also proved beneficial 'for chronic diarrhoea – dysentery and catarrhs' and is still prescribed for these today.

A similar substance, known as Pale Catechu, is extracted from the Gambir or Gambier Plant (*Uncaria gambier*, syn. *Terra japonica* or *Ourouparia gambir*), a stout climbing shrub common to much of India and Burma and the surrounding regions, where it is cultivated in plantations. The round branches bear smooth ovate leaves and loose heads of green and pink flowers. The leaves and shoots of this perennial plant were simply boiled in water and the resulting liquid poured into wooden trays. When set, this was cut up into brownish looking cubes (although reddish inside) and exported to many countries, mainly from Singapore. The Pale Catechu, like the Black Catechu, is very astringent in action, and after dissolving the required amount in boiling water was prescribed for 'affections of the mouth – as a stomachic in dyspeptic complaints, especially when accompanied with pyrosis' and again like the previous plant 'for chronic diarrhoea and dysentery'. It is still prescribed today in the form of Catechu Lozenges, although now its principal use is in tanning.

During the nineteenth century the juice of the Egyptian Thorn (*A. vera*) was popularly prescribed in many countries, including Britain and the United States, in the form of an 'Acacian Balsam'. This sharply spined, withered looking tree or crooked shrub is native to Arabia, but is found wild in several other parts of Asia. It grows 10m/32ft or more high, and bears yellowish globe-shaped

powders, lozenges and solutions, or combined with syrups and decoctions.

Another good source of Acacia Gum was the Gum Acacia or Gum Arabic (*A. senegal*), a small tree native to Africa from Ethiopia to Senegal. Here again the gum exudes of its own accord from the stems, although incisions are made for larger yields. This gum is classed as demulcent and mucilaginous and was often added to other medicinal compounds in the treatment of diarrhoea, dysentery, coughs and fevers. In all about 40 species of Acacia yielding gums of varying grades are still employed in commerce, especially in dyeing and printing. The finest is known as Kordofan Gum.

The bark of two other species, *A. arabica* and *A. decurrens*, from the drier areas of Africa, India and other tropical countries are used in the tanning industry today under the name of Acacia or Babul Bark.

Several of the Australian Acacias provide 'tanbark', while the durable wood of others is employed in the manufacture of tool handles,

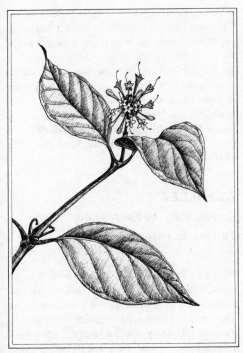

Uncaria gambier

flowers, followed by long pods containing many flat, brownish seeds.

The medicinal part of the plant, a form of Gum Arabic, exudes naturally from the bark of the trees in the wild, although this is often encouraged by making incisions in the trunk; the more cuts, the more gum it expels, which on exposure to the air hardens into yellowish-white transparent beads. These are collected and in many cases powdered down. When mixed with its own weight in water, the powder forms into 'a thick mucilaginous solution considered as nutritive and demulcent, exerting 'a remarkably soothing influence upon irritated or inflamed mucous surfaces', and removing 'griping and painful stools, in catarrh, cough, hoarseness, consumption, gonorrhoea'. For diseases of the lungs it was regarded as an especial and 'indispensable vehicle in which to carry the necessary curative and powerful corrective agents, while at the same time its nutritive qualities also exert a good influence, often supplying the place of food where the stomach is too weak to partake of anything else.' It was given alone in

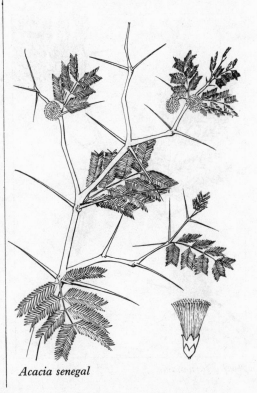

Acacia senegal

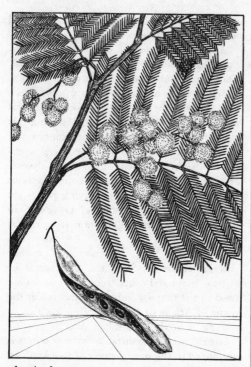

Acacia decurrens

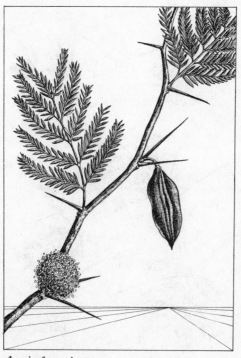

Acacia farnesiana

cabinets, furniture, etc. Although the Popinac (*A. farnesiana*), a much-branched shrub or small tree about 6m/19ft high, is native to the West Indies, it is grown commercially in France for its very fragrant flowers which are used in perfumery. This species is also known as Opopanax, Cassie or Huisache.

Acacia, the botanical name of the genus, is derived from the Greek word *akakia* – a point, referring to the thorns borne by some of the species.

ACHILLEA
Compositae, the Daisy family
Yarrow, Sneezewort

About 40 species of Achillea grow in Europe alone, although only two of these were employed to any extent in medieval medicine. The most commonly prescribed was the Yarrow (*A. millefolium*) a hardy, rather variable species, inhabiting much of Europe, including the British Isles, although now found in many other parts of the world such as Canada and the United States, Australia and New Zealand.

This erect-growing perennial, often known as Milfoil or Thousand Seal, referring to its finely divided, feathery leaves (as does millefolium, its specific name), has simple stems reaching 10–50cm/3–20in. high, bearing from early summer onwards flat-topped clusters of small but numerous white, or cream to pink flowers. In the wild it is found in pastures and meadows, on cultivated land as well as by the wayside, where it grows freely in almost any soil.

As a medicinal herb Yarrow has been administered from ancient times. Its generic name is believed to refer to Achilles, the legendary Greek hero, who apparently made an ointment from the leaves, using it to treat his warriors wounded in the siege of Troy. Other accounts state the word Achillea is derived from Achillo, an ancient Greek doctor, who employed the herb to cure a warrior named Teleph of his serious wounds. Several of the Yarrow's more common names – Staunchgrass, Bloodwort, Knight's Milfoil,

Herbe Militaris, Sanguinary and Soldier's Woundwort – actually point to its value on the battlefield, with the leaves simply 'being expectorated and applied to the place'.

By the 1450s, the herb had become so popular and was used for so many purposes throughout Europe, that it was commonly grown in gardens and taken or applied for all manner of complaints, from a hair wash for preventing baldness to the sweating out of virulent fevers, while in Sweden it was added to one of their bitter beers to increase the

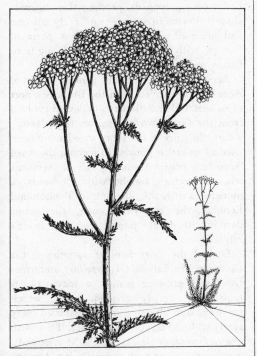

Achillea millefolium

inebriating effect. The 'tuthache' sufferers of this period were always advised to chew the green leaves of Yarrow to try to avoid the agony of having the offending tooth pulled. This remedy, still occasionally used in Norway, was repeated later by Gerard, who writes: 'The juice mixed with vinegar and holden in the mouth, easeth much pain of the toothache.' He also recommended the herb for headache: 'The leaves being put into the nose, do cause it to bleed and easeth the paine of the megrin . . .' hence Nosebleed, another of its common names. The dried powdered

leaves in the form of a snuff were usually given for this purpose.

Early in the seventeenth century 'the juice applied' was considered as one of the better cures for 'septic wound or running sore'. Drayton mentions it in his *Polyolbion* of 1622: 'The Yarrow, wherewithall he stops the wound made gore' adding 'the healing tutsan and plantane for a sore'. Soon after, Culpeper informs us that as a medicine Yarrow is 'drying and binding' and 'is excellent for the piles' either 'drunk plentifully' in a strong tea or applied in a poultice mixed with pomatum (apples) and Toad Flax. He also writes 'an ointment of the leaves cures wounds, and is good for inflammations, ulcers, fistulas and all such runnings as abound with moisture.'

When introduced to North America by the early settlers, the plant soon escaped and rapidly established itself in the wild. It was prescribed there in herbal medicine much as it had been in Europe – 'as efficacious in bleeding from the lungs and other internal hemorhages – incontinence of urine – dysentery – suppressed or restrained menses – flatulence – lack of appetite – and various spasmodic diseases'. Achilleine, the active principle of the herb, was frequently prescribed late into the nineteenth century as a substitute for quinia, in the treatment of intermittent fevers, mostly in southern Europe.

Although the common Achillea is still prescribed for its diaphoretic, stimulant and tonic effects, mainly in warm infusions as a way of opening the pores to induce perspiration in the treatment of colds and influenza, its excessive internal use is not advised, as it can cause headache and dizziness. Used externally the juice makes a useful hairwash and in a facewash will clear the skin. In several countries of northern Europe the dried leaves, made into a tea, are still taken for the relief of depression and melancholy. At one time the shoots of this plant were added in small amounts to cattle fodder, which was supposed to help the animals' digestion.

The second species of Achillea also common to much of Europe, including Britain, is the Sneezewort (*A. ptarmica*), which, like the

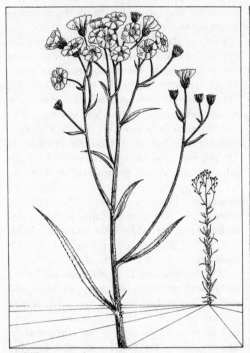

Achillea ptarmica

Yarrow, has been introduced to numerous other countries. This erect hardy perennial, with its finely saw-toothed, lance-shaped, hairless leaves, grows from 20–60cm/7–23in. high, has angular hairy stems and produces its white or pinkish flowers in loose flat-topped clusters and is normally found in meadows and by the sides of roads.

As Gerard's name of Neesewort implies, this was the 'herbe which procureth sneesing' and 'neese exceedingly'. Culpeper, who knew the plant as Bastard Pellitory, also recommended the powder of the herb 'snuffed' up the nose to cause sneezing and to cleanse 'the head of tough slimy humours'. The bruised root held in the mouth, or the leaves chewed and applied, would help the toothache by, it was commonly believed, 'evacuating the rheum' a remedy that would 'bring mightely forth the slimy flegme from the brain'. The young shoots were included as a matter of course in salads 'to correct the coldness of other herbs' and to excite the flow of saliva, while a tea of the leaves would 'counteract immoderate fluxes of the bowels and other parts' as well as help 'female weakness'. The same was regarded as a tonic for 'nervous debility', for which it is still occasionally prescribed. The whole of the plant yields an essential oil sometimes used in medicine.

ACONITUM
Ranunculaceae, the Buttercup family
Monkshood, Wolfsbane

These handsome but very poisonous, hardy herbaceous perennials, produce their helmet-shaped flowers in summer and early autumn and are native mainly to various parts of Europe, with one or two species coming from China and Japan.

According to Pliny, the generic name of Aconitum is derived from the Black Sea port of Aconis. Other authorities believe it evolved from the Greek word *akoniton*, from 'akon', a dart, the juice of the roots once having been used as an arrow poison. In legend, the word Aconitum comes from the hill of Aconitus where Hercules fought with Cerberus, a monstrous dog, the offspring of Typhon and Echidna the serpent woman, the genus deriving its deadly poison from the beast's saliva.

One of the more familiar varieties is the Common Monkshood (*A. napellus*), an attractive erect growing plant, 50–100cm/1½–3ft high, with deeply divided leaves, which produces dull blue or purplish coloured (very rarely whitish) flowers in summer. This, with one or two other closely related Monkshoods, such as the plant now generally listed as the Wolfsbane (*A. vulparia*, syn. *A. lyoctonum*) with its spikes of attractive yellow flowers, has been employed since classical times as a sure method to dispose of an unwanted spouse, although in several countries they were considered 'vulgar poisons' and far better put down in 'woolf's baite'. There were exceptions to this, as on the ancient Greek island of Kos, where officials prescribed simple draughts of Aconite as a quick way to rid themselves of their troublesome aged and infirm. As a poison it was surely abused in the time of the Roman Emperor Trajan, for he forbade the growing of Aconitum by law and made it an offence punishable by death. It was known to the Anglo-Saxons as *Thung* – meaning very poisonous, and they used it on their weapons. The most virulent part of the plant however is the root.

Although *A. vulparia* was mentioned in one or two of the earlier English herbals, it was not recorded as a herb in general cultivation there until the 1550s, when Turner warned of the danger of this 'most hastie poyson'. Yet three hundred years before, during the thirteenth century, the Physicians of Myddval in Wales had considered the Monkshood a herb that every physician should grow.

It appears that if any part of the plant was eaten it could kill. After a few minutes the unfortunate victim would get the 'icy cold sweats and a shaking' quickly followed by 'a burning tingling' spreading throughout the body. Then came 'a burning fire in mouth and throat – a deathly chill thereafter – with anguish and torments in the head, the neck and back and sometimes blindness'. At this latter stage death would probably result within three to four hours. Even so, small portions of the thick and blackish fleshy roots were frequently but very carefully administered in witchcraft rites to numb the taker's senses and give a sensation of flying.

In medicine the root and leaves were classed as sedative, anodyne and febrifuge and were prescribed in England as in the rest of Europe, 'for febrile and inflammatory diseases – scarletina – bad cases of tonsillitis – croup – and spasms of the heart'. It was imported to North America by the early settlers who grew the plant in their gardens, using it much as above, for 'acute rheumatism – pneumonia – peritonitis – gastritis – and other disorders'. Its action was recorded 'to be more especially displayed in the highest grades of fever and inflammation'. The best extracts were prepared by evaporating a tincture made of one pound of Aconite and a quart of alcohol. Most writers of the period stress that overdoses should be avoided, for no certain antidote was known. If the worst came to the worst, a mixture of sal-volatile and brandy was generally administered to the patient.

The common Monkshood is still valued in medicine today. Extracts and tinctures of the roots and leaves, when properly prescribed by doctors, can slow a quick heart and help reduce blood pressure, while a painkiller for relieving neuralgia and rheumatism is extracted from the roots. The active constituent is an alkaloid known as Aconitine.

Other species are known to have been used medicinally in the Far East, possibly the Indian Aconite Root (*A. deinorhizum*) or the Japanese Aconite Root (*A. uncinatum*). This genus was also listed in *Pen Tsao* the Great Herbal of ancient China. One of the authors of this work, which is still used in China, was the Emperor Shen Nung, who lived about 3000 years B.C. This great man raised and carefully cultivated the majority of the herbs then known and for many years is believed to have experimented on himself, discovering in

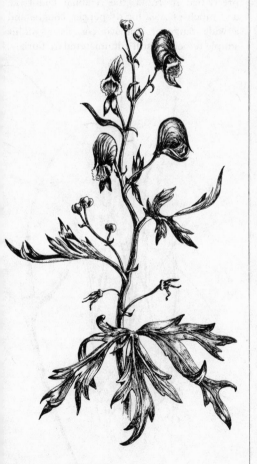

Aconitum napellus

the process a large number of drugs and poisons.

Other names for the common Monkshood include Friar's Cap, Blue Rocket, Helmet Flower, Chariot and Horses, Grannies Nightcap and Luckie's Mutch. In Scotland it is known as Auld Wife's Huid.

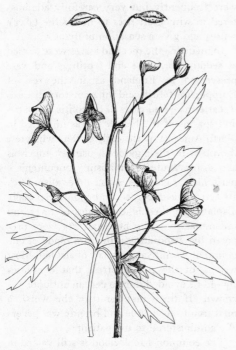

Aconitum uncinatum

ACORUS
Aracea, the Arum family
Sweet Flag

Only two or three species of Acorus are recognized throughout the world, and only one, the Sweet Flag (*A. calamus*, syn. *Calamus aromaticus*), a handsome, hardy, herbaceous aquatic perennial, was used to any extent in medicine. It has upright, sword-shaped leaves 1m/3ft or more in height and produces tiny, densely packed, greenish-yellow flowers, on a short spike-like branch (or spadix) which projects out and upwards about three-quarters of the way along the leaf-like stalk. Although

native to parts of Asia and North and Central America, the Sweet Flag is now naturalized in many other countries of the world, including the British Isles and most of Europe, where it was introduced by the late 1550s. It is common in the mud of marshes and swamps and in shallow water by the margins of rivers and ponds.

The specific name of this plant, *calamus*, is derived either from the Greek *kalamos* or the Sanskrit *kalamas* both words meaning stalk or reed, the glossy yellow-green leaves once having been employed in thatching, and indoors for 'strewing floors'.

The pungent-tasting rootstocks with their sweet, aromatic scent were valued mainly when fresh for their carminative and stomachic effects. These were usually candied and prescribed in India, the Arabian countries, and much of Asia for dyspepsia, coughs and a wide range of stomach complaints. This simple remedy is still administered in Turkey.

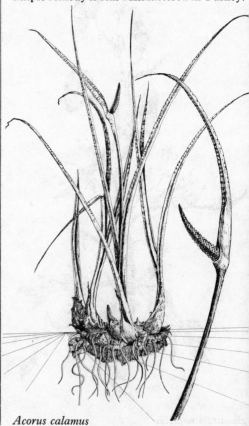

Acorus calamus

The ancient Greeks used the plant when treating eye afflictions. The generic name, Acorus derives from *kore*, a pupil.

The North American Indians valued the rhizomes of the species, which grow in matted masses, again for their stomachic and carminative principles, often simply pulling up and chewing a piece of it. Alternatively, they sometimes dug up the underground parts, roasted them over a fire and ate them as vegetables. The Indians of northern Canada extracted the oil from the roots, taking it internally to induce visual hallucinations. This oil from the fresh green plant smells of tangerine when bruised and is nowadays used in perfumery. It is also added to gin to correct its flavour and to beer for added fragrance.

Infusions of the root are still prescribed in parts of Asia and Europe for dyspepsia, and during the nineteenth century it was taken in teacupful doses as 'a useful remedy for the ague'.

Other common names for the Sweet Flag include Calamus Root, Myrtle Sedge and Sweet Sedge.

ADIANTUM
Polypodiaceae, the Polypody family
Venus Hair, Common Maidenhair

Many kinds of Adiantum, a large genus of graceful ferns, are known. The majority are native to tropical countries, principally America, from where over the years many forms have been developed for use as pot plants in the home and conservatory, or as florist's green. Only a few of the species can be classed as hardy; of these two have long been prescribed in herbal medicine.

The first – the Venus Hair, Maidenhair or Rock Fern (*A. capillus-veneris*), a small evergreen perennial 15–25cm/5–9in. tall, with fan-shaped leaflets on blackish wiry stalks – is native to southern Europe, where it is found in moist, sheltered places, such as rocks and cliffs. It is now naturalized in many other countries, like the British Isles, where it grows locally by the sea. There are also many attractive forms and varieties of this species,

some of which are now found as far apart as Canada and the United States, South America, Australia, New Zealand and even China.

In medicine the leaves of the plant were generally infused and prescribed for their expectorant, pectoral and mucilaginous effects, mainly for easing throat infections, bronchial and other chest conditions. The herb was

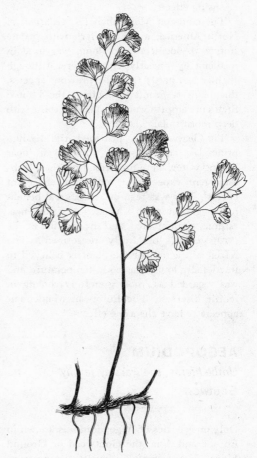

Adiantum capillus-veneris

never boiled, but added to boiling water and then allowed to cool; otherwise its healing properties were said 'to evaporate'. The resulting mixture was sweetened with honey or sugar and taken in wineglassful doses. The unsweetened infusion was at one time popular as a hair wash and even as 'a restorer of hair'. Culpeper tells us: 'This is a good remedy for coughs, asthmas, pleurisy, etc. and on account of its being a gentle diuretic, also, in the jaundice, gravel and other impurities of the kidneys.'

At one time in France large quantities of the leaves were made into a syrup, the 'Sirop de Capillare', which was taken for many of the complaints listed above. Some herbalists still prescribe the species for its diuretic and cleansing effects.

The common Maidenhair (*A. pedatum*) of North America, a delicate fern with pedate fronds 30–60cm/11–23in. long, was used in medicine by the early settlers there. Although slightly less hardy than the previous species, this plant is found throughout the United States in dampish woods, especially those with deep moist soils.

The leaves again provided the healing principles, and, on their infusion in near boiling water, were prescribed for their 'subastringent, expectorant, tonic and refrigerant effects'. This was regarded as 'a great benefit in coughs, catarrh, hoarseness, influenza, asthma, pleurisy etc.', and the mixture or the syrup could 'be freely prescribed'. The refrigerant action of the plant is believed to fractionally lower the body temperature and was regarded as 'most gratefully cooling in febrile diseases'. The European Maidenhair appears to have the same effects.

AEGOPODIUM
Umbelliferae, the Parsley family
Goutwort

Only one species of Aegopodium is known in Europe and Asia, the Goutweed or Ground Elder (*A. podograria*), a hairless leafy perennial, with erect hollow grooved stems 50cm– 1m/1½–3ft high, bearing umbels of white flowers in summer. It is a common carpet-forming herb, found on banks, in hedges, shady places under trees and along the sides of rivers and streams. In gardens the Goutwort is generally classed as an unwelcome and persistent weed, and Gerard was certainly right when he wrote, it 'groweth of itselfe in gardens without setting or sowing and is so

fruitful in his increase, that where it hath once taken root, it will hardly be gotten out againe. . . .'

The generic name of this plant, Aegopodium, refers to the shape of its leaves, and is derived from the Greek *aigos* or *aix* – a goat, and *pous* or *podium* – a foot, whence Goat's Foot or Goat's Herb, two more common names. Podograria is thought to draw attention to the herb's ability to relieve the symptoms of the gout, which in turn gave rise to the name of Gout Weed. Other names include Ash Weed, Bishop's Weed, Dog Elder, Ground Ash, Herb Guard and Gout Herb.

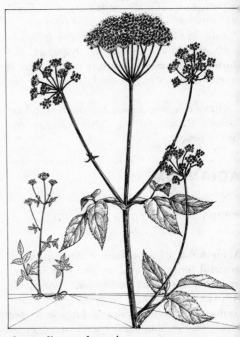

Aegopodium podograria

The Gout Weed is believed to have been introduced into England from the Continent shortly after the Norman Conquest and was grown at first in monastery gardens, the monks making good use of the leaves as a pot herb. From several accounts it appears that a number of these pious men were afflicted with gout, and had prayed to St Gerard for some form of relief. After taking the herb with their daily meals for some time, the monks finally came to the conclusion that it was actually suppressing their painful symptoms, and assumed that St Gerard had answered their prayers. Before very long the species was renamed Herb Gerard in the Saint's honour. Bishop's Weed also refers to its use in relieving the goutiness of the religious.

No doubt due to the Gout Weed's vigorous cultivation in England at that time and partly to its rapid habit of growth, the plant soon escaped from its monastic confines and firmly established itself in the wild, much as it did later on in North America when introduced there.

Herbalists still prescribe the plant, generally under the name of Ground Elder, as a diuretic and sedative. In the form of a tea, the leaves and saline tasting root are useful as a diuretic. As a poultice, hot fomentations of the leaves can be applied to rheumatic or swollen joints. In certain parts of Europe the more tender leaves, which contain a high percentage of Vitamin C, are included in salads, or boiled and eaten like spinach. However, they do tend to have a strong and sometimes disagreeable flavour.

AGRIMONIA
Rosaceae, the Rose family
Cockleburr

The Agrimonias are a genus of hardy perennial herbs, native to much of the northern temperate zone. The most familiar species, the Cockleburr (*A. eupatoria*), has upright stems and hairy leaves. It is commonly found in fields, open woods, hedgerows, by the wayside and similar places, in all the countries of Europe (excepting Iceland) as well as in Asia, Canada and the United States. It grows to a height of 50–60cm/19–23in. producing in summer many small star-like yellow flowers, placed one above the other on long slender tapering spikes.

As a medicinal herb the use of this Agrimonia goes back to the time of the ancient Greeks, when, as *argemone*, it was prescribed with other similar plants in the treatment of eye complaints. It was certainly known to Pliny who extolled it as a 'herb of sovereign

power'. He emphasized that if the seed was taken in wine, it was a singular remedy for dysentery and the bloody flux. In old French writings it appears under the name of *aigregmoine*, which evolved by the early medieval period to Agrimony, its familiar and current name. The specific name of *eupatoria* points to the similarity between this species

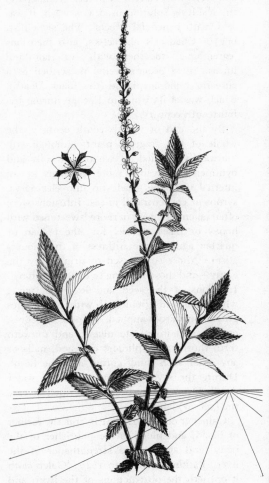

Agrimonia eupatoria

and the Hemp Agrimony (*Eupatorium cannabinum*), a medicinal herb belonging to the Daisy family. Its other common names include Yellow Agrimony, Eupator's Agrimony, European Agrimony, Church Steeples (alluding to the flowers) and Stickwort, referring to the hooked bristles of the fruits, which when ripe stick to animal fur and clothing.

During the Anglo-Saxon period, Agrimony was principally employed in Europe as a wound herb (often under the name of Garclive) for which it was still prescribed in Chaucer's England. For 'alle woundes and bad back', and similar ailments, the leaves and seeds were soaked in water, strained, and the resulting solution used as a wash, it was said 'with beneficial effects'. The alchemist, one of Chaucer's characters, also mentions 'egremogne' together with 'valerian and lunaria' in a useless recipe prescribed as a cure for bubonic plague (the Black Death), which was at its worst in Europe during the fourteenth century.

By the end of the sixteenth century, the whole of this fragrant plant, although still 'outwardly applied to wounds in oils and oyntments', became more popular as an internal medicine, made up into electuarys, syrups or concentrated juices. Infusions were often taken for a year or more 'sweetened with honey or black treacle' for 'the tertian or quartan agues – the stiffness of the rheumatism – those suppressed of urine – by the gouty – and those wanting to expel the stone'. Infusions of the seed and leaves in wine, when 'stamped [pounded] with old swines grease' outwardly applied, 'helpeth old sores, cancers and inveterate ulcers, and draweth forth thorns and splinters of wood, nails or any other such thing gotten into the flesh'. During the seventeenth century, the water distilled from the herb was prescribed 'to ease the (yellow) jaundice'.

Culpeper observed: 'The liver is the former of blood, and blood is the nourisher of the body, and agrimony a strengthener of the liver.' Parkinson wrote in 1640: 'Galen saith it openeth the obstructions of the liver, and clenseth it, it helpeth the jaundice and strengthened the inward parts – and is very beneficial to the bowels.' Hill, however, informs us in the 1750s that 'although Agrimony was greatly recommended by the ancients', it is 'very much neglected in the present practice'.

In Canada and the United States, the Agrimony was prescribed late into the nine-teenth century in the treatment of 'certain cutaneous diseases, chronic affections of the digestive organs, chronic mucous diseases leucorrhoea', and was considered 'useful in bowel complaints, gravel, asthma, coughs obstructed menstruation and as a gargle for a sore throat or mouth'.

Infusions of the whole herb, described as mildly tonic, astringent and alterative, are still prescribed taken over a period of time, to cleanse the blood, as a general tonic, and to a lesser degree to relieve simple diarrhoea.

The plant is also grown commercially for its yellow dye, which is extracted for use in the textile trade.

ALCHEMILLA
Rosaceae, the Rose family
Lady's Mantle, Parsley Piert

Most of the members of this family are summer-flowering, hardy evergreen perennial or annual herbs, native principally to the mountain areas of Europe, Central America and other countries. At least 118 species are listed for Europe alone, while numerous microspecies have also been described.

Two of the better known species were popularly included in the medieval medicine of Europe. The first, the Lady's Mantle (*A. vulgaris*) in all its forms, was valued mainly for its 'astringent and styptic principles'. This perennial herb, with its woody rootstock, has erect or spreading stems up to 50cm/19in. tall, bearing tiny green petalless flowers in small clusters from about May to September. It is native to most of Europe, including the British Isles, where it is found in damp meadows, open woods and rocky places. Its common name of Lady's Mantle refers to the shape of the leaves, said to resemble the cloaks worn by the more wealthy ladies of the medieval period. Alchemilla, the generic name, is derived from the Arabic *alkmelyeh* or *alkemelych* and is so-called because some of these plants were thought to possess certain 'alchemical virtues' and were included in all manner of magic potions and spells. Hence the name 'Alchemists Herb',

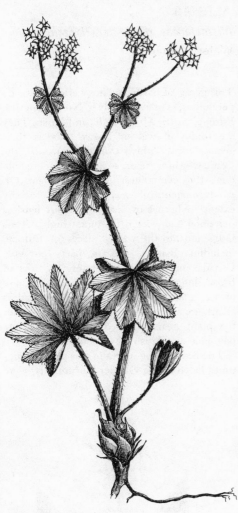

Alchemilla vulgaris

conception, and to retain the birth, if the woman do sometimes sit in a bath made of the decoction of the herb.'

Infusions of the herb, which is sometimes known as Lion's Foot, are still prescribed as a cure for excessive menstruation.

The second species of Alchemilla to be popularly included in early medieval European medicine was the Parsley Piert (*A. arvensis*, syn. *Aphanes arvensis*), a small, hairy, branching and spreading leafy annual or biennial 5–20cm/2–7in. high, with short-stalked fan-shaped leaves. This widely distributed plant is also native to much of Europe, including the British Isles, and is found in bare and fallow land, where it produces its tiny green flowers from May to August.

In medicine the whole of this plant was put to good use. Strong infusions of the freshly gathered herb, 'being demulcent and diuretic in action', were regarded as best 'for jaundice – and other complaints arising from obstructions of the liver – and again for the gravel and stone' by 'acting directly on those parts effected by expelling urine'. The dried herbs, taken in white wine or made into a syrup – 'would also bring the gravel away from the kidneys – help the stranguary – and the complaints of the bladder'.

Infusions are still given by herbalists, mainly as listed above for kidney and bladder complaints.

ALETRIS
Liliaceae, the Lily family
Unicorn Root

Although several members of this genus are said to possess similar properties, the species mainly prescribed in medicine was the Unicorn Root (*A. farinosa*). This native of the United States is found from Maine to Minnesota and south to Florida and Louisiana growing in sandy soils as by the edge of woods. Its smooth-ribbed leaves form on the ground, producing in early summer, simple slender stems 30–90cm/11–35in. high, terminating in a spike-like raceme of white or yellowish bell-shaped flowers.

which covers several plants of this order. Vulgaris, the specific name of the Lady's Mantle, simply means that this is the most common species.

Culpeper prescribes the Lady's Mantle principally as a wound-herb, but observes that it was also 'effectual to stay bleedings, vomitings and fluxes of all sorts, bruises by falls or otherwise, and helps ruptures, and women who have over-flagging breasts, causing them to grow less and hard, both when drank and outwardly applied; the distilled water drank for twenty days together, helps

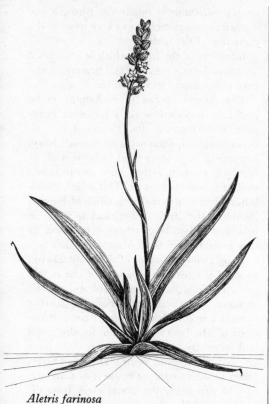

Aletris farinosa

The fibrous roots, when thoroughly dried, were prescribed, mainly in Canada and the United States, as an intensely bitter tonic and stomachic, and these 'in decoction or tincture are of great utility in dyspepsia, general or local debility, flatulence, colic, hysteria, etc.' It was administered under various names, such as Colic Root, Ague Root, Crow Corn, Blazing Star and Star Grass as a 'strengthener of the female generative organs', a 'protection against miscarriage' and also in 'chlorosis, amenorrhoea, dysmenorrhoea, engorged conditions of the uterus, prolapses of that organ' and for various 'other women's complaints'.

An intense bitter known as Aletrim is still extracted from the roots of this species and used medicinally as a stomachic and tonic. It is mostly given in small doses as a tonic for women, mainly in cases of debility. Larger doses cause sickness accompanied by dizziness.

ALISMA
Alismataceae, the Water-Plantain family
Water Plantain

This genus of hardy aquatic, generally weedy perennials, is native chiefly to North America, Europe, North Africa, India and Japan. They are found in wet or boggy soils as their generic name, which evolved from *alis*, the Celtic word for water, suggests. Of these only one, the commonest Water Plantain (*A. plantago-aquatica*), was prescribed to any extent in herbal medicine. A stout hairless perennial 40–100cm/15–39in. high, it is indigenous to the watery places of Europe, including Britain, and to parts of Asia, Canada and the United States. Its tufts of broad, long stalked leaves, ribbed like those of the Plantain, together with the leafless stems, are carried above the water. In summer the plant bears whorled spikes of delicate pale-lilac or whitish three-petalled flowers.

The acid-tasting leaves of this plant, sometimes listed as the Greater Thrumwort, were

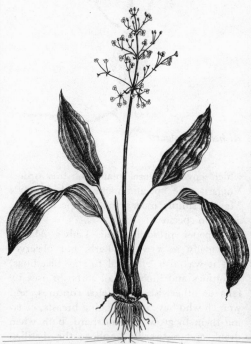

Alisma plantago-aquatica

the parts prescribed in medicine, principally for their diuretic and diaphoretic effects as an excellent way 'of ridding the body of gravel and stone – and for relieving kidney and urinary affections', such as the 'hotness and the pains of passing water' and 'for the pains in the loins'. The leaves were simply collected, dried and then carefully powdered down. This, when infused in the proportion one ounce to a pint of boiling water and taken three or four times a day in wineglassful doses, was said to be 'very efficacious' for the above complaints, and was prescribed as a popular remedy not only in Europe but in Canada and the United States, especially during the eighteenth and nineteenth centuries.

At one time the common Water Plantain was considered as 'a capital remedy' in Russia in the treatment cf hydrophobia. As the infection inevitably resulted from the bite of a rabid dog, this species, which supposedly possessed the power to cure it, became known as Mad-Dog Weed.

The dried powdered leaves are still occasionally prescribed by herbalists, usually in the form of an infusion, in the treatment of various urinary infections.

ALNUS
Betulaceae, the Birch family
Tag Alder, Common Alder

The majority of the Alnus genus consists of a group of hardy deciduous, catkin-bearing trees or shrubs, most of which flourish in moist or boggy soils, and are native to the cold and temperate regions of North America, Europe, Asia and North Africa. Their generic name of Alnus appears to have been taken from *Alr*, an Anglo-Saxon term of uncertain meaning. From several such forms as *Aelr* and *Aler*, it gradually evolved over the years to *Aller* or *Aldir* and eventually, during the medieval period, to their collective and familiar present-day name of Alder.

Although several sorts of Alnus are known to have been used in the medicine of medieval Europe, the species principally employed was the one referred to as the Alder, or the Common Alder (*A. glutinosa*) which is native to the whole of Europe (except Iceland) and much of Asia, and is now found naturalized in parts of eastern North America, where it was formerly used by the settlers in their medicine. In its natural habitat, this water-loving Alder is generally found in marshes and similar swampy places where it often forms small woods, with individual trees sometimes exceeding 20m/65ft in height, but in more porous soils it merely forms large bushes.

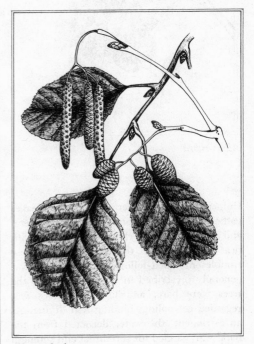

Alnus glutinosa

The parts of the tree prescribed in healing were either the dark brown fissured bark, or the rounded leaves, to which the specific name *glutinosa* meaning sticky or gluey refers. They were applied externally when young and fresh 'to dissolveth swellings and stay the hardness of inflammations'. Decoctions 'of the leaves or the distilled water thereof' also made 'an excellent wash for burnings and inflammations – either with wounds or without'.

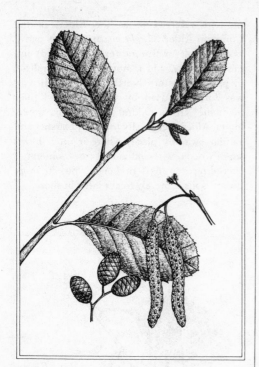

Alnus rubra

explosives, for which it was grown as a coppice tree.

The bark of another familiar species, the Tag Alder (*A. rubra*, syn. *A. serrulata*), was valued for its alterative, astringent and tonic effects. This Alder is common in Europe, including the British Isles, and parts of North America, and is found either as a medium-sized tree, or as a shrub with numerous stems often growing as a clump, forming thickets in swamps, or by the banks of ponds or rivers.

The bitter-tasting bark of this tree was prescribed infused 'for the debility of the stomach caused by indigestion – and for diarrhoea and similar afflictions of the bowels and belly'. It was still popularly administered both in England and the United States during the nineteenth and early part of the twentieth centuries, and it was 'universally acknowledged to be alterative and emetic, and is especially recommended for scrofula, secondary syphilis' and for 'other eruptions and cutaneous diseases of the skin'. The active medicinal principle prepared from the bark was known as Alnuin, although this rarely appears to be used nowadays.

The Tag Alder's other common names include Smooth Alder, Red Alder and, like the previous species, Common Alder.

ALTHAEA
Malvaceae, the Mallow family
Marsh Mallow, Hollyhock

Culpeper tells of another use: 'The said leaves gathered while the morning dew is on them, and brought into a chamber troubled with fleas ... will rid the chamber of these troublesome bed-fellows.' The bark was generally prescribed in the winter when the trees were bare, and like the leaves was regarded as cooling, binding and drying. As an astringent 'the water decocted from the bark' was 'gargled for sorethroat and soreneth of the throat and gums'.

Nowadays this species, which is sometimes known as the English Alder, is little used in herbal medicine, although its wood has several uses. This is white when alive, red on exposure to the air, changing to pink when dry, and since it is very durable in water it is frequently used in the making of stakes and piles. It is also light and easily worked, and so is used in general turnery, in the making of plywood, brush backs, cabinets, soles for clogs etc., and at one time was held in high repute in making the best charcoal for

Most of the species belonging to this genus are non-woody, downy or bristly haired, erect biennial or perennial plants, native to China, Asia (including Siberia) and much of Europe. Of these one or two containing 'an abundance of mucilage' were prescribed in ancient medicine. Althaea, their generic name, evolved from the Greek *althaia* or *altho* meaning to cure or heal.

The most popular species, the Marsh Mallow (*A. officinalis*), is a hardy, somewhat hoary-looking little branched perennial, native to most of Europe, where it is found in salt-rich places near the sea, by dykes and the banks of tidal rivers and estuaries. It grows

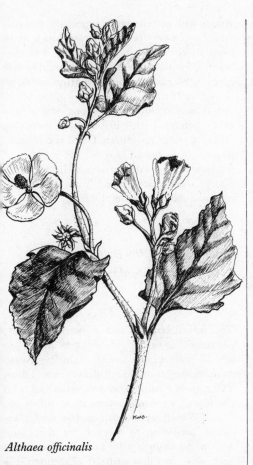

Althaea officinalis

in clumps up to 2m/6ft high, has broad, greyish-green shallow lobed leaves, and bears soft pale pink or mauve flowers from about June to September.

Like the Common Mallow (see Malva), the Marsh Mallow was once eaten as a food. The Romans, for example, regarded it as a succulent vegetable dish, although some of the writers of the period warned of its laxative effects. The leaves can still be used for this purpose, while the fresh young tops make a useful addition to spring salads which, with a syrup made from the roots, is still taken in France to stimulate the kidneys. The seed also had its uses and was served in oil at the tables of the ancient Greeks as a 'highly tonic' dish.

In medicine the Marsh Mallow was usually prescribed because it contained more healing mucilage than any other Mallow, 'being far superior to other kinds'. Of its early history in Britain and France little is known, although the Romans probably used it. It was certainly known and used by the Anglo-Saxons. By the medieval period it had become a very popular healing herb and was widely administered for its 'emollient principles' which were mainly 'derived from the roots'. The latter are described by Culpeper in the 1640s as 'of a whitish yellow colour on the outside, and white within, full of a slimy juice, which if laid in water will thicken, as if it were a jelly'. Decoctions of the root 'or the juice thereof in wine' was 'taken inwardly for coughs and colds, hoarsness, and wheezings with shortness of breath' and by those 'that are wounded and faint through loss of blood'. At the same time for 'wounds and tears in the skin' it was 'mixed with honey and rosin' and 'applied direct'. The juice 'doth also relieve excoriations, the phthisis, pleurisy and other such chest diseases – and will help women to a speedy delivery of child' as well as 'give an abundance of milk to nurses and mothers'. Decoctions of the seed in milk or wine were prescribed for the same conditions. The bruised leaves, or the roots in ointments or plasters, with Oil of Roses added were regarded 'applied thereto' as 'an especial remedy for the relieving and the easing of pain in hard tumours – inflammations – swellings – imposthumes in the private parts – ruptures and cramps – the swellings of women's breasts' as for 'hurts by falls – swelling pains – bruises by falls or blows – disjointed limbs – aches of the sinews and muscles – and for the place stung by a bee or wasp'.

The seed first boiled in oil was often applied to 'take away roughness in the skin, scurf or dry scabby heads – and to heal burns and scalds' while the seed 'green and dry' mixed with vinegar 'cleanseth the skin from morphew'. The flowers alone first boiled in oil or water, with honey or alum added 'makes an excellent gargle to heal a sore throat or mouth'. For septic sores the root was crushed and 'anointed hot to the place', while the bed-ridden were given the shoots to eat as a reliable preventative against bed sores, this particular species then becoming well known as the Mortification Root. Its other names include Mallards, Mauls and Cheeses (referring to the shape of the seeds), Guimauve and Schloss Tea.

The leaves and root of the Marsh Mallow are classed as demulcent and emollient, and are still prescribed by herbalists, mainly for soothing coughs and bronchitis, inflammations of the digestive and urinary organs, including cystitis, and in ointments with other herbs for treating burns and minor skin infections. For chest complaints it can be taken in a pleasant tasting syrup. Grown commercially, the dried and finely powdered root is added to Marshmallow confections, to lozenges and pastes (Pâté de Guimauve). The latter makes a useful emollient for soothing hoarseness, coughs and other chest complaints.

The Marsh Mallow was one of the herbs grown in the New World by Cotton Mather (1662–1727) the New England Puritan and colonial magistrate, after its introduction from Europe. It has since become naturalized there in certain regions, including the salt marshes along the coasts of New England and New York and in Michigan and Arkansas.

The common Hollyhock (*Althaea rosea*, syn. *Alcea rosea*), now a familiar sight in many gardens, was formerly prescribed for its demulcent, diuretic and emollient effects. A handsome perennial plant with strong growing stems up to 2½m/8ft high, it has rough heart-shaped lobed or angled leaves, usually bearing pink but sometimes white or violet close-set flowers in summer, borne on long temporal spikes. Although the exact origin of this species is unknown, it is believed by some authorities to have originated in China, although now grown as an ornamental all over the world, including North America, Asia and much of Europe, where in certain areas it is found in the wild.

This plant's familiar name of Hollyhock is derived from the Anglo-Saxon *halig* – meaning holy, and *hoc* – a mallow, thus *halighoc*, because it was believed to have been introduced into Europe from the Holy Land itself. By the Middle English period this spelling had evolved to *holihoc* and *holihocce* and in time to Hollyhock.

The whole of the plant was said to have a rough and austere taste, especially the root and: 'is of a very binding nature, and may be used to advantage both inwardly and outwardly, for incontinence of urine, immoderate menses, bleeding wounds, spitting of blood, the bloody flux, and other fluxes of the belly.' It was 'also of efficacy in a spongy state of the gums, attended with looseness of the teeth, and soreness of the mouth. Dried and reduced to powder, or boiled in wine, and partaken of freely, it prevents miscarriage, helps ruptures, dissolves coagulated blood from falls, blows, etc., and kills worms in children.'

ANEMONE

Ranunculaceae, the Buttercup family
Wood Anemone, Pasque Flower, Liverwort

This mixed genus of rather charming, hardy, perennial flowering plants are native to several parts of the world, including North America, Japan and much of Europe and Asia. Their generic name Anemone is derived from the Greek word *anemos* meaning the wind. Hence Windflower, their common name, 'so-called' according to Gerard 'for the floure doth never open it selfe but when the wind doth blow, as Pliny writeth: whereupon it is named of divers, Herba venti: in English Wind-floure.'

One of the better known species to be prescribed in the medieval medicine of Europe was the Wood Anemone (*A. nemorosa*) which is common to much of Europe and parts of the United States, where it grows in colonies in woods and similar shady places, especially in limestone or alkaline soils. This delicate but very pretty little plant spreads itself by means of creeping rhizomes, producing in early spring solitary drooping whitish coloured flowers, often tinged with pink or purple, on short, unbranched stems.

During the early part of the medieval period the bitter acrid juice of this particular herb was prescribed for leprosy, often under the names of Smell Fox or Wood Crowfoot, throughout much of Europe and Asia. The affected part was simply 'bathed' with a strong

Althaea rosea

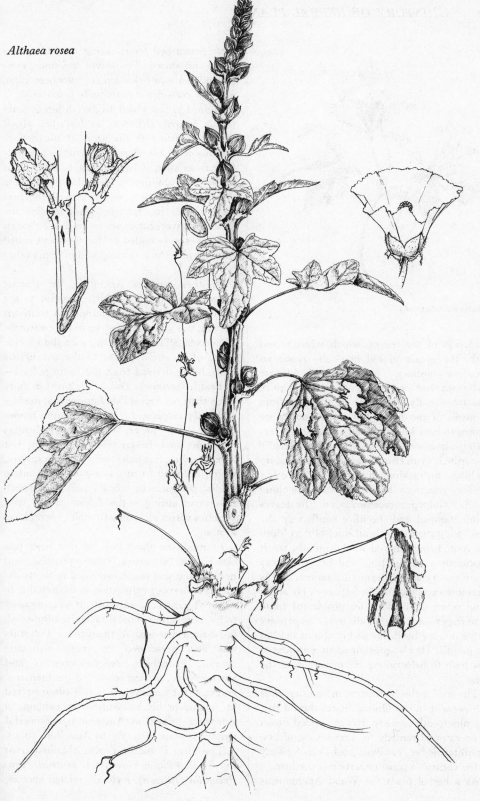

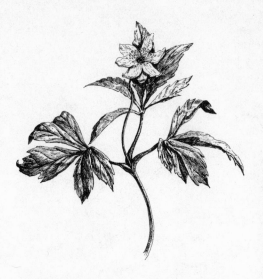

Anemone nemorosa

decoction of the leaves, which when mixed with 'the grease of old hog' also made an excellent ointment 'good for to cleanse malignant and corroding ulcers'. The juice was occasionally given to those suffering from paralysis of the body, but strong doses are known to have killed as well as cured. Nevertheless, later on, decoctions were internally prescribed 'as an emmenagogue for secondary syphilis – for rackings of the chest – and other similar afflictions such as the whooping cough'. Culpeper recommended 'the leaves being stamped and the juice snuffed up the nose' to 'purgeth the head mightily' as 'doth the root, being chewed in the mouth, for it procureth much spitting, and bringeth away many watery and phlegmatic humors, and is therefore excellent for the lethargy'. He adds: 'And when all is done let physicians prate what they please, all the pills in the dispensary purge not the head like so hot things held in the mouth.' He also prescribed an ointment of this herb to help relieve inflammation of the eyes.

The use of the 'Anemone in solution' was still popular in the United States during the, late nineteenth century. It was applied direct as an external remedy to treat scalds, ulcers, syphilitic nodes, paralysis and even 'opacity of the cornea', a most uncertain procedure.

As a herbal plant the Wood Anemone is little prescribed today, being unstable when dried and stored. The leaves and juice, containing a substance known as Protoanemonine, are now considered potentially poisonous.

Gerard raised about twelve different sorts in his garden, although he described about thirty according to his ideas of distinction. Parkinson in his *Paradisus* writes of Windflowers as such delightful plants that . . . it passed his abilities to describe the infinite varieties: 'I think it would grovell the best experienced in Europe.' Apparently the Anemones were little used in his day, although the leaves were added to 'the ointment called Marciatum, which is composed of many other hot herbs . . .'

Another type of Anemone, the Pasque Flower (*A. pulsatilla*) which is native to the Soviet Union, central Europe to southern Britain, was at one time given in the treatment of nervous afflictions. In this case the specific name of *pulsatilla* points to the use of the herb, being derived from the Latin *pulsare* – to beat (overcome). Today, the plant is more often than not found listed under that name – *Pulsatilla vulgaris*. Its other common names include Passe Flower, Wind Flower, Meadow Anemone and Easter Flower. As the last name implies, this hairy, very variable species, which is found in meadows, on hills and in glades, produces its solitary pale or purplish flowers in spring – the colour of the wild varieties varies according to their geographical location.

In medicine the whole of this herb was classed as alterative, antispasmodic and nervine and was much esteemed in the treatment of nervous exhaustion in women due to various menstrual complaints. It was supposed to be more 'efficacious' if taken by blue-eyed, fair-haired women. A tincture of Pulsatilla was also prescribed 'to sooth asthmatic coughs, bronchitis, relieve catarrhs and amenorrhoae, or suppression of the menses – and cure the measles'. It is still administered in homoeopathic medicines. It contains a substance known as Anemonin, a powerful irritant similar in action to Aconitum (q.v.).

The drug Pulsatilla is also obtained from the Small Pasque Flower (*A. pratensis*, syn. *Pulsatilla pratensis*), a closely related species,

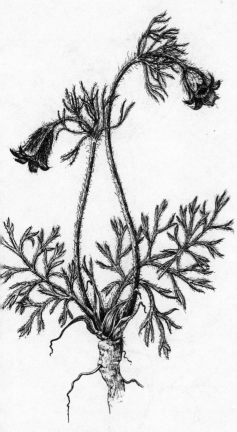

Anemone pulsatilla

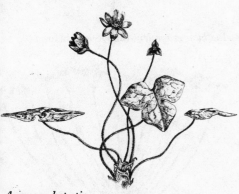

Anemone hepatica

(*A. hepatica*, syn. *Hepatica nobilus* or *H. triloba*), was also prescribed during the medieval period in Europe, where it still grows in shady woods and copses, forming dense tufts of three to five lobed leaves supposedly liver-shaped and of a smooth leathery nature. These usually appear after the whitish-pink or whitish-blue flowers have faded, and remain green during the winter months. This species is also common in the United States where it is often found in early spring pushing its flowers through the snow. It is best known there under the names of Choisy, Kidneywort or Liverleaf, and sometimes Round-Leaved Hepatica, Noble Liverwort Trefoil, Herb Trinity and Edellebere.

As might be guessed, this was one of the principal plants prescribed 'for all diseases of the liver for to cool and cleanse – to help inflammations of any part – to fortify and strengthen – and is for those that have livers corrupted by surfeits'. To a lesser degree the extracted juice in an ointment was 'helpful to stay the spreading of tetters, fretting or running sores – the scab and the itch of ringworm'. In England it was mentioned by Gardiner in 1440 and again by Turner in the 1550s, who tells us: 'The later writers hold that this herbe is good for the liver, and especially for the liver of new married yong men, which are desyrous of childer.'

Popular as the Liverwort was, towards the end of the seventeenth century it slowly slipped from favour, and in Europe is little used in herbal medicine today. In England, where this species was rarely found in the wild, it had to be grown in gardens, becoming known in certain areas as the Trinity Flower. Infusions are still prescribed in parts of the United States, for the herb's mildly astringent, tonic and pectoral effects – it contains tannin and sugar. The juice was also applied at one time for freckles and sunburn.

Another species belonging to this genus, *A. cylindrica*, which is native to parts of the United States, was used by the Indians there as a cure for rattlesnake bite. They chewed the tops off the plant, swallowing a little of the juice, then applied the wet mixture direct to the bite. It was supposed to render the poison harmless within a few minutes.

native mainly to Germany, Italy and Denmark, where it is still occasionally prescribed in an ointment for treating certain eye complaints.

A third Anemone, the Common Liverwort

ANETHUM

Umbelliferae, the Parsley family
Dill

The Dill (*A. graveolens*, syn. *Peucedanum graveolens*) is an aromatic, rather dark green, feathery leaved annual, with a spindle-like root, native to the Mediterranean and Black Sea regions, where it grows in fields and similar places. It reaches 25–100cm/9–39in. high and produces broad flattened umbels of small yellow flowers in early summer.

The first mention of this plant appeared in an Egyptian list some 5,000 years ago, thus making it one of the oldest known medicinal herbs. Some authorities believed it to be the Anise of the Bible (Matthew, xxiii, 23) which is known to have been widely cultivated in Palestine at that time. It was certainly known to Pliny and Dioscorides, who wrote 'it stayeth the hickets [hiccough]'. The herb's more familiar name of Dill apparently evolved from the Anglo-Saxon *Dylle* or *Dylla*, which had changed by the medieval period to *Dille* and later to *Dill* – meaning lull, probably referring to its principal use as a carminative for relieving wind and colic in infants. By the fifteenth and sixteenth centuries it had become a very common plant indeed and was employed throughout Europe, including England, where it was grown in every kitchen garden, for hindering 'witches of their will', as a charm 'against witchcraft and enchantments'. It was also a popular ingredient in potions and magic spells.

During the seventeenth century most of these superstitious uses were forgotten as the herb became more frequently prescribed in simple medicine, usually as in ancient times 'for flatulence – as a gallant expeller of wind – and especially so for the mother and child'. It was sometimes 'smelled unto being boiled in wine and tied in a cloth'.

The fruit was regarded as the most effective part. It is most 'effectual to digest raw and viscous humours, and is used in medicines that serve to expel wind, and the pains proceeding thereof.' Culpeper notes that they were added to 'oils or plaisters' to dissolve

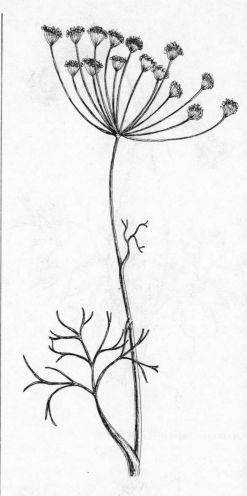

Anethum graveolens (above and below)

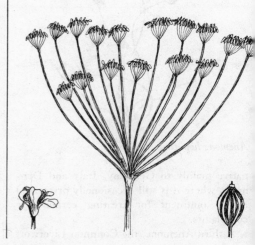

'the imposthumes in the fundament' and to 'drieth up all moist ulcers especially in that part'. He adds: 'The decoction of Dill, be it herb or seed, (only if you boil the seed you must bruise it) in white wine, being drunk, it is a gallant expeller of wind and provoker of terms.' Mothers-to-be who were 'troubled' were often recommended 'to sit therein a decoction to rid them of their pains'.

Nowadays the Dill is widely cultivated in countries as far apart as England, Roumania, Germany, Spain, South Africa, America, Japan and India (as Soyah) much as it was in Europe and the Mediterranean region during the medieval period, for the sake of its fruits, which contain an essential oil with carminative, stimulant and aromatic properties. Even today, most mothers have at one time or another resorted to Gripe or Dill Water to relieve flatulence and other digestive disorders in their children. The fruit, known medicinally as *Fructus Anethi*, is sometimes made up into little cakes which are very soothing for teething babies to chew on, while in France they are added as a matter of course to flavour bread, cakes and sauces, and the leaves to soups and stews.

Dill seed is also well known as one of the main ingredients in cucumber and gherkin pickles, one of its chief modern uses. These, together with Dill vinegar, probably date back in England to the early seventeenth century. Evelyn, writing in 1680, lists a recipe for 'Dill and Collyflower Pickle', in his *Acetaria*, a 'book about Sallets' (salads). This plant was introduced to the New World by the early settlers from Europe and was one of the herbs grown there by John Winthrop (1605–76). In certain areas, like the West Indies, it has since become naturalized. The extracted oil of Dill is also extensively used in commerce for scenting soap.

At one time the Dill was commonly known as False Fennel, and was attributed with similar properties as that closely related species *Foeniculum vulgare*.

ANGELICA
Umbelliferae, the Parsley family
Garden Angelica, Wild Angelica, American Angelica

The principal species of this genus to be prescribed in Anglo-Saxon Europe was the Common or Garden Angelica (*A. archangelica*, syn. *Archangelica officinalis*). A robust aro-

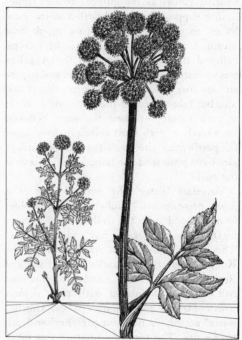

Angelica archangelica

matic biennial or perennial herb, it is believed to be native to northern Europe, including Iceland, Greenland, Lithuania and central Russia, where it is found in damp soils, as in meadows, marshes, by the riverside and other such watery places. In such situations, the hollow jointed stems of the plant often reach 2–3m/6–9ft high, the large, broad and pointed leaves are divided into smaller numerous leaflets with finely serrated edges, and the small but numerous green or greenish-white flowers, in somewhat globular umbels are produced in July.

Little is known of this herb's early history,

other than the fact that when it was introduced to the warmer countries of Europe, it was found to flower on 8 May, St Michael the Archangel's Day, hence its use as the 'Root or Herb of the Holy Ghost' in many rituals, chiefly as a preventative against witches and their spells. It appears to have been introduced to England by the 1550s, where, as in other European countries, it soon became naturalized. By the end of that century it had become a very common garden plant and was widely regarded as 'the antidote' to the Plague, having supposedly been revealed as the cure by an angel who appeared to a monk in a dream. Unfortunately the people of Europe believed the monk's tale, and the Angelica was soon included in many useless and superstitious cures. Even Gerard writes that if one 'doe but take a piece of the roote and holde it in your mouth, or chew the same between your teeth, it doth most certainly drive away the pestilentiall aire, yea although the corrupt aire have possessed the hart, yet it driveth it out again.

'Angelica Water' also formed part of a royal prescription, published in pamphlet form in London by the College of Physicians in 1665, the year of the city's Great Plague. This official prescription was entitled: 'The King's Majesty's [Charles II] Excellent Recipe for the Plague', and recommended half an ounce of nutmeg, with 'three pennyworth of treacle and a quarter of best Angelica water' added, to be 'beat together' and put over a fire. The resulting mixture was taken twice a day by thousands of desperate Londoners to stave off the dreaded sickness.

The thick yellowish juice from the aromatic and fleshy, spindle-shaped roots, with a warm and agreeable if somewhat bitter taste, was often included in a recipe for 'Carmelite Water'. If 'habitually taken by distinguished people' this 'sovereign remedy' was firmly believed to 'ensure long life' as well as protect against 'enchantyments, poysons and the spells of wytches', an echo of the plant's more superstitious past.

For other medicinal uses, the root was powdered or shredded, decocted in wine and taken internally for 'the ague fitt – the bites of mad doggs – pains of the cholic – the strang-

uary – stoppage of the urine – pleurisy – the cough – shortness of breath – and other diseases of the lungs', and 'to procureth women's courses – expel the afterbirth – and openeth the stoppages of the liver and spleen'. At the same time, the water distilled from the root, steeped in wine 'relieves the pain and torments coming of all cold windes'. The 'herb in a Syrup was also recommended as 'good for digestion – as a remedy for a surfeit – and for chest disease' while the juice alone dropped in the ears 'helps dimness of sight and deafness'. The same if placed in 'the hollow of the teeth easeth their pain' and 'put into filthy dead ulcers' or the powder of the root 'doth clean and cause them to heal quickly, by covering the naked bones with flesh'. For the bite of a mad dog, the root was applied to the wound well mixed in with a little pitch.

By the end of the seventeenth century the use of the Garden Angelica, as a medicinal plant had faded away, although it was still prescribed to a certain extent to relieve flatulence, or 'corrupt air' as it was known, and it probably worked 'if the bruised root was infused and partaken of warm after meals'. A tea of the leaves is often taken for this purpose, although the nicest way of consuming the herb is in the form of the sweetmeat known as Angelica Candy. This is made much as it was in London in the early 1600s, where the species was especially grown for this purpose. Much of the Angelica now used for flavouring and decorating cakes and other confections is grown commercially in Spain and the south of France.

As a culinary herb the more tender stems can be chopped up and added to salads. Both the seeds and the roots are rich in essential oils. The former are included in the preparation of Vermouth and Chartreuse, while the oil of the seed is used in the manufacture of perfume. The roots are used either together with Juniper berries in the making of gin, or as a substitute for them. Roots can also be dried and powdered and made into a form of bread, as in Norway, while in Finland the young stems baked in ashes are regarded as a great delicacy.

In the 1934 edition of the *British Pharma-*

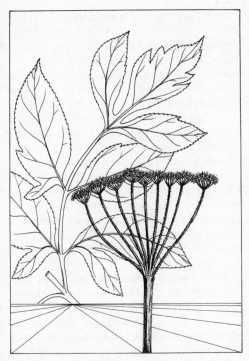

Angelica atropurpurea

grows in damp places, reaches a height of about 2m/6ft and produces its umbels of greenish white flowers from about May to August.

For medicinal purposes, it was regarded as 'aromatic, stimulant, carminative, diaphoretic, expectorant, diuretic and emmenagogue' and was given principally 'in flatulent colic and heartburn' and as serviceable 'in diseases of the urinary organs'. The normal dosage was two to four ounces of the decoction, or between thirty to sixty grains of the powder. John Clayton writing to a friend in 1686 mentions a Virginian Angelica and observed that the Indians knew it as Hunting or Fishing Root, because if rubbed on the hands the smell of it attracted fish and game. The plant he describes is probably *A. atropurpurea*, which grows from Newfoundland to Iowa, for it certainly has a peculiar, although not unpleasant, odour and a warm, sweetish taste.

ANTHEMIS
Compositae, the Daisy family
Chamomile, Mayweed, German Chamomile

At least 50 species of this genus are known to be native to various parts of Europe, North Africa and the temperate regions of Asia.

The Roman or True Chamomile (*A. nobilis*, syn. *Chamaemelum nobile*) has been included in the medicine of the Mediterranean region now for well over two thousand years and is still commonly prescribed today. This hairy, pleasantly scented, but bitter-tasting perennial has feathery fern-like leaves and branching stems of a creeping habit 10–30cm/3–11in. long, which root as the plant spreads along, bearing in summer its daisy-like flowers, consisting of a yellow centre, surrounded by white florets. Although native to the cornfields, heaths and other grassy places of western Europe, including Britain, the Chamomile is now found naturalized in many other countries, having escaped from cultivation.

Chamomile, or Camomile, the herb's common name, is derived from the Greek

ceutical Codex, the fruits were listed as an ingredient in Warburg's Tincture, which was prescribed as an antispasmodic. In certain other European Pharmacopoeias, such as the Austrian, German and Swiss, only the root of the plant was listed as official. Its other common names include Officinal Angelica and European Angelica.

The Garden Angelica should not be confused with the Wild Angelica or Jack-jump-About (*A. sylvestris*) which although found in a similar habitat, such as damp meadows and fens, has purplish coloured stems producing umbels of white or pinkish-white flowers from July to September. This common herb is native to the whole of Europe, and although prescribed in medicine, was not regarded as highly as the Garden Angelica. It also yields a good yellow dye.

Another species was found growing in Maine by the settlers, where it became known as the American Angelica or Masterwort (*A. atropurpurea*). It is less branched and slightly paler in colour than the European kind and has a purplish-coloured root. This herb also

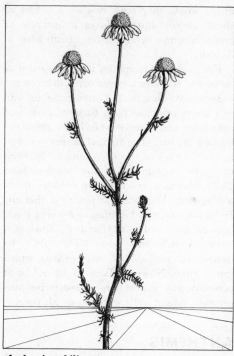

Anthemis nobilis

word *chamaimelon* – *chamai* meaning on the ground, and *melon* an apple, referring to its distinctive smell when fresh. The Spaniards call it *Manzanilla* – little apple – and still add it as a flavouring to one of their lighter sherries of that name. The generic name of Anthemis derives from the Greek word *anthos* – a flower. The plant's specific name of *nobilis* – noble or noted – refers perhaps to its healing virtues, which are known to have been employed by the Ancient Egyptians. Certain Moorish herbals also mention the plant and its use in relieving sprains and strains of the muscles and similar pains including cramps. The Saxons certainly used it, for they referred to it as *Maythen* in an ancient document, which still exists, as one of their nine sacred herbs. It was first recorded in England as a cultivated plant in 1265 and was later mentioned in the wardrobe accounts of King Edward II (1307–27). By this period, due no doubt to its pungent smell when crushed, the Chamomile had become a favourite strewing herb for floors throughout Europe, and was even on occasions burnt to

help rid homes 'of the foulness of offending odours'. During the Tudor period it was often grown instead of grass on lawns, and as a low creeping cover for alleys, walks and banks, where, according to Falstaff in Shakespeare's *Henry IV*, the more it was trodden upon the faster it grew, which no doubt gave rise to the 'Herb of Humility' – another common name. Sir Francis Drake is believed to have been playing bowls on such a green in July 1588, when informed that the Spanish Armada was approaching the English Channel. Cultivated out of doors the Chamomile was also regarded as the 'plants' physician' or tonic, a reputation it still has in several countries, and if set near a sickly plant or shrub, it was supposed to rapidly revive and help its recovery.

The Chamomile had many medicinal uses. Decoctions of the whole herb – the flowers boiled as a posset – syrups of the juice – the oil of the flower – or the flower in wine – all were taken or applied throughout the whole of Europe, from Greece to Sweden, for the relief of complaints from 'the wind and pains and torments of the belly – the pain of the colic and stone – as a mollifyer of swellings and sinews that be over strained – inflammation of the bowels – cramps and aches all over – pains and stiches in the side – including the region of the liver and spleen – for cases of weak or irritable stomachs – as a provoker of lusty urine – and for intermittent and typhoid fevers'. One of the herb's principal uses was in the treatment of agues. As Culpeper puts it, 'if the part grieved be anointed with that oil, taken from the flowers, from the crown of the head to the sole of the foot, and afterward laid to sweat in bed, and he sweats well.' The oil was also regarded 'as profitable for all sorts of agues that come either from phlegm or melancholy, or from an inflammation of the bowels . . .' Turner agrees and writes: 'Thys herbe was conserated by the wyse men of Egypt unto the Sonne and was rekened to be the only remedy of all agues.'

On the Chamomile's introduction to the United States, it was prescribed much as in Europe as a stomachic, tonic and antispasmodic. It was occasionally made into a poultice which was said to prevent gangrene 'and remove it when present'. Used this way or in the form of a lotion, it certainly deadens pain if applied direct to toothache, earache and even neuralgia. The flowers are still prescribed by herbalists in teas and infusions, which, when taken internally, have a sedative as well as a tonic effect on the body. They are excellent for soothing the nerves and ensuring a good night's sleep – an extremely useful and very ancient remedy for women suffering from hysterical and other nervous complaints, including nightmare. A good herb beer can also be made from this species.

The *British Pharmacopoeia* directs that the Chamomile flowers used for medicinal purposes should be those of the cultivated, double flowering form, which was introduced into Germany from Spain, probably during the sixteenth century. It is now commercially grown in several European countries, including Belgium and France and to a certain extent in England. The oil of Chamomile, a beautiful blue when first distilled later turning a greenish-brown, is still used in hair shampoos.

The Mayweed or Dog Fennel (*A. cotula*, syn. *Maruta cotula* or *Maruta foetida*) was also prescribed for its medicinal effects during the medieval period, although slightly less commonly than the above species. This herb, a fetid, much branched annual up to 50cm/19in. tall, has finely divided leaves, and bears from May to September, solitary terminal flower heads of white ray petals surrounding a yellow disc. It is found in cornfields, waste places and by habitation. Although native to the whole of Europe (except Iceland) and parts of Asia, this species is now naturalized in several other parts of the world, including the United States.

In medicine the flowers and leaves of this disagreeable and acrid-tasting plant, which Gerard tells us has 'a naughty smell', are described 'as tonic, antispasmodic, emmenagogue and emetic' and were administered for 'the headache – those recovering from fevers – scrofula – dysentery – amenorrhoea and dysmennorrhoea'. Culpeper writes: 'The flowers have, but in a very inferior degree, some of the virtues of camomile, and are far more disagreeable in taste. The leaves operate

by urine, and in some constitutions by stool; but both ways roughly, and should be very cautiously tampered with.' Joseph Miller observes: 'Mr. Ray says it is sometimes made use of in scrofulous cases, and Tournefort, That about Paris they use it in Fomentations for pains and swellings of the Haemorrhoides.'

The herb's other common names include Cotula, Wild Chamomile, Dog Chamomile, Stinking Mayweed, Foetid Chamomile, Stinking Chamomile, Maroute, Maithes, Maithen or Mathor. It is rarely prescribed nowadays, although sometimes used as an insecticide.

The Yellow Chamomile (*A. tinctoria*), a stiff, branched, woolly-haired perennial, which bears solitary, yellow, long-stalked flower heads in July and August, is native to the dry and rocky waste places of much of Europe. It was sometimes substituted for the above species.

Another species, the Corn Chamomile (*A. arvensis*), an erect, branching annual or perennial, with grey downy stems and deeply cut leaves, downy underneath, is found throughout the whole of Europe, in both

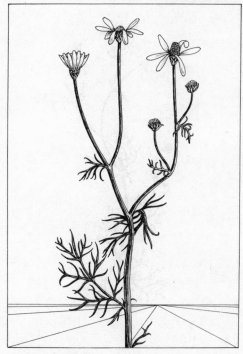

Anthemis cotula

arable and waste ground and by the wayside, and is still prescribed in France as a febrifuge.

The German Chamomile, known as the Wild or Single Chamomile, or Pin Heads (*Matricaria recutita*, syn. *M. chamomilla*) a closely related plant, listed under a different genus in the Compositae Order, was and still is given for its carminative, sedative and tonic effects. This aromatic annual reaches 15–60cm/5–23in. tall, has hairless, erect or prostrate branching stems with feathery leaves, bearing daisy-like flowers in summer, and is found in cultivated ground, waste places and by tracksides. Although native to Europe, including the British Isles and western Asia, it is also found wild in parts of the United States, India, Australia and various other countries, having escaped from cultivation.

This herb's generic name, Matricaria, refers to one of its principal uses in the medieval period, when the flowers were used as a fomentation in treating a range of uterine complaints, being derived from the Latin *matrix* (*-icis*) meaning womb, while *recutita*

alludes to the white, reflexed ray florets of the flowers themselves. These were also given in the treatment of childrens' ailments, in cases of earache caused by teething, stomach disorders and neuralgic pains, for which teas and infusions are still prescribed. In Finland infusions of the Corn Feverfew or Scentless Mayweed (*M. inodora*) were formerly prescribed in consumption.

APOCYNUM
Apocynaceae, the Dogbane family
Bitter Root, Canadian Hemp

Most of the Apocynums, a small genus of shrubby and perennial herbs containing a milky juice, which exudes from the plant if wounded, are found in the northern temperate regions.

The first, the Bitter Root (*A. androsaemifolium*), a smooth elegant plant 1½–2m/5–6½ft high, with ovate leaves, pale beneath and dark green above, bears clusters of dainty

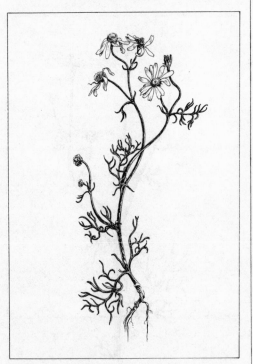

Matricaria recutita

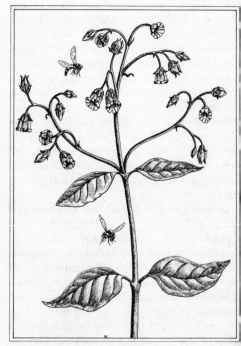

Apocynum androsaemifolium

pinkish-white flowers from about May to August, followed by pairs of long slender pods. Common to much of North America, especially from Maine to Florida, it is found in dry sandy soils especially by the edges of woods and, to a lesser extent, in parts of the mountainous regions of Europe.

The large milky root of this bitter tasting herb, from which the names of Bitter Root and Milk-Weed derive, was prescribed in medicine for its cathartic, diuretic, emetic, laxative and tonic effects 'after yielding them to water'. This liquid was taken internally for 'all liver and hepatic affections – is excellent in dyspepsia in a powder of four or five grains, three times a day – in amenorrhoea – dropsy – and as a laxative for constipation'.

Although basically an American herb, the Bitter Root was certainly known and used in England during the seventeenth century, for Parkinson writes that it was a 'soveraine remedy against all poysons – and against the biting of a mad dogge', hence another common name, that of Dogsbane. The generic name of *Apocynum* also refers to this and is derived from the Greek *apokynon*, *apo* meaning from or away, and *kyon* or *kynos*, a dog. Parkinson goes on: 'The downe that is found in the cods of these herbes [it was also known as Wild Cotton] doe make farre softer stuffing for cushions or pillows or the like than thistle downe, which is much used in some places for the like purposes.' The Indians of North America also used the bark of this and one or two other species as a Hemp substitute in the making of linen, twine and fishing nets.

In both Canada and the United States during the nineteenth century the Bitter Root was prescribed: 'When it is required to promptly empty the stomach, without causing much nausea or a relaxed condition of the muscular system ... It is also useful as an alterative in rheumatism, scrofula and syphilis.' The same was often administered in England as a heart stimulant and was regarded as 'of an admirable value in cardiac dropsy'.

The powdered root is still prescribed mainly as an alterative in the treatment of rheumatism and scrofula, and in dropsy as a

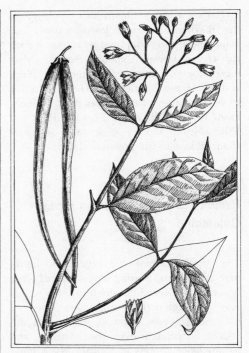

Apocynum cannabinum

hydragogue. Its use can, however, cause nausea and poisoning effects. Another name for this plant, Fly Trap, refers to its flowers, which attract and imprison insects.

The roots and rhizomes of the Canadian Hemp (*A. cannabinum*, syn. *A. pubescens*), another native of the United States and Canada, closely resemble the previous species. It has upright stems and branches with nearly sessile leaves, and grows in sandy and gravelly soils, especially by water. It was prescribed for its diaphoretic, diuretic, emetic and expectorant effects. In small amounts it was said to be good 'for intermittent and remittent fevers – amenorrhoea – leucorrhoea – other women's complaints – and as beneficial in the dropsy'. As 'a sure and reliable emetic' ten to thirty grains of the powdered root was prescribed in wine.

The dried roots are still carefully prescribed today usually in tinctures or liquid extracts, as a heart tonic and for dropsy. If taken in too large a dose or allowed to accumulate in the body, violent sickness will occur, with poisoning similar to that of the Foxglove.

The Canadian Hemp is also employed in the making of coarse linen, twines and fishing nets, and should not be confused with the Indian Hemp (*Cannabis indica*). Other names for the former plant include: Black Indian Hemp, American Hemp, Indian Physic, Bowman's Root, Bitter Root, Rheumatism Weed, Milk-Weed, Choctaw Root and Wild Cotton, though these may be interchangeable with the previous plant.

AQUILEGIA
Ranunculacea, the Buttercup family
Columbine

The Aquilegias make up a genus of hardy perennial plants, bearing long-spurred, often beautifully coloured flowers from May to late July. Although native to the cooler regions of both hemispheres, most of the species are widely distributed over the northern and mountainous regions of Canada, the United States, Europe and temperate Asia, including Siberia.

Of these, several species are believed to have been used in ancient medicine, but the plant chiefly prescribed was the common Columbine (*A. vulgaris*), a native of much of Europe, including the British Isles, but introduced elsewhere. Found locally in chalky soils, in woods, mountain pastures and rocky places, its slender stalks reach 30–80cm/ 11–31in. high, and bear compound leaves and in early summer violet-blue, but occasionally pink or white, flowers.

The generic name of this very variable species is derived from the Latin *aquila*, meaning eagle, and refers to the spur-like petals of the flowers. Its common name of Columbine, according to Tournefort, comes from *columba* – a dove, again alluding to the shape of the flowers, which are 'composed of plain petals intermixed with others that are hollow and horned, so that they imitate a Pidgeon with expanded Wings'. The Anglo-Saxon name of Culvertwort refers to much the same thing – *culfre* meaning pigeon – thus Pidgeon Wort or Plant. According to Gerard this species was also known as *Herba Leonis*

or the herb wherein the 'Lion doth delight', although he gives no explanation for this.

Of its early medicinal uses little appears to be known, other than that during the thirteenth century the juice was prescribed in several European countries in a useless effort to combat the all too frequent plagues.

In England, the common Columbine was first mentioned in a poem written in about 1310, and later Chaucer, Skelton and Shakespeare all write about it. By the end of the

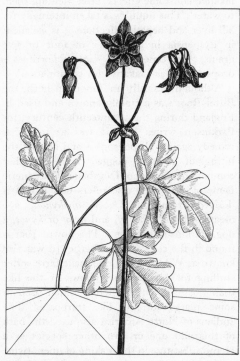

Aquilegia vulgaris

sixteenth century it had become a very popular garden plant, with several varieties of the species being grown in cottage gardens (sometimes as a protection against witches and their spells).

During the sixteenth and seventeenth centuries, the leaves of the Columbine were generally prescribed in lotions 'with good success for sore throats and mouths' while the extracted and very acrid-tasting juice was applied direct to wounds and various skin eruptions. The seed which Turner describes as 'like unto fleas' was usually crushed and administered a dram at a time in wine with a little Saffron added 'to relieve the complaints of the spleen, the liver, the bladder and the dropsy'. The same remedy was also 'good for the yellow jaundice, if the person after the taking thereof be laid to sweat well in bed'. Culpeper observed: 'The Spaniards used to eat a piece of the root thereof in a morning fasting, many days together, to help them when troubled with stone in the reins or kidneys.' The seed was still given during the eighteenth century, for Tournefort in his *Herbal* writes, that it was 'in frequent use among women, in driving out the measles and the smallpox'. The same in wine was sometimes administered to bring about a speedy delivery to women in childbirth, of which Culpeper had previously written, 'if one draught suffice not let her drink a second, and it will be found effectual'. Later on, however, Linnaeus warns that he had known children die through eating the herb.

The Columbine's active constituent has still to be identified. Although very similar to that of Aconitum, it is rarely given as an internal medicine in herbalism today.

ARISTOLOCHIA
Aristolachiaceae, the Birthwort family
Birthwort, Long Birthwort, Virginian Snake Root, Texas Snake Root

Most of the species belonging to this large genus are woody, twining climbers, although a few are non-climbing herbaceous plants. The majority are found in tropical countries, such as Brazil, Mexico, Guatemala, West Africa and the Philippines; others are native to the temperate regions of the southern parts of the United States, Europe and China.

The roots of several of the European species were once used in medicine there to help childbirth. This use is referred to in *Aristolochia*, the generic name, derived from the Greek *aristolocheia* with *aristos*, meaning best, and *locheia*, childbirth, hence Birthwort, the common and collective name. Dioscorides prescribed the dried roots as an internal medicine in wine to bring away both the

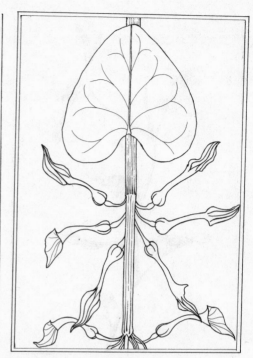

Aristolochia clematitis

child and afterbirth.

One of the more familiar Birthworts (*A. clematitis*) is known to have been employed in Greece at least three or four hundred years before the birth of Christ to help women in labour, and later as a cure for snakebite. This species is a strong-smelling hairless perennial, with creeping roots and unbranched stems 30–90cm/11–35in. high, bearing small clusters of pale yellow, erect, tubular or irregularly trumpet shaped flowers in the axils of the heart-shaped upper leaves, from about May to August. Although native to south-eastern Europe this plant is now naturalized as a result of cultivation, especially during the medieval period, in much of Europe, including parts of the British Isles, where it is found in hedges, woods, old ruins and by habitation.

The Long Birthwort (*A. longa*), a native of the Mediterranean region, which is now found wild in several other European countries, was also prescribed with the species listed above. This plant has somewhat cylindrical tubers, stems up to 60cm/23in. tall, with alternate ivy-like leaves and bears long, hollow, tube-

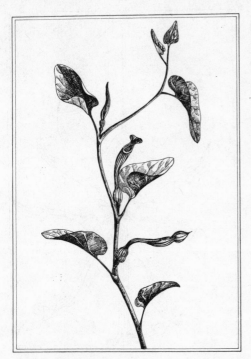

Aristolochia longa

bite. A perennial herb, it has short horizontal rhizomes with long slender roots below, bearing small brownish-purple coloured flowers produced close to the ground. Thomas Johnson noted: 'The root of the Virginian Pistolochia, which is of a strong and aromatick sent, is a singular and much used antidote against the bite of the Rattlesnake, or rather Adder or Viper, whose bite is very deadly . . . if any be bitten they chew [this root] and apply to the wound, and also swallow some of it downe, by which means they quickly overcome the malignitie of this poisonous bite . . .'

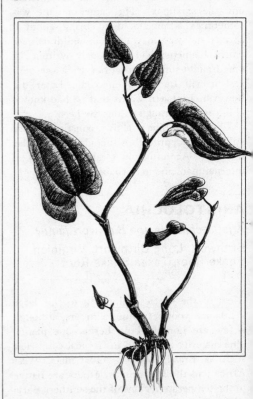

Aristolochia serpentaria

shaped brownish-yellow or greenish flowers. Gerard observes: 'The root is long, thick, of the colour of box, of a strong savour and bitter taste . . . Dioscorides writeth, That a dram weight of long Birthwoort drunke with wine and so applied, is good against serpents and deadly things.' From the seventeenth to the early part of the twentieth century the roots were regarded as aromatic and stimulant and were prescribed with other species for the rheumatism and gout. Joseph Miller writes that the same: 'Cleanses the stomach and lungs of tough phlegm' while 'outwardly it is useful in cleansing sordid ulcers.' The recommended dose was the same as prescribed by Dioscorides centuries earlier.

The root of another European species, the Round Aristolochia (*A. rotunda*), 'doth beautifie, clense and fasten the teeth if they be often fretted or rubbed with the pouder thereof.'

During the early seventeenth century in America a species then listed as *Pistolchia cretica*, but today known as Virginian Snakeroot (*A. serpentaria*), was used to treat snake-

The Texas Snake Root (*A. reticulata*), a similar plant native to the south-western part of the United States, was also prescribed for snakebite. The branching aromatic roots of this herb known as Red River, Serpentary or Texan Snake Root, have a bitterish camphorlike taste, and were administered for their anodyne, antispasmodic, diaphoretic, nervine, stimulant and tonic effects, mainly in fevers, including typhus and typhoid, and sometimes in place of or in combination with Peruvian Bark. Some herbalists still prescribe them for bilious complaints or to promote perspiration. The Virginian Snake Root was often substituted for the Texas Snake Root.

Other species known to have been used as antidotes for snakebite include *A. maxima* in South America and *A. sempervirens* in the Middle East where it was also prescribed as a counter-poison. In Egypt the juice of *A. anguicida* was not only administered for snakebite, but to subdue or stupefy snakes when their handlers wanted to hold them. Other medicinal species include *A. foetida*, which in Mexico was applied externally to ulcers and sores; *A. argentina*, used in the Argentine for its diuretic and diaphoretic effects, mainly in the treatment of rheumatism; and *A. indica* of the East Indies, valued as a stomachic, purgative and vermifuge as well as for its uses in the treatment of arthritis and rheumatism. *A. cymbifera* was at one time valued in Mexico and Brazil for its

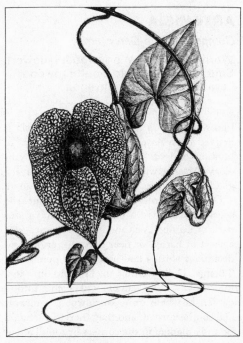

Aristolochia grandiflora

reputed aphrodisiac effects, although it is nowadays mainly prescribed in the treatment of pruritis and neuralgia. A few of the Birthworts are still prescribed today.

The flowers of several Aristolochias emit a most unpleasant odour to attract pollinating insects, which become imprisoned in their strangely bent calyx tubes. One of the more remarkable kinds, the Pelican Flower (*A. grandiflora*, syn. *A. gigas*, var. 'Sturtevantii'), a woody climber native to the West Indies, produces curious whitish-purple spotted flowers often 45cm/17in. in diameter, with tails up to 90cm/35in. long.

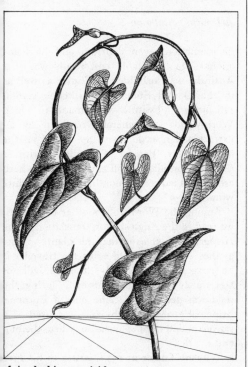

Aristolochia anguicida

ARTEMISIA

Compositae, the Daisy family

Wormwood, Sea Wormwood, Mugwort,
Southernwood, Field Southernwood,
Levant-Wormseed, Tarragon

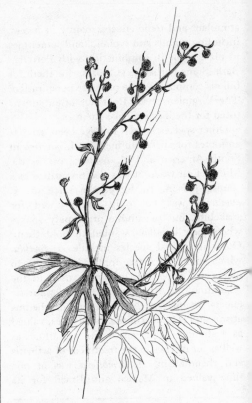

Artemisia absinthium

Pliny informs us that the word Artemisia is derived from Artemis, the Greek goddess of hunting and of chastity. In Roman mythology, Artemis was identified with Diana, the goddess of nature, the forests and the moon.

Of the Artemisias themselves about 180 species are known. Most are native to various parts of Europe, Asia and North America, and consist of hardy, or near hardy, evergreen or deciduous shrubs and herbaceous perennials. Thomas Hyll, writing in England in 1568, informs us: 'No adder will come into a garden in which grow wormwood, mugwort and southernwood' and they therefore 'should be aptly planted in the corners or round about the garden'.

The first species he mentions, the true Wormwood (*A. absinthium*), is a hardy, much-branched, very aromatic shrub-like perennial 30–100cm/11–39in. tall, with grooved stems and deeply cut silver-grey hairy leaves. It bears small flowers of greenish-yellow in summer, and is native to the whole of Europe (except Iceland) and parts of northern Asia, including Siberia, although now naturalized elsewhere including North America.

The use of this particular Wormwood in medicine dates back some four to five hundred years before the birth of Christ, and was a plant highly esteemed by Hippocrates and the Greeks, who claimed it restored disorders of the brain. They also infused the leaves in wine to supposedly lessen the intoxicating effects of alcohol. Pliny also mentions an artificial wine known as *absinthites*. The principal extract of the herb, a bitter, dark green oil, once formed the main ingredient of Absinthe, an aromatic liqueur popular in France. Unfortunately, drinking Absinthe was like drinking a slow-acting poison. In time it upset the nervous system, irritated the stomach and increased the action of the heart. If taken in quantity, or too often, it caused disorientation, even delirium and hallucinations. The inevitable end result was that Absinthe was forbidden in France as well as in the United States. Nevertheless certain satisfactory substitutes were made, in which Wormwood was generally replaced by an extract of Aniseed. These are found on the market today. 'Pernod', a popular aperitif, is the most familiar. Small amounts of the herb are still added to Vermouth, a fortified white wine.

Among the Wormwood's other early uses, we read in the Anglo-Saxon translation of the *Herbarium of Apuleius* that this plant, or wort as they called it, would assist the traveller if he carried it in his hand – 'then he will not feel much toil in his journey'. During the medieval period it became one of Europe's principal strewing herbs and was used as a powerful deterrent against 'body lice, the bug and the flea'.

William Tusser in 1573, writes in his *Five Hundred Pointes of Good Husbandrie*:

While wormwood hath seed get a handful
    or twain,
To save against March, to make flea to
    refraine,
Where the chamber is swept and the
    wormwood is strowne,
No flea for his life dare abide to be
    knowne.

Turner, repeating the ancient Greeks, tells us that if the herb was mixed and 'dronken' with vinegar 'it remedieth the strangling that cometh of eating of Todestoles.' Gerard writes: 'Being taken in wine it is good against the poison of Ixia, and of Hemlock and against the biting of the shrew mouse and of the sea dragon.' The same was often prescribed for 'the sickness of the sea'.

During the seventeenth century the leaves and flowers of this species were administered internally 'in slight infusions' for treating all manner of complaints, from jaundice to indigestion and hysterics. The leaves, boiled and strained, were occasionally 'applied with success' as a fomentation to 'spreading gangrenes'. Boiled in grease, balm or wine, the leaves made a useful poultice for 'applying to white swellings'. Joseph Miller in 1722, mentions: 'a Cataplasm of the green leaves beat up with Hog's Lard was commended to Mr. Ray by Dr. Hulse as a good external remedy against the swellings of the Tonsils and Quinzy.'

In the 1770s, Hill in his *Herbal* recommended the infused flowers taken in brandy to prevent the formation of gravel and as helpful in relieving the pain of gout. This common Wormwood (also known as Ajenjo or Green Ginger, the latter referring perhaps to its root) was employed in the United States during the nineteenth century as an 'anthelmintic, tonic and narcotic'. The leaves were also used externally 'as a fomentation for sprains, bruises and local inflammations'.

Infusions of the leaves and flowers are still prescribed by herbalists for their anthelmintic, febrifuge, stomachic and tonic effects, mainly as a tonic for loss of appetite and debility and in the treatment of worms.

Several other species of Wormwood were used in the herbal medicine of medieval Europe and western Asia, including the Sea Wormwood or Old Woman (*A. maritima*), an aromatic, downy perennial, reaching about 30cm/11in. high, having silvery-grey leaves and bearing yellowish-brown sometimes drooping flowers. In its various forms it is native to the coasts and salty inland regions of most of Europe, including the Mediterranean, and to the Caspian Sea, western Asia, the Soviet Union, central Siberia through to Mongolia.

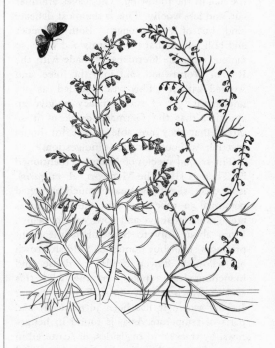

Artemisia maritima (left) and *Artemisia campestris* (right)

Culpeper observes that this species 'is a very noble bitter, and succeeds in procuring an appetite, better than common Wormwood, which is best to assist digestion'. The young leaves and the shoots were infused in boiling water, which when taken internally were said to be excellent for the stomach. Culpeper recommends a tincture made with brandy, and tells us that 'Hysteric complaints' had been completely cured by its constant use. He goes on: 'In the scurvy, and in the hypochondriacal disorders of studious sedentary men, few things have greater effect, for these it is best in strong infusions.' He warns, however: 'The whole blood, and all the juices of the body, are effected by taking this herb' and that it 'turns the milk bitter in the breasts of nurses, if taken when suckling'.

The fresh tops of the Roman Wormwood (*A. pontica*), a native of southern Europe, were used 'to strengthen the stomach – remove obstructions of liver and spleen – and to relax the pains of the gout'. Culpeper writes: 'The Roman Wormwood differs from the Sea in the following. The leaves are finer cut, and less woolly. This is the most delicate kind, but of least strength.' Both Culpeper and Hill tell us that the Wormwood wine 'so famous with the Germans, is made with the Roman Wormwood, put into the juice, and worked with it'. This was regarded 'as not unpleasant, yet of such efficacy to give an appetite, that the Germans drink of it so often, that they are able to eat for hours together, without sickness or indigestion.'

The second species of Artemisia mentioned by Thomas Hyll, the Mugwort (*A. vulgaris*), is an erect, slightly aromatic, much branched perennial 50–120cm/19–47in. tall. The leaves are dark green above and downy white below. From about July to September, the plant produces small but numerous reddish-brown or yellowish flower heads in dense and branching leafy spikes. In the wild this species, which is native to all Europe (except Iceland where it has been introduced) and parts of temperate Asia, is found in hedgerows, by tracks and roadsides, or scattered in waste places. It has also become naturalized in parts of Canada and the United States, having escaped from cultivation.

In medieval Europe, the Mugwort was closely associated with witchcraft and superstition and in many cases is found listed as *Cingulum Sancti Johannis* (St John's Belt), for it was believed that John the Baptist, wore a girdle of its leaves when in the wilderness. It was said that if the herb was hung above a door on Midsummer Day, it would preserve the house and the people inside from lightning, while a spray inside would keep the devil away. The *Grete Herbal* advises that should the herb be laid under the entrance door, 'man nor woman can not anoy in that

hous'. At the same time the powdered leaves could be soaked overnight in water, and if this liquid was applied the following morning to the nape and the back of the neck 'as a wash' it was said to 'strengthen miraculously for the rest of the day'. Gerard writes: 'Pliny

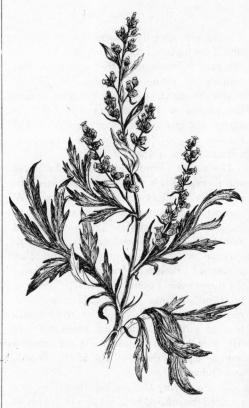

Artemisia vulgaris

saith, That the traveller or wayfaring man that hath the herbe tied about him feeleth no wearisomenesse at all; and that he who hath it about him can be hurt by no poysonsome medicines, nor by any wilde beast, neither yet by the sun itself; and also that it is drunke against Opium, or the juyce of blacke Poppy.'

During the sixteenth and seventeenth centuries, the rather bitter leaves and flowering tops of this plant were generally infused and taken in wineglassful doses two or three times a day, for treating a fairly wide range of 'female complaints'. A 'tea of Mugwort' was popularly prescribed in parts of England, as n Cornwall 'to relieve general body pain' and n other places as a nervine for 'the fit, the hakes and the epileptic' or as Gerard writes, o 'cureth the shakings of the joynts inclining o the Palsie . . .' Used externally the boiled eaves were regarded as useful in most women's complaints'. The juice of the root n wine, 'helpeth the fitte and expelleth the vorme of the childe'.

In the 1620s the Mugwort was recorded as an herb of Venus' and therefore as 'most xcellent and safe in female disorders' with Drayton writing in his *Polyolbion*: 'The belly urt by birth, by mugwort to make sound.' Not long after Culpeper tells us that if the uice was: 'Made up with hog's grease into an ointment, it takes away wens, hard knots and kernals that grow about the neck'.

In the 1650s, the silvery down or the 'moxa', obtained from the undersides of the eaves of this plant was employed as a cure or the pain of gout 'by burning the part ffected', a painful remedy which originated n ancient China. A similar ritual was carried out in Japan for relieving rheumatism, the apanese using the downy moxa obtained from the shrub of that name, *Artemisia moxa*, as well as a second species, *A. sinensis*.

Herbalists still prescribe infusions of Mugwort for its diaphoretic, diuretic, emmenagogue and slightly tonic effects, mainly in women's complaints, as in cases of obstructed menstruation. Sometimes in such infusions it is combined with Pennyroyal and Southernwood. The common Mugwort or Felon Herb is better known on the Continent as St John's Plant, or the Herb of St John the Baptist.

The third plant mentioned by Thomas Hyll, the Southernwood (*A. abrotanum*) a native of the Mediterranean region, has, like the previous species, been cultivated for its medicinal value certainly as far back as Roman times. John Josselyn records its introduction to New England in 1672. It is a smallish grey-green, shrubby perennial, 60–90cm/23–35in. high, bearing small loose panicles of yellowish flowers in summer.

Dioscorides described the Southernwood as having very small hair-like leaves, these having an apple-like scent, while later on in the ninth century Walafred Strabo, a Benedictine monk from St Gall in Switzerland, writes that this herb has 'many virtues' and in his time was used to cure fevers and wounds. During the medieval period the seed and the leaves were prescribed throughout most of Europe, including the British Isles (where it rarely flowers), for complaints similar to the Mugwort.

Turner, writing of the Southernwood in 1551, says 'it is good for them that shake or shudder with colde, sodden in oyle and lyde upon the body' adding 'that some holde that this herbe layde but under a mannes bolster provoketh men to the multiplying of their kind.' The use of the oil was at one time regarded 'as a singular remedy for treating agues'. Culpeper prescribed the oil in much the same way, and goes on 'it removes inflammations in the eyes, if part of a roasted quince, and a few crumbs of bread be boiled and added. Boiled with barley-meal, it removes pimples, and wheals from the face, or other parts of the body.' He also tells us: 'The ashes mingled with old salad oil, helps those that are bald, causing the hair to grow again on the head or beard.'

In the house the leaves of the herb were once used to dye wool a deep yellow and to keep moths away from clothes, thus *Garde Robe* one of its commoner French names, while as a strewing herb the plant found its way into bedrooms, for many people believed it to possess certain aphrodisiac properties. Its other names include Old Man, Boy's Love, Lad's Love, God's Tree, Appleringie and Maiden's Ruin.

The shoots of the garden Southernwood are still prescribed by herbalists in liquid extracts and infusions for their antiseptic detergent, emmenagogue and stimulant effects.

Culpeper also made use of the Field Southernwood (*A. campestris*), a woody-based, erect-growing perennial 30–150cm/11–59in. high, which he informs us has flowers that 'stand in thick spikes at the tops of the branches; and they are small and brown'. This somewhat variable species is found in most of Europe (apart from Ireland and Iceland) and in parts of Asia. It grows in sandy places, among rocks and similar areas of waste ground and uncultivated soil.

Of its medicinal uses Culpeper writes: 'It is a powerful diuretic and is good in hysteric cases. The best way of using it is in conserve made of the fresh tops, beaten up with twice their weight of sugar. One thing in its favour in particular, it is a composer, and always disposes to sleep.' Hill writes that while 'Opiates weaken the stomach and must not be given often where we wish for their assistance; this possesses the soothing quality without the mischief.' As a medicinal herb the Field Southernwood is little used nowadays.

All three Artemisias mentioned by Thomas Hyll – the common Wormwood, the Mugwort and the Southernwood – were being cultivated in English gardens by the early 1440s.

The flowerheads of another species, the Levant Wormseed or Santonica (*A. cina* syn. *A. santonicum* or *A. chamaemelifolia*, including several others), have been employed in the treatment of worms from before the time of Dioscorides. Santonica, one of the plant's more common names, refers to Santones in Gaul, its ancient habitat. It is also common to much of Iran, northern Turkestan, Siberia and Mongolia, where the minute flowerheads, which are generally known as seeds (*flos cinae*), are collected and marketed to many other countries for the extraction of the drug known as Santonin. This is made into lozenge or tablet form by druggists and prescribed almost specifically by doctors, taken night and morning, to paralyse and expel both round and thread worms from the digestive system, although it appears to have little effect on tape worms. Herbalists also prescribe the seeds as a vermifuge, generally mixed with honey or treacle, but care has to be taken as large doses are known to have seriously poisoned or killed the patient. Even in small amounts Santonin can cause a feeling of sickness, with vomiting and headache. Large doses will cause convulsions and upset the vision, causing the sight to appear tinged with yellow. Parkinson, during the seventeenth century, mentions the Wormseed as a children's vermifuge although he rarely used it in other medicine.

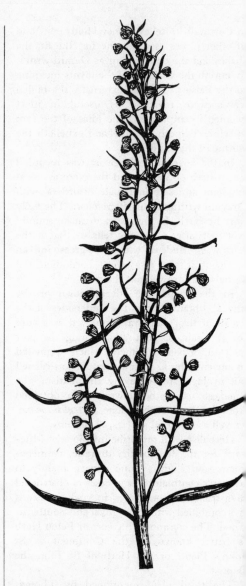

Artemisia cina

The fragrant leaves of the Tarragon (*A. dracunculus*) have always been used, as they still are, for seasoning and flavouring. This herb, a bushy perennial 60–150cm/23–59in high, has woody stems with slender branching shoots and smooth, narrow, hairless, olive-green leaves. The small and inconspicuous whitish-green flowerheads in drooping, lax branched clusters appear in August. Although native to Asia, this species has been cultivated for many years in western and central Europe

specially in France, for its use in flavouring
inegar, to season pickles and salads, and as
n essential ingredient of French mustard and
artare sauce.

According to Gerard: 'It is called in Latine,
Draco; in French, Dragon; in English Tar-
agon.' These three names together with the
French Estragon or Esdragon, from which its
pecific name 'dracunculus' – a little dragon –
derived, suggests that the 'Oil of Tarragon'
as at one time used for treating snakebite
nd the bite of other venomous serpents. It
as certainly applied to the bites of mad dogs.
nother source says the name of the plant
efers to the root, which supposedly coils
ack like a dragon. The root itself was once
applied for relieving toothache. In the United
tates, Rudy Favretti lists the Tarragon
mong the plants known to have been growing
a New England before 1800.

A similar species, the False or Russian
Tarragon (*A. dracunculoides*) which has
ightly rougher leaves of a brighter green,
as occasionally substituted for the French
r True Tarragon.

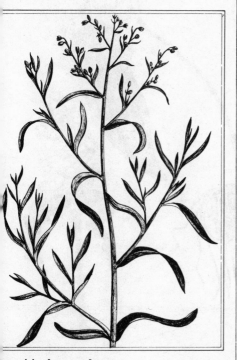

rtemisia dracunculus

ARUM

Araceae, the Arum family
Cuckoo Pint, Dragon Arum, Indian Turnip

These bulbous or tuberous rooted plants with
their large and conspicuous funnel-shaped
flower spathes, borne on fleshy spikes, are
native to North and South America, much of
Europe, the Mediterranean region and parts
of Asia, where they are mainly found in
woods and bushy places.

Of the more familiar species, the tuber-
forming Cuckoo Pint (*A. maculatum*) has been
employed as a medicine at least since the
time of the Romans. This common hedgerow
plant is found in most of Europe, including
the British Isles. In April and May it produces
an erect, pale greenish-yellow spathe, edged
and often spotted with purple, about 15–
25cm/6–10in. high. Within the spathe itself
grows a dull purple, although occasionally a
yellowish, club-shaped spadix, the lower part
of which bears the flowering organs, followed
by green berries turning to scarlet in the
autumn.

In the distant past, the long-stalked dark
and glossy leaves of this species were prescribed for their diaphoretic and expectorant
principles. They were first carefully dried and
boiled in water and the resulting liquid taken
as an internal medicine, which on occasion
caused death. Perhaps the plant's generic
name of Arum points to this possible danger,
as the Greek word *aron* is believed to refer to
certain poisonous plants. The herb's specific
name of *maculatum* is derived from the Latin
macula, a spot, and alludes to the black
blemishes sometimes found on the leaves.
Dioscorides is known to have used the leaves
of an Arum species, prepared as above, as an
internal remedy. He also prescribed the
crushed root mixed with cow dung as an
external application against the pains of gout.

In Europe during the medieval period, a
dram weight of the ground up herb, either
green or dried, was thought to be a useful
remedy against poison and plague. The juice
was regarded as having the same effect with

Arum maculatum

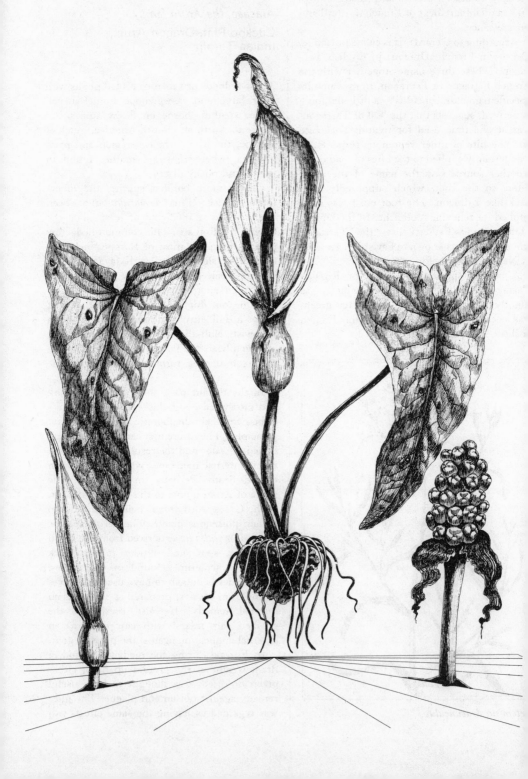

vinegar added to remove some of its acrid taste, while the fresh bruised leaves laid on boils or plague sores was thought 'a wonderful helpe to break and drive forth the poison'. The sweetened powder of the dried root often formed part of a 'licking electuary' taken to relieve 'those that are pursy and short winded – as also those that have phlegm coughs of the stomach and lungs'. The roots boiled in milk and the milk taken as medicine was 'effectual for the same purposes afore-said'.

During the sixteenth and seventeenth centuries little of the plant was wasted: the juice of the herbe – the water distilled from the herb – the green root – the green or dried leaves – the juice or powder of the berries – the berries and roots together' were all prescribed outwardly and inwardly in the treatment of a whole range of complaints from 'inward ulcers of the bowels, ruptures, the cleansing of rotten and filthy ulcers, waterings and redness of the eyes, earache, sore throat and jaw, gout and the piles and the falling down of the fundament'. The latter complaint could be eased according to Culpeper by 'sitting over the hot fumes thereof'. He goes on to tell us: 'The fresh roots bruised and distilled with a little milk, yieldeth a most sovereign water to cleanse the skin from scurf, freckles, spots, or blemishes, whatsoever therein.'

Gerard noted that: 'The most pure and white starch is made of the roots of Cuckow-pint ...' This was employed to starch the ruffs worn by both men and women during the sixteenth and seventeenth centuries. But, as Gerard also observed, it was 'most hurtfull to the hands of the Laundresse that hath the handling of it, for it choppeth, blistereth, and maketh the hands rough and rugged, and withall smarting.'

It later became known as British Arrowroot or Portland Sago, and although little used now was at one time eaten as a foodstuff. The powdered root, which was occasionally used in the treatment of sore throat, was formerly listed in the Dublin *Pharmacopoeia*.

Other names for the plant include Wild Arum, Lords and Ladies, Starchwort, Wake Robin, Ramp, Alron, Janus, Barba-Aran, Priest's Pintle, Parson and Clerk, Quaker, Kings and Queens, Bobbins and Adder's Root.

A second species of Araceae, the Dragon Arum (*A. dracunculus*) or Snake Plant, now listed as *Dracunculus vulgaris*, was formerly prescribed, rather drastically, 'as an inward scourer and cleanser'. This tuberous-rooted leafy perennial gives off at certain stages a disagreeable smell. It is native to southern Europe, where it grows to a height of about 1m/3ft, producing from April to June a large chocolate-purple spathe with a wavy margin, up to 35cm/14in. long, containing a thick fleshy spadix of a similar colour inside. In this case the herb's name of Snake Plant refers to the mottled stalks, which were likened to the skin of a snake, as does Dracunculus, a Latin word coming from *draco* or dragon, the spotted or mottled stems being likened to a serpent's belly. Because of these conspicuous markings, Pliny and Dioscorides firmly believed that 'no Venemous creature or serpent would go near or meddle with any person carrying this plant about him.' During the medieval period this 'Great Dragon' due to its 'violent purging nature' was regarded as an outward medicine only. Mixed with vinegar it helped 'freckles – morphew – and the sun burn' while in ointments it 'consumed cankers' and was 'good for wounds and ulcers'. Another old name for this species, Nedder's Tongue, is derived from *nedderis*, adder. One ancient English manuscript asserts that if one washes one's hands in the juice of this plant 'you shall Nedderis withoutyn peryle gaderyn and handelyn hem at thi wylle.' As a medicinal herb the Dragon Arum is rarely used nowadays.

A third Arum, known as the Dragon Root or Indian Turnip (*A. triphyllum*, syn. *Arisaema triphyllum*), inhabits the moist woods of parts of both North and South America. The root was prescribed for its expectorant and diaphoretic effects. This species has compound leaves and a strong fleshy stem about 90cm/35in. high, and produces a greenish flower spathe striped with purple, enfolding the spadix (or jack) arching above it like the canopy of a pulpit, thus Jack-in-the-Pulpit, another common

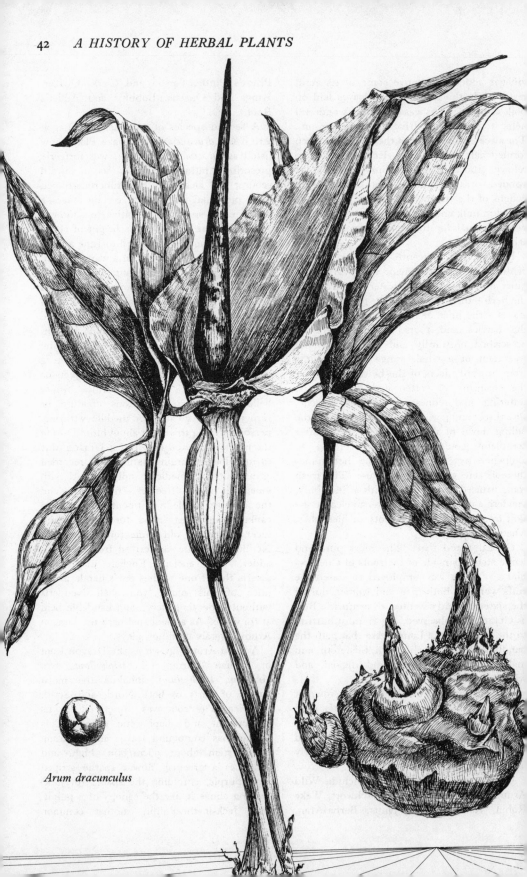

Arum dracunculus

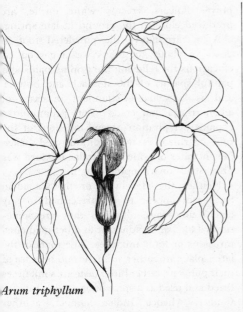

Arum triphyllum

name. The flowers are again situated at the base of the club-shaped spadix and these develop by the autumn into a cluster of scarlet berries which, with the acrid-tasting corms, were boiled and eaten as a food by the American Indians.

In medicine only the roots were employed and only then after being partly dried off first, being much too fierce to use when fresh. After this drying the root yielded 'a pure and delicate, very white amylaceous matter' resembling arrowroot, that was said 'to be very nutritive'. In many illnesses the powdered root was prescribed 'in syrup or mucilage' as in the treatment of 'asthma, whooping cough, chronic bronchitis, chronic rheumatism, pains in the chest, colic, low stages of typhus and general debility' and 'externally in scrofulous tumors, scald heads and various skin diseases'. It is still prescribed for its stimulant, diaphoretic and expectorant principles as in the treatment of coughs, asthma and hoarseness. Other names for the plant include American Wake Robin, Wild Turnip, Pepper Turnip and Devil's Ear.

The roots of a species from India, *A. montanum*, are believed to have been formerly used to poison tigers.

ASARUM
Aristolochiaceae, the Birthwort family
Asarabacca, Canadian Snakeroot

The majority of the plants belonging to this genus of stemless perennial herbs are native to Canada and the United States and only one to Europe. All have at one time or other been prescribed, if only to a small extent, in medicine. Their collective name, Asarabacca, is derived from the Greek word *asaron* or the Latin *asarum*, the meaning of which is obscure, and the Latin *bacca*, berry. The word Asarone or Asarin is generally used nowadays to refer to the crystallized substance known as 'Camphor of Asarum', usually obtained from the European species.

One of the more familiar species of Asarabacca, the Hazelwort or Wild Nard (*A. europaeum*), is found wild in open woods and similar shady places in much of Europe, Siberia and the Caucasus. It has dark ever-

Asarum europaeum

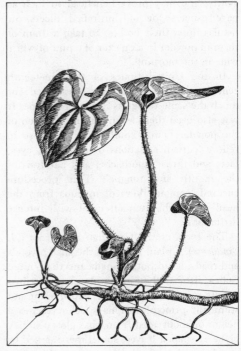

green kidney-shaped leaves, on downy stalks from 3–10cm/1–3in. tall, and bears close to the ground, solitary three-lobed bell-shaped, drooping, greenish-purple coloured flowers, generally from about March to May.

In medicine the leaves and root of this species were prescribed for their emetic, purgative, cathartic and sternatatory effects. Culpeper tells us that: 'The common use hereof is to take the juice of five or seven leaves in a little drink to cause vomiting; the roots have also the same virtue, though do not operate so forcibly; they are very effectual against the biting of serpents, and therefore are put in as an ingredient both into Mithridate and Venice treacle.' A similar remedy was used in France by drunks to induce vomiting. Both the roots and leaves steeped in wine 'purgeth the body downwards – by urine also – rids the body of choler and phlegm – is profitable for the jaundice – for removing obstructions of liver and spleen' and will 'helpeth to relieve the continued ague'. Culpeper discouraged the excessive use of the leaves; for, as he said: 'the roots purge more gently, and may prove beneficial to such as have cancers, or old putrefied ulcers, or fistulas upon their bodies, to take a dram of them in powder in a quarter of a pint of white wine in the morning.'

In the United States of the nineteenth century the Hazelwort was prescribed for much the same things as it was in Europe. It was also used there as an errhine, a pinch of the powder being 'snuffed' up the nose to relieve 'certain affections of the brain, eyes, face, and throat, toothache, and paralysis of the mouth and tongue'. This procedure ensured 'copious flows of mucous from the head' although often attended with intense 'irritations'.

The roots of the Canadian Snakeroot (*A. canadense*), a plant native to the shady woods and roadsides of both Canada and the United States, also had their uses and were prescribed mainly for their carminative, expectorant and stimulant principles. This species reaches a height of about 30cm/11in., has glossy kidney or heart-shaped leaves, sometimes marked or mottled with curious patterns something like a Cyclamen leaf. The dull brown or brownish-

purple flowers, creamy white inside, are produced close to the ground in late spring.

As a carminative the powdered root in doses of about 20 grains was regarded 'as efficacious for relieving the griping pains and painful spasms of the stomach and bowels' and as 'a valuable stimulant in cases of amenorrhoea and colds'. For 'promoting a copious perspiration' strong infusions of the root or rhizomes were administered 'taken hot in water or wine'. A similar mixture was prescribed for whooping cough.

Neither the Hazelwort or the Canadian Snakeroot appear to be prescribed to any extent nowadays, although they are sometimes added as an adjuvant to other medicinal infusions or tonic mixtures. The roots of the latter plant are rather aromatic and because of their pungent, rather bitter taste are sometimes dried and used as a spice or as a substitute for Ginger, whence Indian Ginger, another common name.

The roots of a similar North American species, the Heart Snakeroot (*A. virginicum*), are also employed as a spice. This Asarum has thick leathery leaves, with the upper surface mottled with white.

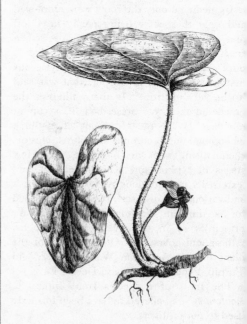

Asarum canadense

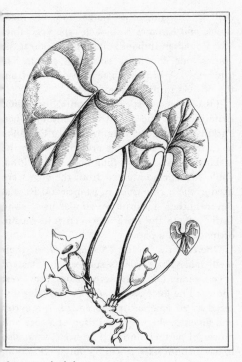

Asarum virginicum

ASCLEPIAS
Asclepiadaceae, the Milkweed family
Pleurisy Root, Swamp Milkweed,
Silkweed

Most of the plants belonging to the Milkweed family are erect and coarse growing perennials with attractive flowers ranging from white to pink to orange, followed by seed pods or follicles, containing numerous flat seeds. The majority are native to both North and South America, principally to the United States, with others native to Africa.

One of the more familiar species of Asclepias, the Pleurisy Root (*A. tuberosa*) a native of the United States, was formerly used by the American Indians, both in cooking – they ate the roots, pods and stems as a vegetable – and in medicine for treating a range of chest complaints. This plant is commonly found in dry fields, especially in gravelly and dry sandy soils, from Maine to Minnesota, and south to Texas and Arizona.

It has a large fleshy perennial root, with a knotty crown, and branching, leafy, hairy stems 30–90cm/11–35in. high, bearing from July to September numerous bright orange to yellow flowers, followed by long seed pods tufted with silky hairs. The flowers themselves are very attractive to butterflies, thus Butterfly Weed, another common name. Other names include Wind Root, Tuber Root and Swallow-wort.

Only the roots of the plant, which is often grown as an ornamental in gardens, were used in medicine and these were classed as antispasmodic, diaphoretic, expectorant and tonic, and to a lesser degree as cathartic and carminative. As the name Pleurisy Root suggests, it was most efficacious in that disease for 'mitigating the pain and for relieving the difficulty of the breathing'. It was also regarded 'as very valuable in assisting all other chest complaints' and was prescribed decocted or infused for 'promoting perspiration and expectoration in diseases of the respiratory organs' ... Acute rheumatism, fevers and dysentery were all believed to

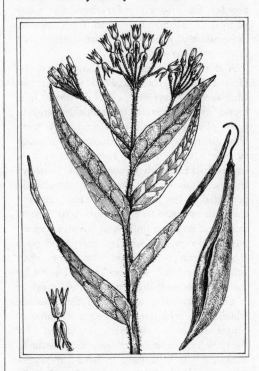

Asclepias tuberosa

benefit 'from a free use of the warm infusion'. It was 'also highly efficacious in some cases of dyspepsia' while in 'uterine difficulties' it had been found 'of great value'.

The active principle of the root, which has a slightly disagreeable taste when fresh, is known as 'Asclepin'. This is still popularly prescribed in the southern part of the United States in the form of a fluid extract mainly in the treatment of chest complaints.

The hard knotty rhizomes and the rootlets of another species indigenous to the United States, the Swamp Milkweed (*A. incarnata*), also had their uses in herbal medicine, because of their emetic and cathartic effects. As the first part of its common name suggests, this herb is a waterside plant. Its long leaves and leafy stems reach 90cm/35in. and it bears umbels of rosy-purple flowers in pairs. Its other names include Swamp Silkweed and Flesh or Rose Coloured Silkweed.

As a medicine the powdered root was infused and the resulting liquid taken internally, either hot or cold, as a fast-acting diuretic and as a reliable stomachic. The powder was also given for rheumatic complaints, as a vermifuge, and for catarrhal, asthmatic and other chest complaints, much as the previous species.

A third species native to Canada and the United States, the Silkweed or Common Milkweed (*A. syriaca*, syn. *A. cornuti*), is found in orchards, along roadsides and in waste places, mainly in rich sandy soils from New Brunswick to Saskatchewan then south to North Carolina and Kansas. It is now naturalized in much of central and southern Europe. This stoutly stemmed unbranched perennial, 1–2m/3–6ft high, has long tapering leaves in opposite pairs, and bears from June to August nodding umbels of sweetly scented purple flowers, followed by warty seed pods about 7–12cm/2–4in. long. The latter, when young and tender, were cooked and eaten by the Platte River Indians with buffalo meat.

The milky juice or latex of this species, which gives this genus its common name of Milkweed, was formerly prescribed for treating lung complaints, including asthma, although it is little used in herbal medicine nowadays. The more tender plants may be boiled, changing the water two or three times, and eaten as a spinach-type vegetable. The Canadian Indians still prepare and eat the young tops and more succulent shoots like asparagus. A brown sugar is also made from the flowers in that region.

This particular species was introduced into Britain during the seventeenth century, when Parkinson named it Virginian Silk. The silky hairs from the seed pods are still used in the making of hats, for stuffing beds and pillows, while the fibres obtained from the stems are used in the textile trade in France and Russia. Several other species have similar uses, as in India, where the fibre is woven into muslin or made into a paper.

One or two other Asclepias had their medicinal values, plants such as the Bastard Ipecacuanha (*A. curassavica*) from the West Indies. The juice of this species was administered as an emetic, or was added to a syrup and given to the negro children as a sure and powerful anthelmintic. The root was also prescribed for its very strong purgative action.

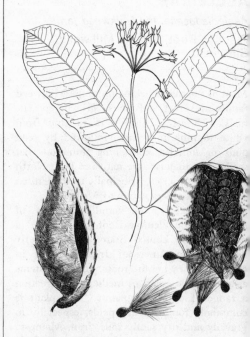

Asclepias syriaca

ASPERULA

Rubiaceae, the Madder family
Woodruff, Squinancy Wort

At least 50 species of this very variable genus of low growing annual and perennial plants are known to grow wild in Europe and parts of Asia.

One of the more common species, the Sweet Woodruff (*A. odorata*, syn. *Galium odoratum*), which is native in Asia and Europe including the British Isles, was formerly regarded 'as very serviceable in tonics – as a vulnery herb' and as 'having valuable domestic virtues in the house'. In the wild this pretty little perennial is found in shady places where the starry-white flowers, borne on slender quadrangular stems 10–30cm/3–11in. tall, smother the ground in May. Its natural habitat is referred to in Woodruff its common name, and this is derived from the Anglo-Saxon *wude-rofe*, with *wude* meaning a wood, while the *rofe* part has possibly evolved from the French *roue* or wheel, to the present ruff – both these words alluding to the way the herb's narrow leaves are arranged in whorls on the stems. The generic name of Asperula comes from the word *asper* or *asperulous* meaning slightly rough to the touch, referring to the texture of the leaves.

During the medieval period in Europe (it was introduced to England in 1440), the Woodruff was principally used for strewing floors, especially bedchambers, for stuffing mattresses and was placed in linen cupboards to keep 'mawths from cloaths'. Although the herb is scentless when fresh, if cut and dried it gives off a fragrance something like Sweet Clover and new mown hay. According to Gerard, bunches were 'hanged up in houses in the heate of the sommer' where they 'doth very well attemper the aire, coole and make fresh the place . . .'

Turner recorded that the herb received 'great commendation for making the herte merry, and for helping of the lyver'. The whole of the plant was simply steeped in wine for a time and the wine then taken. Culpeper

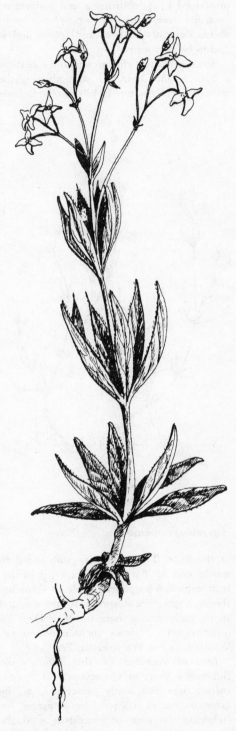

Asperula odorata

prescribed it as 'nourishing and restorative, good for weak consumptive people: it opens obstructions of the liver and spleen and is said to be provocative to venery.'

Some herbalists still prescribe the herb as a diuretic and tonic, for strengthening the stomach and for removing biliary obstructions

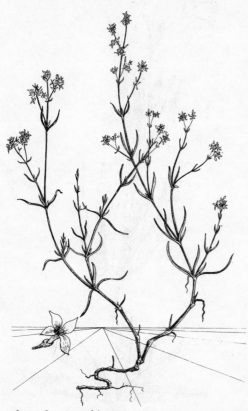

Asperula cynanchica

of the liver. The leaves are still added to snuffs and to flavour beverages, liqueurs, fruit cups and potpourri, while in Germany the fresh sprigs are steeped in Rhine wine and traditionally drunk there on May Day. Its other common names include Woodroof, Wood-Rova and Waldmeister Tea.

Another member of this family, the Squinancy Wort or Quinsywort (*A. cynanchica*), was frequently prescribed, as its common names suggest, as a gargle for 'relieving the pain of sorethroat, and the quinsy' although rarely used nowadays. This very variable little perennial is generally found in pastures throughout much of Europe and parts of Asia. It grows up to 40cm/15in. tall, the leaves grow in whorls and sweet-smelling umbels of pinkish-white flowers appear in June. Like the Sweet Woodruff the Squinancy Wort was also administered to 'openeth of obstructions of liver and spleen – was good in jaundice – and all diseases of the stomach and causes appetite', while the green leaves bruised and applied 'heals fresh wounds and cuts'.

A red dye was once produced from the roots of this plant which is sometimes called Woodrow or Woodrowel. The principal species of Asperula employed for colouring cloth was the Dyer's Woodruff (*A. tinctoria*), a common plant widespread throughout most of Europe, the roots of which are actually red. A similar dye was extracted from the roots of the Blue Woodruff (*A. arvensis*), an annual native to the central Mediterranean region and south east Europe, where it is mostly found in cornfields and cultivated soils. This species was introduced into England before 1596 and has since become naturalized there.

ATROPA
Solanaceae, the Nightshade family
Deadly Nightshade

The most familiar species of this small genus of hardy herbaceous perennials is the Deadly Nightshade (*A. belladonna*), a herb native to central and southern Europe, North Africa and from western Asia to Iran, where it is found in woods and thickets. Its branching stems, which reach 1–1½m./3–5ft, carry large green oval leaves and bear from about June to the end of summer brownish-purple or greenish-purple flowers. These are followed by green berries, soon turning to red and then to a shiny black.

In Britain the Deadly Nightshade is often found wild in waste and similar places, as it is in Russia, France and North America, where it is sometimes cultivated as a source of Atropine, which in former times was much misused as a poison. The generic name of the species actually refers to its evil nature, and is derived from the Greek Atropos, who was one of the three Parcae or fates whose duty was to cut the thread of human life. Belladonna, formerly the plant's common and now its specific name, means fair or beautiful lady, referring to the old custom of putting drops of the juice in the eyes to dilate the pupils and so enhance their beauty.

In medieval Europe the purple-black berries were widely employed to promote madness, produce hallucinations and occasionally death in witchcraft rites, which gave the plant such names as Enchanter's Nightshade, Devil's Herb (or Cherry), Sorcerer's Herb

and Apples of Sodom. More often than not it was regarded as the Devil's own herb, as he supposedly tended it himself. On taking the juice, the unfortunate victim first became talkative and very cheerful and in many cases started to sing and dance, although a confused state would follow shortly after, often accompanied by loss of speech, at which stage he or she would act as if mad and do whatever told.

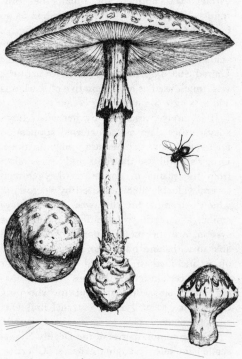

Amanita muscaria

This would be followed by outbursts of mania and delirium, ending in violent convulsions and finally sleep or possibly death, from respiratory failure. The antidote is supposed to be found in the Fly Agaric (*Amanita muscaria*), itself a deadly fungus containing a poison known as Muscarine, which affects the heart. Muscarine poisoning in turn can be counteracted by Atropine, although the exact balance between the two is unknown.

Culpeper recorded: 'Only a part of this plant has its uses. This Nightshade bears a very bad character as being of a poisonous nature.' He employed it as an external remedy, as did most apothecaries of his time,

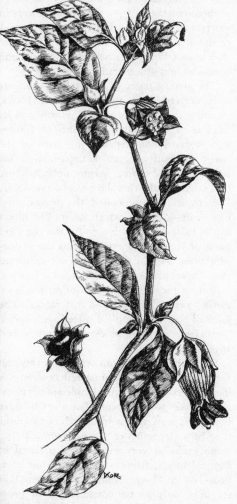

Atropa belladonna

using the leaves and roots 'applied outwardly, by way of poultice' to ease 'inflammatory swellings ... with good success', while the bruised leaves alone laid on women's breasts 'will dissipate any hard swellings of those parts'. For 'hard ill-conditioned tumours and foul ulcers' the roots were boiled in milk and laid on the part affected. The juice of the plant 'evaporated to the consistence of an extract' was applied for much the same things. When the herb was prescribed as an internal medicine 'by the educated herbal physician' it was recorded as 'exceedingly valuable in all convulsive diseases' and in the United States during the nineteenth century, was 'much used as a preventative of scarlatina and as a cure for whooping cough'.

It is rarely prescribed by herbalists nowadays, other than as an external application for gouty and rheumatic inflammations. Druggists still use the roots and leaves taken from the plants in flower, as they contain several valuable alkaloids used by doctors, of which Atropine for the eyes and Hyoscyamine, a narcotic which affects the nervous system, are the most important. These are able to withstand boiling and drying and are often included in internal medicines for relieving certain febrile diseases, for suppressing glandular secretions and in whooping cough, etc., as well as for external liniments and ointments.

Other common names of the Deadly Nightshade include Naughty man's Cherries, Great Morel, Black Cherry, Banewort, Dwayberry, Divale and Dwale. The latter is an Anglo-Saxon or Scandinavian term alluding to the power of the plant to dull the senses and cause a trance-like sleep. Thomas Lupton referred to this use in 1585: 'Dwale makes one to sleep while he is cut or burnt by cauterizing.'

In 1597 Gerard recorded that the leaves of this plant, which he listed as Sleeping Nightshade, moistened with wine vinegar and then laid on the head 'would induce sleep'.

(For the Black and Woody Nightshade, see Solanum.)

BALLOTA
Labiatea, the Mint family
Black Horehound

All the species of this genus are native principally to Europe and parts of Asia. A least one, the Black or Black Stinking Horehound (*B. nigra*, syn. *Marrubium nigram*), was formerly 'extolled' in the medicine of southern Europe and the Mediterranean region. This dark green, hairy, disagreeable smelling perennial, reaches from 30–100cm/11–39in high. It has stalked, toothed, pointed wrinkled oval leaves, and bears from June onwards numerous whorls of purplish-pink flowers in clusters in the axils of the upper leaves. A common and untidy looking herb, it is found throughout Europe in hedges, by tracks and roadsides and other similar places.

The generic name of this species – Ballota – is derived from the Greek word *ballo* meaning to strike the senses, referring to its unpleasant smell. Both the ancient Greeks and Romans administered the juice of the herb, primarily as an antispasmodic, for preventing and curing spasms, such as those that might result from the bite of a rabid dog. Dioscorides recommended the leaves, first beaten up with salt, which he applied direct to the infected bites. No doubt the common name of Horehound points to this use as does Madweed, for the leaves and the extracted juice were prescribed in much of Europe, including the British Isles, during medieval times 'to cure those afflicted with rabies'. The juice of the herb, applied mixed with honey 'also cleanseth the foulness from rotting and stinking ulcers'.

During the seventeenth century in England the juice was often administered as a remedy 'against hysteric and hypochondriac affections' and 'other womens complaints'. Culpeper writes: 'It is an intense bitter, which bespeaks it to be a strengthener of weak stomachs ... some praise it very much as a pectoral in coughs and shortness of breath; but it is necessary to observe some caution, viz. that it ought only to be administered to gross phlegmatic people, and not to thin plethoric persons . . . It is also good to kill worms.'

It is still prescribed by herbalists, generally in the form of a liquid extract for its antispasmodic, stimulant and vermifuge effects, mainly to correct menstrual disorders.

The dried sepals (calices) of another species, *Ballota acetabulosa*, which is native to Greece, are used there as wicks for oil lamps, especially in the Orthodox churches.

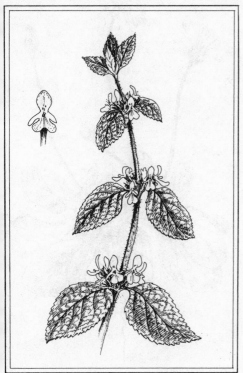

Ballota nigra

BAPTISIA
Leguminosae, the Pea family
Wild Indigo

The Baptisias are hardy herbaceous or shrubby plants, varying in height from 60–120cm/23–47in., and native to North America.

The roots and leaves of one of the more shrubby types, the Wild Indigo (*B. tinctoria* syn. *Sophora tinctoria* or *Podalyria tinctoria*), which is found in the dry soils of hilly woods

from Canada to Carolina, were formerly prescribed for their 'antiseptic, astringent, emetic, emmenagogue and purgative effects'. This is a perennial plant with a black and woody root, and a smooth, round muchbranched stem 60–90cm/23–35in. high, having small alternate leaves, bearing from July to September small loose terminal racemes of bright yellow flowers, followed by short oblong pods containing bluish-black seeds.

In North America during the nineteenth century the decocted bark of the root of this plant was regarded as a 'highly esteemed antiseptic' and as 'efficacious' in 'the cure of all kinds of external sores and ulcerations' and was often used 'in the form of an injection for foul discharges', while the leaves alone as a fomentation made 'a useful application in ulcers and tumours – and for the sore breasts or cracked nipples in nursing mothers'.

For its cathartic effects, the young shoots were decocted and taken in small amounts 'as a powerful laxative', although some writers warn of the 'drastic purgations' caused by prescribing the shoots 'after they acquire a

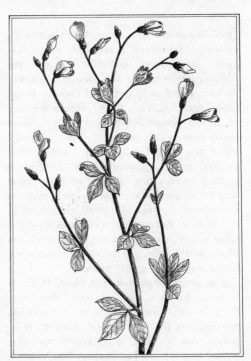

Baptisia tinctoria

green colour'. Decoctions of the bitter roots were also given, often in the form of a syrup, 'for scarlatina, typhus and all cases where there is a tendency to putrescency'.

The leaves and the bark of the root of the Wild Indigo are still occasionally prescribed decocted, or in fluid extracts, in the treatment of rheumatism, or as an ointment for applying to ulcers and sores.

The herb's other common names include Horsefly Weed, Rattlebush, Baptisia and Indigo Weed. The latter refers to its use as a dye, which can be extracted from any part of the plant if dried. Baptisia, the generic name, means much the same and is derived from the Greek *baptein*, to dye. This blue colouring matter is not rated as high as that from the true Indigo obtained from the plant of that name, *Indigofera tinctoria* (Syn. *Pigmentum indicum*).

BELLIS
Compositae, the Daisy family
Common Daisy

Only one species of this small genus of low-growing herbaceous perennials, which are native to Europe, including Britain, the Mediterranean region and western Asia was prescribed in medicine: the Common Daisy (*Bellis perennis*). This downy, rosette forming plant has spoon-shaped leaves, and bears pretty flowers consisting of white ray florets sometimes tinged with pink, with yellow centres, each produced singly on leafless stalks 3–15cm/1–6in. tall, mainly from about March to November, but in mild winters throughout the year. Although indigenous to the whole of Europe, and western Asia, it has since become naturalized in many other parts of the world, where it is found in meadows, lawns and similar grassy places.

The generic name of this plant, Bellis, is believed to have evolved from the Latin *bellus* or *bella*, meaning pretty or beautiful, referring to the flowers, or possibly from *bellum*, war, alluding to its ancient use as a wound herb on the battlefield, while *perennis*, the specific name, denotes its perennial habit.

Other authorities suggest that Bellis is derived from Belides, the name of a wood nymph in Greek mythology who died in fear of Vertumnus, the god of gardens and changing seasons, and who sank to the earth in the form of a daisy.

As to Daisy, the herb's most familiar name,

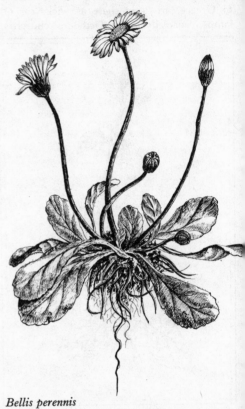

Bellis perennis

this could have evolved from the Anglo-Saxon *daeges*, days and *eage*, meaning eye, thus *Daezeceze* or Day's Eye, referring to the flowers which close at night and open again the following morning. This spelling gradually changed to Daysie or Daysy, then to the Dayses of the fifteenth century, when the plant was listed among the 'herbes for a sallade', and finally to Daisy by Culpeper's time. Chaucer, it seems, left his sick bed especially to see these flowers and he writes: 'That blissful sighte softeneth all my sorwe.'

As a medicinal herb the Daisy was known in Britain for several centuries under the name of Bruisewort and was prescribed as a principal ingredient in ointments 'for application to bruises, wounds, the eyes, gout and similar paines'. Culpeper, referring to it as Little Daisy tells us: 'The leaves, and sometimes the roots, are used, and are reckoned among the traumatic and vulnerary plants, being used in wound drinks, and are accounted good to dissolve congealed and coagulated blood, to help the pleurisy and peripneumonia.' He goes on to recommend infusions 'just boiled in asses milk' as 'very effectual in consumption of the lungs'. Decoctions of the whole herb taken inwardly, and cataplasms of the leaves applied, were used in the treatment of 'varicose veins – pains and aches – especially of the liver, including inflammation – and of the joints – fevers – agues – the King's Evil' and a little later on 'for the scurvy'.

By the Elizabethan period several double-flowering varieties of the Common Daisy had been introduced into English gardens, although Gerard points out that the best sort to use in physic was the common daisy of the field. By this time the juice of the herb was frequently prescribed for the migraine, the expectorated juice being 'snuffed up the nose'.

Another early custom practised throughout parts of Europe during the medieval period was to administer milk laced with the juice of the Daisy to puppies 'to keep them small' for use as lap-dogs, or, as Gerard put it, to 'keepeth them from growing great'. This practice of stunting growth had already spread to children. A small child would be kept small on purpose and made to look much older than he really was by regularly feeding him on the juices of the Common Daisy, Dwarf Elder, Knotgrass and several other common herbs.

The Daisy, which is sometimes known as Bairnewort or Herb Margaret, appears to be little prescribed in herbal medicine now, although in some countries the rather acrid-tasting leaves are used as a pot-herb.

BERBERIS
Berberidaceae, the Barberry family
Barberry, American Barberry, Oregon Grape

At least 170 species of this genus are known to be in general cultivation, not counting the innumerable varieties and forms. The species are widely distributed throughout Europe, including Britain, temperate Asia, the Himalayas, China, Japan, North Africa, North America and the Andes of South America.

Of the more familiar species, the Barberry (*B. vulgaris*) was at one time, mainly during the medieval period, prescribed in medicine for its antiseptic, purgative and tonic effects.

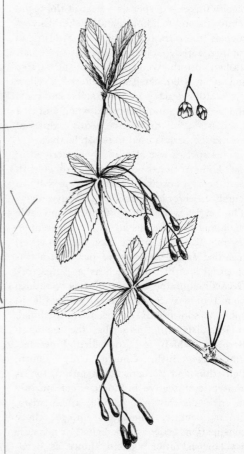

Berberis vulgaris

This is an erect, slender, arched, but densely branched deciduous shrub 1½–3m/5–10ft high, having saw-toothed oval leaves, with three pronged needle-like spines on the stems, which often take the place of the leaves on some of the younger shoots. In early summer small bi-sexual yellow flowers in pendulous racemes appear, followed by orange-red cylindrical berries. Although native to much of Europe and parts of Asia, this sharply spined shrub is now widely naturalized, particularly in North America.

The medicinal parts of the plant were classed as the root, the root bark and the berries, which were made up into various forms and prescribed, generally in white wine, as an internal medicine 'to cleanse the body of choleric humours – bindings of the bowels – yellow jaundice – biles – hot agues – gout – bloody fluxes – dyspepsia – heat of the blood – burning and scaldings', and in skin diseases such as 'the scab, itch, tetters, ringworm and running sores'. Culpeper advised: 'The hair washed with the lye made of ashes of the tree and water, will make it turn yellow.' A yellow dye is still extracted from the stalks and roots and used on cotton, linen and wool, and as a wood stain in marquetry work, while in Poland the bark is used to polish leather.

This species was also widely prescribed in the United States during the nineteenth century as a laxative and tonic, especially in jaundice, chronic diarrhoea and dysentery. The berries were said to 'form an agreeable acidulous draught, useful as a refrigerant in fevers.' The bark of the root was, however, regarded as the most active part and a tea-spoonful of this 'will act as a purgative'. Decoctions of the bark or berries were also 'found of service as a wash or gargle in aphthous sore mouth and chronic ophthalmia'.

Herbalists still prescribe the common Berberis, which is also called Piperidge, Pipperidge Bush, Gouan, Holy Thorn, Berberidis and Berberis Dumetorum, for its antiseptic, purgative and tonic effects, mainly in liver disorders, dyspepsia, rheumatism, general debility, biliousness and to relieve constipation. Its active medicinal principal is a yellowish, bitter alkaloid known as Berberine, Berberina or Berberis.

Farmers regard this Barbery as a potentially harmful shrub, as it is the alternative host of the Wheat Rust Fungus, or Rust Disease (*Puccinia graminis*), which can spread from infected shrubs to the corn crop.

The American Barberry (*B. canadensis*), common to the mountains from Virginia to Georgia, is a similar but slightly smaller shrub to that described above and was also prescribed, although to a lesser degree, in the herbal medicine of the United States. The fruits of this plant ripen in early autumn and are shorter and a little more oval than those of the previous species. They are still used to make a refreshing but slightly acid drink for giving to feverish patients. The fruits of both plants were and still are added to jellies and preserves, as are the berries of the Red-Fruited Barberry (*B. haematocarpa*, syn. *Odostemon haematocarpus*), a shrub indigenous to Arizona and New Mexico.

The roots of the Oregon or Mountain Grape (*B. aquifolium*, syn. *Odostemon aquifolium*), a species native to western North America, had several medicinal uses. It is usually found listed nowadays as *Mahonia aquifolium*, a stoloniferous, little branched evergreen shrub with spineless stems ½–1m/1½–3ft high. It has thick holly-like evergreen and pinnate leaves, producing in spring terminal racemes of scented greenish-yellow flowers, followed by roundish purple or blue-black berries with a whitish bloom. This little shrub is found from the Rocky Mountains through to Oregon, California and British Columbia to the Pacific Coast and has since naturalized itself in several parts of Europe, including the British Isles, where it was introduced in the early 1820s.

In the United States the bitter roots of this plant were prescribed decocted, sometimes under the name of the Holly-Leaved Barberry, for their alterative and tonic principles as 'an aid to digestion – for cleansing the blood – for scrofula – and skin diseases of a scaly nature' as well as for 'syphilis – psoriasis – and chronic mucous complaints'.

It is still prescribed by herbalists, mostly in the form of a fluid extract. These fruits too can be made into a jelly, or taken as a beverage

The root-bark of an Indian species known

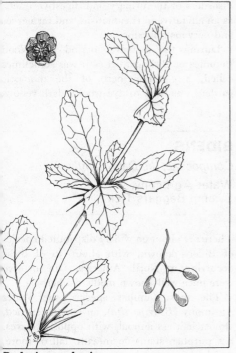

Berberis canadensis

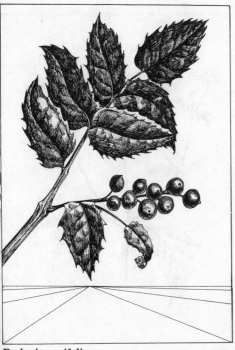

Berberis aquifolium

as Rusot or Indian Barberry (*B. asiatica*) made up into a bitter-tasting extract with the consistency of Opium, is still prescribed there for its very astringent principles. The stem of the Darlahad Barberry (*B. aristata*), indigenous to India and Ceylon, is also given in powders or tinctures for its bitter tonic effects in the treatment of intermittent fevers and as an antiperiodic. This is often listed as the Nepal or Ophthalmic Barberry.

BETONICA
Labiatae, the Mint family
Betony

Most of the Betonicas are now described under the generic name of Stachys, while the Betony or Wood Betony (*B. officinalis*, syn. *Stachys officinalis* or *Stachys betonica*) mentioned here, once a herbal plant held in high repute, appears to be listed equally between the two.

This hairy, usually unbranched perennial, which is native to the heaths and bushy places of Europe and Asia Minor, produces most of its leaves in the form of a basal rosette. Its erect and slender sparsely leaved stems reach 20–60cm/7–23in. tall, and bear from June to the autumn oblong spikes of bright reddish-purple (or rarely white) flowers in whorls.

According to Pliny, Betonica, this species' generic name, originated from *Vettonica* – a plant of the *Vettones* an ancient tribe from Gaul. This gradually evolved into the Old French word *Beteine* and to Betony, its familiar present-day name, by the medieval period. The Latin *officinalis*, the Betony's specific name, refers to the plant's authorized use in medicine. Other authorities believe that Betonica is derived from *bentonic*, a Celtic word, with *ben*, meaning a head, and *ton*, either good or tonic, the plant therefore being good for complaints of the head.

Many of the more ancient writers on medicine including Dioscorides and Galen, extolled the use of this plant as a panacea. Apulius claimed it was used in the treatment of forty-six serious and incurable diseases, including paralysis of the body and the

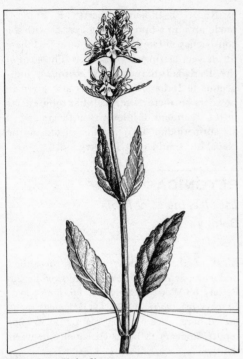

Betonica officinalis

disorders of the urinary and digestive tracts, as an alterative in rheumatism, and for nerves and nervous migraine.

During the medieval period the Wood Betonica or Bishopswort as it was sometimes called, a common herb of the monastic garden, was used to dye wool a dark yellow.

BIDENS
Compositae, the Daisy family

Water Agrimony,
Swamp Beggars Tick

There are about 90 widely distributed species of Bidens known, with about 30 of these occurring in North America. One or two were once well-known medicinal herbs.

The most familiar species, the Water Agrimony (*B. tripartita*), an erect branched, almost hairless annual, with opposite leaves, has purplish stems 60cm/23in. tall or more, which bear unrayed nearly erect, round topped brownish-yellow button-like flowers

dreaded rabies. According to Culpeper: 'Antonius Musa, physician to the Emperor Agustus Caeser', thought highly of the herb.

The *Grete Herbal* recommended a powder of Betony 'for them that be fearful'. Later, Gerard, writing of its habitat, observes: 'Betony loves shadowie woods, hedge-rowes, and copses, the borders of pastures, and such like places.'

Parkinson, like Culpeper, quoted from the writings of Antonius Musa that 'it is said also to hinder drunkenness being taken before-hand and quickly to expel it afterwards ...' The powdered leaves were often 'snuffed' at this time 'to provoketh sneezing – and relieve the hiccough' and are still employed today in 'Ersatz Snuff' as a means to clear the head in colds and influenza. The root is little used now, as it has a rather unpleasant flavour and if taken in quantity can cause vomiting. The leaves are still prescribed for their aromatic, astringent and alterative effects and are some-times combined with other herbs, as a tonic in dyspepsia, for inflammations and con-gestive conditions such as asthma, catarrhal

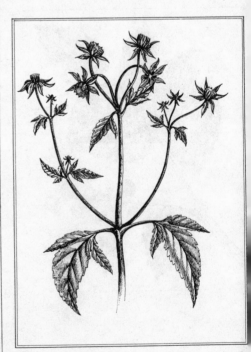

Bidens tripartita

from about July to the autumn. It is found throughout Europe, including the British Isles, and parts of Asia, growing mostly by water or on the beds of dried up ponds and ditches. Culpeper wrote of its common names: 'It is called in some countries Water Hemp, Bastard Hemp, and Bastard Agrimony; Eupatorium and Hipatorium, because it strengthens the liver.' Nowadays it is generally listed as Trifid or Tripartite Bur-Marigold, with *tripartita* the specific name referring to its leaves, which are divided into three parts nearly to the base, while Bidens the generic name has evolved from the Latin *bis*, meaning double, and *dens*, a tooth, referring to the burr-like fruits.

The whole of the herb was administered in Europe, principally during the sixteenth and seventeenth centuries, for its astringent, diaphoretic and diuretic properties. Culpeper summed up its 'Virtues' when he wrote, agreeing with nearly all the other apothecaries of his time: 'It healeth and drieth, cutteth and cleanseth thick and tough humours of the breast ... it helps the cachexia or evil disposition of the body, the dropsy and the yellow jaundice; it opens the obstructions of the liver, mollifies the hardness of the spleen, being applied outwardly; it breaks imposthumes, taken inwardly; it provokes urine and the terms: it kills worms, and cleanseth the body of sharp humours, which are the cause of itch and scabs; the herb being burnt, the smoke thereof drives away flies, wasps, etc.: It strengthens the lungs exceedingly . . . . Country people give it to their cattle when they are troubled with the cough, or broken winded.' It was also prescribed for 'the fever – the gravel or stone of both kidney and bladder' and as a 'styptic in bleedings'.

Infusions of the whole plant are still prescribed by herbalists for bleeding of the respiratory organs, and for uterine haemorrhage.

In the United States, the root and seed of a second species, the Swamp Beggar's Tick (*B. connata*), were employed for their emmenagogue and expectorant effects. This common weed has a smooth stem from 30–90cm/ 11–35in. high, opposite, lanceolate serrate leaves, and bears in August terminal flowers in yellow florets. It grows in wet soils, rich fields, marshes, swamps and ditches, from New England to New Missouri.

During the nineteenth century the seed of this plant in powder or tincture was prescribed 'for suppression of the menses – amenorrhoea – dysmenorrhoea – and other uterine derangements', while infusions of the root have 'proved beneficial in severe cough'.

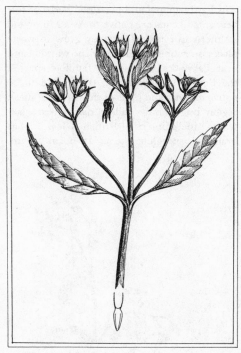

Bidens connata

It was also 'used with great success for palpitation of the heart and for croup'. For the latter, very strong infusions of the leaves sweetened with honey were given to the patient in tablespoonful doses every fifteen minutes until vomiting was produced, and when this happened it was regarded as the cure. In the form of a poultice, the heated leaves of the plant 'laid upon the throat and chest' were 'very beneficial' for 'bronchial and laryngeal attacks from exposure to cold, etc.'

Two other North American species of Bidens, the Beggar's Tick (*B. frondosa*) which is occasionally found wild in Europe, including England, and the Spanish Needles (*B. bipinnata*), were prescribed in the United States as an emmenagogue and in the treatment of laryngeal and chest complaints.

BORAGO
Boraginaceae, the Borage family
Borage

The hardy annual and perennial herbs of this very small genus are native to Asia Minor and southern Europe, where they grow in waste places on rubbish dumps, by the wayside and near habitation. The most familiar species, the Borage (*B. officinalis*), is believed to be native to Syria and parts of the Mediterranean region but is now widely naturalized elsewhere, including the British Isles. It has branched succulent stems 20–60cm/7–23in.

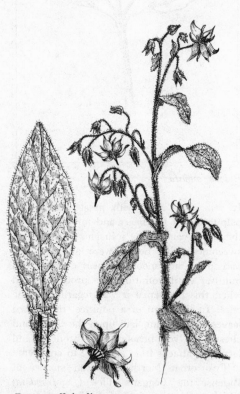

Borago officinalis

high bearing rather rough, bristly, white-haired leaves. Clusters of bright blue starry flowers with blackish-purple anthers are produced from about April to September.

For many centuries this particular annual has been used in medicine for its 'gladdening effects' and in the preparation of various cordials and refreshing cups. Dioscorides and Pliny both had a high opinion of it, the latter observing that its use 'maketh a man merry and joyful'.

During the medieval period, it was prescribed for much the same things as it had been by the Greeks and Romans, and was often given in the form of a courage-giving tea to competitors of tournaments and jousts. In England it appears to have been first mentioned in 1265, and in 1440 was regarded as a common plant, cultivated for the sake of its leaves. These were added as a flavouring, again for their courage-giving effects, to the cordials and beverages of that period. A practice Gerard recommended at the turn of the sixteenth century. He also quotes the now familiar verse, echoing much of the past, 'Ego Borago gaudia semper ago – I Borage bring alwais courage.'

The leaves of the 'Burrage in cordial – the candied flower – the flowers in conserves or wine – the distilled water of the herb' all were prescribed to treat a wide range of complaints such as 'redness and inflammation of the eyes – as a clarifier of the blood – an increaser of milk in women's breasts – and to comfort the heart and spirits of those people that are troubled'. The leaves were sometimes 'mixed, with fumitory, to cool, cleanse and temper the blood thereby; it helpeth the itch, ringworms and tetters, or other spreading scabs or sores.'

Towards the end of the seventeenth century the Borage's medicinal uses gradually dwindled, as the authorities began to express doubts about its effectiveness. At present it is used to a limited extent in the treatment of kidney and bladder disorders, and in France the infused leaves are prescribed for fevers and coughs. The leaves are still popularly added to cordial type drinks, much as they were in 1723 when Millar observed: 'The tops are frequently put into wine and cool tankards.'

The fresh young leaves are often included in salads, having an agreeable cucumber flavour, and the blue flowers make a useful garnish. The mature lower leaves are also cooked and eaten like spinach and contain, as does the rest of the plant, several beneficial vitamins, while the whole herb is rich in calcium and potassium nitrate.

Nowadays the Borage is cultivated in many countries, including the United States, where it was introduced by the early settlers and was one of the herbs listed by John Winthrop. There is a lesser known white flowering variety of this species. Other common names for the Borage include Bee Bread, Cool Tankard and Ox-Tongue.

BRAYERA
Rosaceae, the Rose family
Kousso

The Kousso (*B. anthelmintica*, syn. *Hagenia abyssinica*, or *Banksia abyssinica*) is native to the table-lands of Ethiopia and other parts of north eastern Africa, where it is found at an elevation of about 1,000–2,500m/3,000–8,000 ft. Its round rusty branches reach 6–7m/ 19–22ft high, with crowded alternate leaves with acute and oblong leaflets. The small, unisexual flowers are greenish before turning purple.

These flowers, which are regarded nowadays as principally anthelmintic and purgative in action, have for many years been gathered when in bloom and taken by the natives as a reliable means of expelling tapeworm. The early white explorers, on discovering the value of this tree in the early 1820s, soon dispatched samples of the dried flowers back to their respective countries, where they were found to be very effective in destroying, not only the Pork Tapeworm (*Taenia solium*) and the Beef Tapeworm (*Taenis saginata*), but also the Broad Tapeworm (*Bothriocephalus latus*).

In certain parts of north-east Africa the natives gather the honey from their beehives immediately after the Kousso has flowered, and this taken in small doses as a taenicide

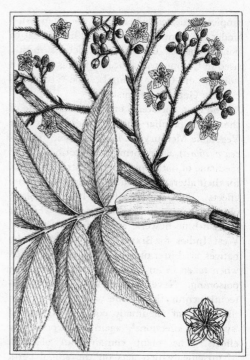

Brayera anthelmintica

is said to be quite effective in poisoning the worms.

One of this tree's generic names, Brayera, is from the name of Dr A. Brayera, a Frenchman who wrote a paper on its use in 1823, France being one of the first of the European countries to make good use of the flowers. Hagenia, another of its botanical names, refers to the German botanist K. G. Hagen of Konigsberg who died in 1829. The common name of Kousso is also spelt as Kooso, Kusso, Kosso, Cosoo and Cusso.

BRUNFELSIA
Solanaceae, the Nightshade family
Manaca

Most of the Brunfelsias are evergreen flowering shrubs or small trees, having woody stems and large oval leaves, with white to yellow, light blue to purple, often richly scented flowers borne in terminal clusters. They are native to Jamaica, the West Indies and tropical America, where they are often listed under the name of Franciscea. The alternative generic name, Brunfelsia, which is mostly used in Europe, was allocated to this family in honour of Otto Brunfels, the sixteenth-century German botanist.

The root, the stems or the leaves of one of the more familiar species, the Manaca or Vegetable Mercury (*B. hopeana*, syn. *Franciscea uniflora*), were formerly prescribed in the medicine of both South and Central America, for their alterative, antirheumatic and diuretic effects. This slender shrub has lanceolate, oblong dark green leaves, produces white or whitish-blue flowers, and is found from the West Indies to Brazil. It was used by the natives as a bitter purgative and emetic, which when taken in any amount often resulted in poisoning. Nevertheless during the nineteenth century it became valued not only in the 'cure' of rheumatic complaints, but of 'syphilitic affections', again with poisoning effects. The plant contains an alkaloid, Mannacine, which acts on the spinal cord, first stimulating then causing lassitude, with

loss of motor co-ordination. Its use also stimulates various glands, including the kidneys, induces perspiration and, if the dose is large enough, a loose greenish discharge. The root is still prescribed in liquid extracts or decoctions, mainly as an alterative in the treatment of rheumatic arthritis.

Several other species of Brunfelsia are known to have been taken by the South American Indians, with other herbs, in an intoxicating beverage known as *caapi*. In the western Amazon the same was added to the preparation of a hallucinogenic drink. A similar concoction was taken by the Kachinaua Indians of the Brazilian Amazon as a form of hallucinogenic love potion. One of the species used, *Brunfelsia tastevini* (syn. *B. americana*), produces greenish-white then yellow flowers. These are very fragrant, their smell being most noticeable at night, thus Lady of the Night its common name. The juice of its leaves when drunk starts to work on the body in about twenty minutes, the effects lasting about five hours depending on the amount consumed. It causes sleeplessness, accompanied by hallucinations and visions, often of snakes and horrific dragon-like creatures. These are believed to be caused by some as yet unidentified tropanes and the alkaloid Scopoletin.

BRYONIA

Cucurbitaceae, the Gourd family
White Briony, European White Briony

The Bryonies consist of a small genus of fleshy tuberous rooted perennials, with vigorous annual climbing stems and long coiling unbranched tendrils. They are native chiefly to Europe, where they are found in thickets, hedges and rocky places. The most common species, the White Briony (*B. dioica*), was formerly prescribed, principally as 'an outward medicine' throughout much of Europe, including the British Isles. It grows in hedges, which it covers in a rampant growth of rough hairy five-lobed leaves. From May onwards, clusters of small greenish-yellow flowers develop in the axils of the

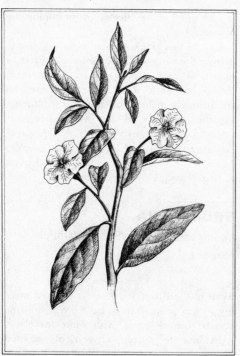

Brunfelsia hopeana

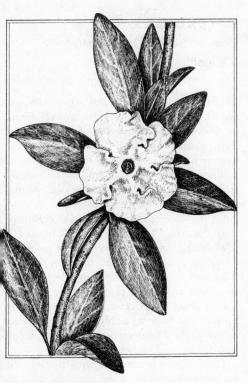

Brunfelsia tastevini

leaves, the male and female on different plants. These are followed by green berries which turn red by the autumn.

A second and closely related species, often known today as the European White Briony or the Black Berried White Briony (*B. alba*), was used in much the same way as the species mentioned above. This herb, native to central and southern Europe, but now naturalized in many other countries, differs little from the former, except that it bears both male and female flowers on the same plant and its fruit turns black when ripe. (Although sometimes known as Tamus, it is not to be confused with the Black Briony (*Tamus communis*) of the Yam family – *Dioscoreaceae*.)

The rampant growth and the large fleshy roots of these plants is referred to in Bryonia their generic name, a Latin word derived from the Greek *bryein* or *bryo* meaning to swell or sprout. Medicinally, the leaves, the ripe fruits and the root were outwardly applied to 'cleanseth old sores – running cankers –

gangrene and the tetters', hence Tetter Berry, another common name. The powdered root alone 'cleanseth the skin of freckles – black or blew spots – the scab and foul ulcers – morphew and manginess – leprosy and other skin deformities', while the root in an ointment of hog's grease applied 'relieves the lumbago – sciatica – and the pains of the joints all over'. Culpeper writes: 'The root bruised and applied of itself to any place where the bones are broken, helpeth to draw them forth, as also splinters and thorns in the flesh; and being applied with a little wine mixed therewith, it breaketh biles, and helpeth whitlows on the joints.'

Of its inward uses Culpeper warns: 'They are furious martial plants. The root of briony purges the belly with great violence, troubling the stomach and burning the liver, and therefore not rashly to be taken.' Even so, 'tinctures of the root, electuaries of the root in honey, or decoctions in wine' were frequently prescribed.

In the fifteenth and sixteenth centuries the roots of the Briony were roughly shaped to

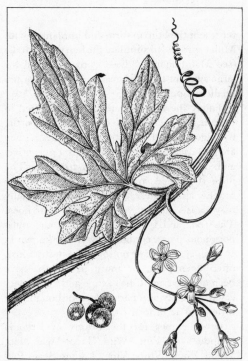

Bryonia dioica

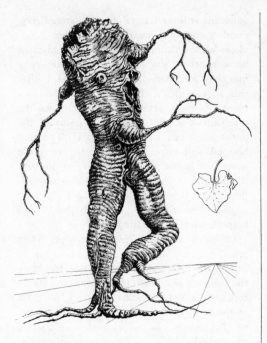

Bryonia dioica (root)

represent the human form and implanted with Millet sprouts, to simulate the hairy Mandrake (see Mandragora). These were then sold for large sums of money because of their reputed medicinal powers.

Today the Brionies are little prescribed in Britain, although regarded as having cathartic, hydragogue and irritating principles. They are still used on the Continent as a purgative, and in small doses for chest troubles. The juice if applied to the skin often produces redness and blistering and if taken internally may cause violent vomiting and diarrhoea. The root and berries, considered the most poisonous parts, contain a glycoside known as Bryonine, an irritant poison. The fleshy roots, often 60cm/23in. or more in length, have been dug up from time to time and mistakenly eaten, possibly as a parsnip, even though very bitter and acrid to the taste.

Other names for the Briony or Bryonia include Wild Vine, Wild Hops, Wild Nep, Wood Vine, White Vine, Ladies Seal, Red Briony, Devil's Turnip and Mandragora.

CALENDULA
Compositae, the Daisy family
Marigold

These very showy annual and perennial plants are native to southern Europe and are found in vineyards, fields and similar places, where they bloom very freely, as Calendula the generic name implies, being derived from the Latin *calendae*, the first day of the month, which is believed to refer to the plant's almost continual flowering habit.

Of the nine species indigenous to Europe only one, the Common or Pot Marigold (*C. officinalis*), was used to any extent in herbal medicine, frequently under the name Golde. This well-known sun-loving perennial grows in almost any soil, has light green alternate leaves, short stems branching from the base up to about 60cm/23in. high, and is probably native to the Mediterranean region, although now naturalized elsewhere.

One fourteenth-century manuscript informs us that: 'Ye odour of ye golde is good to smelle' and if looked upon 'wyscely' in 'erly' morning, would give protection from 'feures' or fevers for the rest of the day. The *Grete Herball* of 1526 refers to the plant under the name of *mary gowles* or *ruddes* and recommends it in garlands for 'feestes and brydeales'.

The use of the petals in a cordial was believed to 'comfort the heart and spirits' and 'expel any malignant or pestilential quality which annoy them.' During the seventeenth century, the petals were administered to poor people as a cheap substitute 'for saffron in the smallpox and the measles' although this was considered as 'less effectual'. The fresh flowers applied, 'soothes bites and insect stings' while the juice from the leaves and flowers taken inwardly 'relieves fevers – ulcers – promotes sweat – and helps the jaundice.' Inward medicines were often made up into a treacle water to take some of the herb's odour and bitter taste away. The Romans also applied the juice externally as an ancient cure for warts, whence *Verrucaria*, its old Latin name. Other names include Jackanapes on Horseback, Garden Marygold,

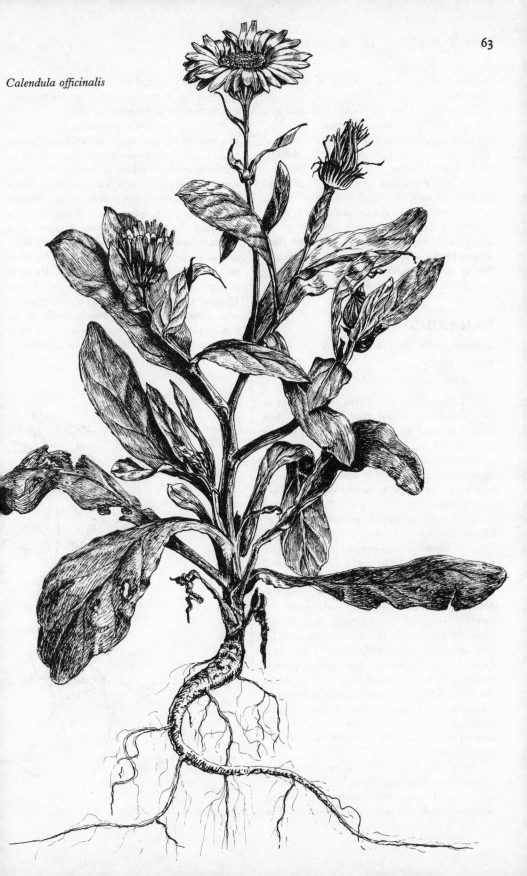

Calendula officinalis

Oculus Christi, Solis Sponsa and Caltha officinalis.

The orange-yellow petals are still used as a potherb, and for colouring butter.

The Marigold was such a useful herb that seed was taken to America by the settlers, where John Josselyn mentions it in his book *New England Rarities Discovered*, published in 1672. During the Civil War there it was used as a styptic by the armies of both sides. In Mexico the herb is regarded as a 'flower of death' and is commonly believed to have sprung from the blood of the natives killed by the Spanish invaders, who in fact actually introduced the plant to that region.

CANNABIS

Cannabaceae, the Hemp family
Indian Hemp

The Indian Hemp (*C. sativa*, syn. *C. indica* or *C. chinense*) is an erect and coarse but elegant annual up to 2½m/8ft tall, having palmate leaves, and bearing in summer branched clusters of small insignificant greenish unisexual flowers, the males drooping and long, the females simple and spur-like. It is probably native to the hilly regions of northern India, although common to much of China, the Soviet Union, the Caucasus and Iran. As a field crop grown for its commercial uses this plant has been, and still is, cultivated in all these countries, as well as in central and south-east Europe, Italy, Spain, Africa, North and South America and Japan. In certain countries, for example the British Isles, its cultivation is presently banned by law, although occasionally found there as a casual weed in hedges and damp places, having possibly set itself from bird-seed. In the United States its commercial cultivation ceased in 1955, since when it has become naturalized in the wild, especially in the alluvial soils along the Missouri and Mississippi rivers.

One of the main reasons for the plant's cultivation was for the sake of the fibrous stem which is still used in the manufacture of string and rope, sacks, cordage and sail-cloth. The seed is also included in bird-seed mixtures. It contains up to 35 per cent of an oil valuable in the making of soap or varnish.

In many countries nowadays, the use or possession of this plant is unlawful, other than for the purposes given, because of its narcotic content, which although not habit-forming in itself, is believed to turn the takers on to stronger drugs, such as the Opium derivatives. Yet, when used in medicine in the past, Indian Hemp was classed as a valuable herb for easing pain, inducing sleep and as a way of soothing people suffering from an assortment of nervous disorders. Its early history can be traced back to the time of the Chinese Emperor Shen Nung, about 2730 B.C. who classed it in his *Pharmocopoeia* as an important medicine. Since then it has been consumed in many different ways, under such

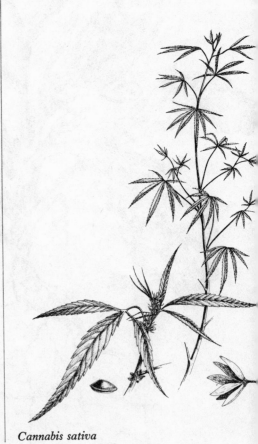

Cannabis sativa

names as Marihuana, Dagga, Bhang, Ganja, Churrus, Guaza, Lamk, Pot, Hashish, Chores, Grass and Hemp among others.

The active constituent of the plant, known as Hemp or Cannabis Resin (or Cannabinone), when extracted was mixed with milk or alcohol and made into greenish pastes, sometimes with human fat, and baked into cakes or added to butter, and this was taken, mostly in eastern countries, for its hallucinatory and exhilarating intoxicating effects and as 'the heavenly guide' and a 'cementer of friendship'. The gummy resinous leaves of the female plant were also smoked, eaten or powdered down and snuffed to obtain the same effect. The most prized variety for producing hallucinations appears to have been cultivated in Yarkand in central Asia, where under the name of Hashish it was made into little flat cakes known as Nasha.

In medieval Europe, the root of the Hemp was prescribed decocted to 'ease the agonies of the gout – pains and the wastings of the sinews – pain of the hip gout' and 'to allay inflammations of the head', while tinctures 'help the birth – menorrhagia – cystitis – and the pains of urinary infections'. The fresh root mixed with a little oil and butter was also regarded as 'a good application' for 'those burns caused by firing and gunpowder blasts'. Decoctions or infusions of the seed, or the emulsion thereof, 'relieves the after pains in the mother – helps the hot or dry cough – the colic – is good for the jaundice – the ague – stays the lax and continual fluxes – bleedings at the mouth, nose, or other places – and opens obstructions of liver and spleen'.

Culpeper noted: 'It is good to kill worms in man or beast; and the juice dropped into the ears kills worms in them, and draws forth earwigs or other living creatures.'

During the nineteenth century the flowering tops and the resin were put to good use in both Europe and North America, for their 'anodyne, antispasmodic and narcotic' effects, which Prof. Phelps Brown recommended for 'gout, neuralgia, rheumatism, locked-jaw, convulsions, chorea, hysteria and uterine haemorrhage.' Adding: 'Its exhilarating qualities are unequalled, and it is a certain restorative in low mental conditions, as well as in

cases of extreme debility and emaciation. In such cases it may be regarded as a real rejuvenator.' At that time, although the plant was extensively cultivated in Europe and Asia, the principle variety used in official medicine came from India, for it was believed the herb's active medicinal properties could only develop fully in the hot climate of Hindustan. Since then active Cannabis from other regions, such as Asia Minor and Africa, have been recognized.

The resin in the form of tinctures and liquid extracts, although carefully controlled, can still be usefully prescribed for relieving depression, easing pain, and to induce sleep in people suffering from nervous disorders.

CARUM
Umbelliferae, the Parsley family
Caraway, Parsley, Yampa

This small genus of hardy, aromatic, biennial or perennial herbs is indigenous to parts of Asia and Europe, where they are found in rocks, mountains, meadows, woods and waste ground. Two species were formerly, and still are to a certain extent, used for their medicinal and flavouring qualities.

The first, the Caraway (*C. carvi*), an erect and hairless biennial, with slender hollow branching stems 25–60cm/9–23in. high, and finely divided leaves, produces umbels of small white flowers in summer, and is widely distributed throughout most of Europe, Siberia, Turkey, Iran, North Africa, India and the Himalayas. Although occasionally found growing wild in parts of the British Isles, it is probably an escape from cultivation. It is also sparingly naturalized in parts of Canada and the United States.

The Arabs are believed to have been one of the first peoples to make use of this herb as a flavouring for their various dishes, the oblong ridged fruits being known at that time as *Karawaya* or *Karwiya*, which is possibly derived from the Greek word *karon* this evolving to the Latin *carvi* and in time to Caraway, its familiar present-day name.

During the medieval period the Caraway

was popularly cultivated in many of the above countries, for use as a flavouring. The spindle-shaped roots mixed with a little milk were made into bread, an old Roman recipe which is still used in Sweden and Norway today, while the young leaves and the seed were used in soups, cheeses and cakes (such as Caraway seed cake) and many other confections. The pleasant tasting seed alone was also sprinkled over cakes, an old custom, or encrusted with honeyed sugar and taken as simple comfits. The latter was very popular in Shakespeare's England and was often eaten with a 'rosted pippin'.

time prescribed the seed as 'conducing to all cold griefs of the head and stomach, bowels, or mother,' and which 'helpeth to sharpen the eye-sight'. The powdered seed in a poultice applied 'taketh away black or blue spots of blows and bruises,' while: 'The herb itself, or with some of the seed bruised and fried, laid hot in a bag or double cloth to the lower parts of the belly, easeth the pains of the wind colic.'

Nowadays only the powdered fruits, which are classed as carminative and stimulant; are used in medicine, and these are prescribed mainly for children's ailments, flatulence and

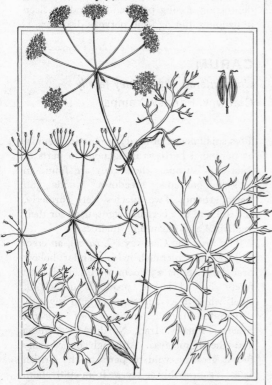

Carum carvi

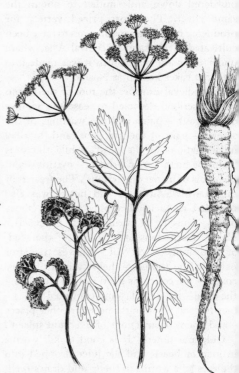

Carum petroselinum

Culpeper writes: 'Carraway seed hath a moderate sharp quality, whereby it breaketh wind and provoketh urine, which also the herb doth. The root is better food than the parsnips; it is pleasant and comfortable to the stomach, and helpeth digestion.' The root alone was often given 'to those people who require their stomachs strengthened.' Culpeper like several other apothecaries of his

stomach complaints. Most of the present-day commercial crops of Caraway, for use as a flavouring agent in cooking and confections, are grown in Holland and to a lesser extent in Morocco, Norway, Finland, Germany and Russia. In the two latter countries the oil from the seed is added to the liqueur known as Kummel.

The second species of Carum prescribed in

herbal medicine was the Parsley (*C. petro-elinum*), sometimes listed as *Petroselinum ativum, P. crispum, P. hortense* or *Apium petroselinum*. An erect, hairless biennial up to 1m/3ft high, it has divided leaves, and in summer bears long stemmed flat-topped umbels of greenish-yellow flowers. The exact origin of this particular plant is unknown, having been cultivated now for many centuries, although it is probably native to southern Europe, where it grows among rocks and stones and in waste places. The word Petroselinum actually refers to its natural habitat, and is derived from the Greek *petros*, meaning rock or stone.

Many forms of this species are known, some having a plain leaf and others a curled, although the latter sort is mostly grown today. Theophrastus the Greek philosopher described both kinds in his *Enquiry into Plants* which was written about 300 B.C. The curled sort was certainly known to Pliny, who extolled its virtues and sprinkled Parsley seed in his fish ponds to cure any sick fish. His fellow countrymen also appreciated the fresh fragrance of the herb and even went so far as to wear its leaves around their necks to ward off intoxication when drinking, and it was the Romans, no doubt, who introduced the plant into several European countries. The seed at this time was also eaten as a way of increasing fertility, both in men and women.

During the eighth century, Charlemagne, the Emperor of the West, is said to have grown this plant in his herb garden, but very little is known about it during this period. According to some authorities it was first cultivated in the British Isles in 1548, although it was probably used by the Romans when they settled there some fourteen hundred years before.

A common superstitition about the plant and dating from the late medieval period, was that when the seed was sown it would go to the devil and back seven times before it actually came up, and that the devil liked it so much he always kept a little. This explained its generally slow and patchy germination. About this time another superstitious rite started, that of sprinkling Parsley seed on one's head as a cure for baldness, a task

advisedly performed at night, a belief that is still occasionally heard of today. Turner goes one better and tells us that if the seed was taken beforehand it would 'helpeth men that have weyke braynes to beare drinks better', which sounds very much like the remedy once used by the Romans.

In the medicine of the sixteenth and seventeenth centuries, the leaves and seeds were inwardly prescribed in various forms to relieve a wide variety of ailments, from coughs and kidney stones to 'the gonorrhoea'. The bruised leaves alone 'applied to women's breasts that are hard through the curding of their milk . . . abates their hardness, and takes away black or blue markes coming of bruises or falls.' The same was applied to 'contusions, swelled breasts, and enlarged glands,' and if 'applied to the breasts of wet nurses dries up their milk.'

An oily non-volatile liquid known as Apiol is nowadays extracted from the roots and seeds of cultivated crops of caraway, which is given in malarial and kidney disorders, and in the treatment of several menstrual complaints. In the United States during the nineteenth century, this essential oil was administered as 'a good substitute for quinia in intermittent fevers, and for ergot as a parturient'. The herb appears to have been first grown there in the late 1600s, and was mentioned by John Josselyn.

The roots, seed and leaves are still used in herbal medicine and are prescribed for their aperient, emmenagogue, but chiefly diuretic principles, in the treatment of gravel, stone, congestion of the kidneys, etc. Both the roots and leaves contain vitamins A, B, and C, the latter mostly in the roots. The fresh leaves are used to flavour soups, stews, sauces, stuffing and as a garnish.

The sweet tasting roots of a third species, known in North America as Yampa, Ipo or Squawroot (*C. gairdneri*), were once eaten as a food by the Indians there. This sparsely leaved, single stemmed plant, produces compound umbels of whitish flowers and is mostly found in the plains and grasslands from British Columbia to California, then east to Colorado and New Mexico. The fleshy tubers were dug up in spring by the

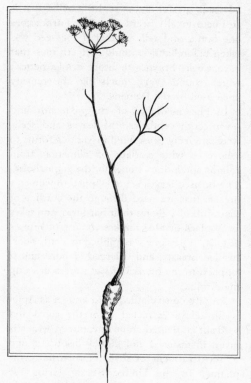

Carum gairdneri

Indians, and either dried and ground into flour for baking into bread and cakes, or were cooked as a vegetable and served with meat. The roots were traded for flour and medicine from the settlers, the settlers themselves using them as the Parsnip is used today.

CHELONE

Scrophulariaceae, the Figwort family
Balmony

The Chelones are a small group of hardy, herbaceous plants, having pointed toothed leaves, and bearing white or purple tubular flowers in crowded terminal spikes, on erect branched stems in summer. They are native to both Canada and the United States, where they are found in swamps, wet woods and along the banks of rivers and streams. Their generic name, Chelone, is the Greek word meaning tortoise, and refers to the lip of the flower which supposedly resembles the head of that reptile, hence Turtle Head or Turtle Bloom their common names.

Of the three species listed, only one appears to have been prescribed in medicine, the Balmony (*C. glabra*). This is found in damp soils and swamps in Canada and the eastern parts of the United States, where it grows from 60–100cm/23–39in. tall, having opposite oblong-lanceolate leaves, and bearing in August and September two-lipped white to purplish to rose-coloured flowers.

The bitter leaves of this plant were first used for their laxative and purgative principles by the North American Indians who then passed on their knowledge to the settlers. By the nineteenth century it had become 'a valuable medicinal plant' and was prescribed for its 'anthelmintic, antibilious, detergent and tonic effects' mainly in 'the jaundice – liver diseases – consumption – and for the removal of worms'. In small doses the powdered leaves were prescribed as 'a good tonic in dyspepsia, debility of the digestive organs' and 'during convalescence from

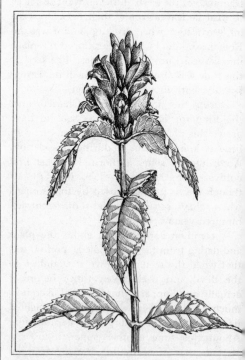

Chelone glabra

ebrile and inflammatory diseases'. A tincture was made by pounding the whole fresh plant to a pulp, which was then prepared with alcohol. In the form of an ointment the fresh leaves were regarded as valuable for applying to 'painful piles – irritable and painful ulcers – and the inflamed breasts of mothers'.

The leaves are still prescribed in powders, infusions or liquid extracts in the treatment of dyspepsia, debility, constipation and liver complaints, and as a reliable remedy for worms in children. The active principle is Chelonine, a bitter brown powder.

This species' common names include Salt Rheum Plant, Snake Head, Bitter Herb, Shellflower, Glatte, Hummingbird Tree, White Chelone and Chelone Obliqua.

CHENOPODIUM

Chenopodiaceae, the Goosefoot family

Good King Henry, Lamb's Quarters, Stinking Orach, Mountain Spinach, Quinoa, American Wormseed

Many of the plants belonging to this variable genus are unattractive weedy annual or perennial, sometimes woody herbs, with flowers in axillary clusters or spikes. They are native to most of Europe, Asia, India, China and to both North and South America.

One of the more familiar species, generally known today as Good King Henry (*C. bonus-henricus*), is a robust perennial up to 60cm/23in. tall, with bright green, broadly tri-angular leaves. From June to September it bears greenish-yellow flowers in long tapering spikes. It is native to most of Europe, including the British Isles, and western Asia, where it is found by the wayside, near habitation and in farmyards. Formerly culti-vated in the kitchen garden for its use as a pot-herb, its succulent leaves were eaten as spinach and its shoots as asparagus, both preparations having a gentle laxative effect. Its commonest name of Good King Henry has nothing to do with Henry VIII of England as is often believed, but was given to this plant, according to Dodoens, to distinguish it from a poisonous one known as *Malus*

Henricus or Bad Henry. Its other common names include All-Good, Good Henry, English Mercury, Marquery, Goosefoot, Wild Spinach and Smearwort.

The generic name of Chenopodium is derived from the Greek *chen* or *chenos*, a goose, and *pous* or *podos*, a foot, thus Goose-foot, referring to the shape of this and the other species' leaves, which supposedly resemble the feet of that bird.

In the medicine of medieval Europe, the young shoots, the leaves and the flowering tops were regarded as 'detersive and diuretic' and were eaten as 'good for the scurvy – as a provoker of urine' and were 'outwardly used in clysters', while 'a cataplasm of the leaves or the ointment thereof, helps the pain of the gout.' When the plant was introduced to America by the early settlers, it soon escaped from the gardens and established itself in the wild, and has since become naturalized, if somewhat sparsely, from Nova Scotia to Ontario, then south to Maryland and Ohio.

Several other Chenopodiums were and still are substituted for the Spinach, including the

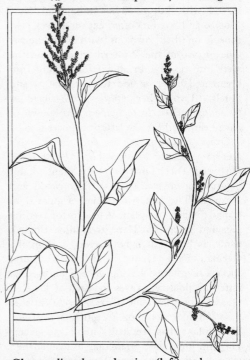

Chenopodium bonus-henricus (left) and *C. vulvaria* (right)

Upright or City Goosefoot (*C. urbicum*) a herb widespread in both North America and Europe, and the Lamb's Quarters (*C. album*). The latter, an annual, is one of the commonest and most variable of the Goosefoots, and although native to Europe and Asia, has naturalized itself throughout much of North America, except the extreme north. It is now almost cosmopolitan, growing in fields and gardens, alongside roads and tracks, on rubbish dumps and compost heaps. Its tough, well-branched stems reach from 10–120cm/3–47in., although sometimes more, have lanceolate-oval to diamond shaped leaves, and bear spikes of tiny greenish coloured, densely clustered flowers, followed by numerous black or brownish to pale-yellowish, smooth flat seeds.

Although little used at present, the peasants of Britain and Europe ate the leaves of this plant as a nutritious pot-herb, or took them for their useful medicinal effects. The young leaves, which are rich in vitamin C, can still be eaten as a vegetable and taste quite palatable if first cooked, chopped up and served with butter. The Indians of New Mexico and Arizona often eat the leaves raw, cooked on their own, or with other herbs. One or two of the Western tribes grind the seed into a meal or flour, for baking into bread and cake, or add them to soups and gruels. Two other species, *Chenopodium fremontii* and *C. leptophyllum*, are known to have been used for the latter purposes also.

Other common names for the Lamb's Quarters include Mutton Tops, Frost Blite, Dirtweed, Dirty Dick (from the plant's habit of growing on muckheaps), Baconweed and Pigweed. The last two names originated in Canada where the plant is grown for feeding pigs and sheep. Fat Hen, its familiar English name, is believed to have evolved from the German Fette Henne, this and the first species mentioned having once been used to fatten up poultry, as was the seed of the Red Goosefoot or Sowbane (*C. rubrum*), a variable fleshy annual, common to much of Europe. This plant has reddish stems 30–90cm/ 11–35in. high, with triangular to oval shaped leaves, and is often found in farm-yards or growing on manure heaps.

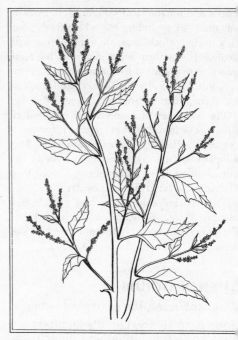

Chenopodium album

Another annual is the much-branched Stinking Orach or Stinking Goosefoot (*C. vulvaria*, syn. *C. olidum*). This mealy looking grey-green, partially prostrate species 10–65cm/3–25in. tall, bears from July to September small clusters of greenish-yellow flowers in the axils of the leaves, and was formerly prescribed for its emmenagogue and anti-spasmodic effects, mostly 'for the complaints of the mother'. As its name suggests this plant tends to smell rather strongly of rotten fish and is native to most of Europe including the British Isles. It grows by road-sides and on dry waste land, especially by the sea.

Gerard tells us: 'It is an hearbe for a yeare which springeth up, and when the seed is ripe it perisheth, and recovereth it selfe againe of his owne seed ... It groweth in the most filthy places that may bee found. Sometimes it is found in places neere Bricke kilns and old walls, which doth somwhat alter his smell which is like tosted cheese: but that which groweth in his natural place smels like stinking salt-fish ...'

The English name, Motherwort, refers to

he herb's use, in the treatment of women's llnesses, from 'barreness to hysteria' to several 'nervous afflictions'. Culpeper writes of its medicinal uses: 'Stinking Arrack is used as a remedy to help women pained, and almost strangled with the mother ... I commend it for a universal medicine of the womb and such a medicine as will easily, safely and speedily cure any disease thereof ... as fits of the mother, dislocation or falling out thereof: it cools the womb being overheated. And let me tell you this, and I will tell you the truth, heat of the womb is one of the greatest causes of hard labour in child-birth. It makes barren women fruitful: it cleanseth the womb if it be foul, and strengthens it exceedingly: it provokes the terms if they be stopped, and stops them if they flow immediately; you can desire no good to your womb but this herb will effect it; therefore if you love children, if you love health, if you love ease, keep a syrup always by you made of the juice of this herb, and sugar or honey, if it be to cleanse the womb; and let such as be rich keep it for their poor neighbours ...'

Culpeper lists this plant as the Wild or Stinking Arrach (botanically as *Atriplex olida*). Its common names of Dog's Arrack, Goat's Arrack or Goat's Orache are believed to point to the unfitness of this plant for use as a pot herb, and at the same time to distinguish it from the true Orache or Mountain Spinach (*Atriplex hortensis*) a closely related annual, native to Tartary, which was introduced into England in 1548 and is also listed under the Natural Order *Chenopodiaceae*. Culpeper refers to the latter as the Garden Arrach: 'Called also Orach and Arage,' and this was prescribed to 'softeneth and looseneth the body of man being eaten' and to 'fortifieth the expulsive faculty in him'. The bruised or boiled herb was applied to the throat as 'excellent good for the swellings' which with the decoction taken and the herb applied to the place ... relieves the pain of the gout.' The decoction was also regarded as 'an excellent remedy for the jaundice'.

The leaves of the Stinking Orach can still be taken infused for relieving nervous debility, colic and menstrual disorders, but because of its very unpleasant odour and taste, is difficult to stomach.

The white or red seeds (depending on the variety grown) of another Chenopodium, *C. quinoa*, are used as a staple food in the Andes of Chile, Peru, Colombia, Bolivia and other parts of South America. This annual, with its many angular branches and dull, glaucous, triangular, long-stalked leaves, grows from 1–2m/3–6ft high and was one of the first cultivated plants found in that region by the Spanish invaders. Its seeds, which are rated

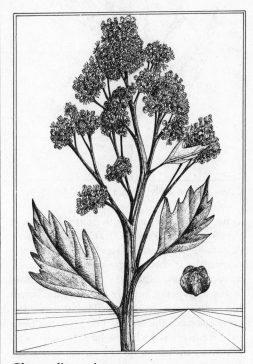

Chenopodium quinoa

highly by the local Indians, are ground into meal for baking into bread, are added to soups and gruel, and fermented with millet seed into local alcoholic brews, such as *chicha*, while the leaves are valued as a potherb, or cooked and eaten on their own as a spinach-type vegetable. As an internal medicine, fairly large quantities of seed were given for their anthelmintic and emetic principles, and these were applied, mostly in the form of a cataplasm, for bruises and sores. The whole of the green plant makes a useful cattle food and the seed is fed to poultry.

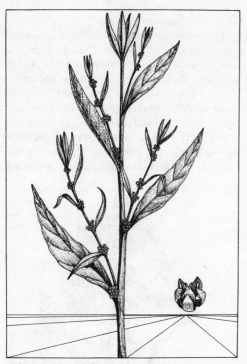

Chenopodium ambrosioides

Another species native to South America is the American Wormseed (*C. ambrosioides*). A coarse, disagreeable smelling, herbaceous perennial, it has erect stems 30–100cm/ 11–39in. high, alternate oblong-lanceolate leaves, and bears from July to September small but numerous greenish-yellow flowers the same colour as the leaves. This, too, has been used for many years by the local Indians as an effective anthelmintic. From the crushed fruit of this plant, which is now widely naturalized in much of the United States, and a variety known as Anthelminticum, often listed as *Chenopodium anthelminticum*, is extracted a drug known as Oil of Chenopodium, or American Wormseed Oil. This is prescribed to expel lumbricoids or round worms from the body, an excellent remedy for treating such infestations in children. The bruised or powdered seeds in the form of an electuary, or an infusion with milk, are given for the same, although overdoses can cause sickness or dizziness.

The herb has also been prescribed as an antispasmodic and as an expectorant in asthma, catarrh and other pectoral complaints and for tapeworm and hookworm. Several Indian tribes of the eastern part of the United States use the whole of the herb decocted to help ease painful menstruation and other female complaints. Although quite common in North America in the wild this plant is regularly cultivated in the state of Maryland as in the East Indies, Mexico and parts of India, for the sake of its oil (which contains among other principles a combination of Ascaridole and Safrol) and this is prescribed in official medicine, again for its important anthelmintic and anti-spasmodic effects.

In New Zealand the American Wormseed is known as Californian Spearmint. Its other names include Herb Sancti Mariae, Jesuit's Tea and Mexican Tea, the last alluding to the use of the leaves as a tea substitute.

A tincture extracted from the Oak-Leaved or Glaucous Goosefoot (*C. glaucum*) found in both North America and much of Europe was also once used for expelling round worms. The Sticky Goosefoot or Feather Geranium (*C. botrys*), a sticky, glandular unpleasant smelling annual, indigenous to much of Europe and parts of Asia, where it is found in sandy soils, was considered to be and prescribed in France as a useful expectorant.

CHIMAPHILA
Pyrolaceae, the Wintergreen family or Ericaceae, the Heath family
Pipsissewa, Spotted Wintergreen

The Chimaphilas are a small genus of dwarf shrubby plants, native to the dry shady woodlands of northern America, Europe, Asia and Japan; of these the Pipsissewa (*C. umbellata* syn. *Pyrola umbellata*) was the species mostly prescribed in medicine. This little evergreen is found in most of the northern latitudes including North America, north and central Europe and the Soviet Union. It consists of a number of creeping rhizomes, producing several erect shoots 10–20cm/4–7in. tall woody at the base, with strongly toothed oblong, wedge-shaped leathery leaves, bearing from about May to August terminal umbels of three to six fragrant pink or pinkish white flowers with spreading petals, borne at the top of long leafless stalks 20–40cm/7–15in. high.

The generic name of this plant, Chimaphila, is derived from the Greek *cheima*, meaning winter, and *philos*, loving, hence winter loving, alluding to its evergreen nature, with *umbellata* the specific name, referring to the shape of its flowers. Pipsissewa, its commonest name, was given to the herb by the Algonquian Indians of Canada. Other names include Umbellate Wintergreen, Wintergreen, Prince's Pine, Ground Holly, Love in Winter, Rheumatism Weed and Butter Winter.

Only the leaves of the plant, which are fragrant when fresh but odourless when dried, were regarded as having any effective value in medicine. These were generally infused in boiling water or alcohol to extract their 'virtues' which during the nineteenth century were known to include 'resin, gum, lignin and saline substances'. They were prescribed for their alterative, astringent, diuretic and tonic effects, 'being especially useful in scrofula and chronic rheumatism' while in 'diseases of the kidneys and dropsy it exerts a decided curative power'. They were also administered 'as advantageous in chronic gonorrhoea – the strangury – catarrh of the bladder' and as 'a cure for ascites' – an accumulation of serous fluid in the abdominal cavity. Besides their internal use, decoctions were often given in the treatment of skin diseases.

The leaves are still prescribed in syrups and fluid extracts for long-standing rheumatic complaints and kidney infections, while one of the active principles, known as Chimaphilin, is described as efficacious in skin diseases.

A second and similar species, the Striped Pipsissewa or Spotted Wintergreen (*C. maculata*) with variegated leaves, was often substituted for the above by the North American Indians in the treatment of scrofula, rheumatism and stomach complaints. They also administered the leaves of this plant as a diuretic in cystitis.

CHRYSANTHEMUM
Compositae, the Daisy family
Feverfew, Ox-Eye Daisy, Tansy, Costmary, Corn Marigold, Dalmatian Pyrethrum

At least 100 species are listed as belonging to this genus of annual or perennial plants. The majority are native to various parts of Europe, North Africa, Asia, China and Japan, although the origin of some of the more popular cultivated sorts is unknown, because of their constant hybridizing over the years.

One of the most valued species was the Feverfew (*C. parthenium*, syn. *Pyrethrum parthenium* or *Matricaria parthenium*) which is native to south-eastern Europe. It is an erect, somewhat downy, leafy branched perennial 25–60cm/10–23in. tall, and in summer bears lax, more-or-less flat-topped clusters of white daisy-like flowers with yellow centres. In the wild this plant, which grows by the wayside, in waste places and by

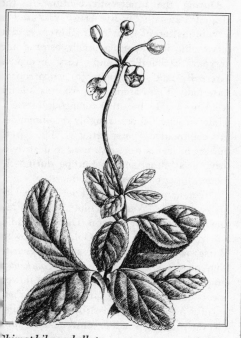

Chimaphila umbellata

habitations, has naturalized itself throughout most of Europe, including the British Isles. It has been introduced to the United States.

According to Plutarch, the Greek biographer, moralist and miscellaneous writer (A.D. c.45–120), this particular herb received its specific name of *parthenium* because it was used to save the life of a man who actually fell from the Parthenon, the principal temple on the Acropolis at Athens, when it was being built between 447–432 B.C. The present name of Feverfew is derived from the Latin *febris*, a fever, and *fugare*, to chase or drive away, so-called because the plant was once prescribed in the cure of fevers and agues. It was known later to the Anglo-Saxons as *feferfuge* or *feferfugia* which had evolved by the early part of the medieval period to *fevyfew* or *feverfue* and in time to Feverfue, Feverfew and Featherfoil.

Of its numerous medicinal uses during the medieval period, it was observed: 'Feverfew is hot in the third degree and dry in the second, it clenseth, purgeth and scoureth, and fully performeth all that bitter things can do.' Gerard writes: 'Feverfew dried and made into pouder and two drams of it taken with honey or sweet wine, purgeth by siege melancholy and flegme; wherefore it is very good for them that are giddie in the head, or which have the turning called Vertigo.'

Warm infusions were prescribed for 'some febrile diseases – hysteria – as a purger of choler – recent colds – stuffings in the chest – for provoking suppression of urine – flatulency – to cleanse the reins and kidneys – bring down women's courses – and as an expeller of worms', while cold infusions 'make a valuable tonic'. It was also regarded as an 'especial remedy to helpe those who have taken Opium too liberally'. The leaves alone in a poultice applied 'restricts the pains and swellings of the bowels' and these applied to the wrists and the decoction taken before 'the coming of the ague fit, does take them away'.

The leaves of the Feverfew are still prescribed by herbalists for their medicinal value, mainly in liquid extracts, or in the form of a tea. Its action is regarded as chiefly tonic, emmenagogue, aperient and stimulant. The

herb's other common names include Flirt wort and Bachelor's Buttons.

The Ox-Eye Daisy (*C. leucanthemum*, syn *Leucanthemum vulgare*) was also widely used in medieval medicine. An erect variable, little branched perennial 20–70cm/7–27in. high, it bears throughout the summer long stalked flower heads of white strap-shaped ray-floret surrounding the yellow disk centres. This is found in grassland, pastures and similar places throughout the whole of Europe including the British Isles, to Russian Asia and Siberia. On the species' introduction to North America, it spread rapidly in the wild and North Carolina adopted it as its State flower.

As a medicine Culpeper tells us that Ox-Eye 'was very fitting to be kept both in oils ointments and plasters, as also in syrup'. It was held to be 'a wound herb of good respect often used in those drinks and salves that are for wounds, either inward or outward', and was prescribed in England at that time in it various forms, for 'the running of the eyes – the heat of the choler – all ulcers and postule in the mouth or tongue' and 'as an application to the secret parts'.

During the nineteenth century in the United States the Ox-Eye Daisy was 'used a a tonic instead of Chamomile flowers, and i serviceable in whooping-cough, asthma and nervous excitability' and 'very beneficial externally and internally in leucorrhoea' Externally it was applied 'to wounds, ulcers scald-head and some other cutaneous diseases' while 'its external use is highly recommended in colliquative perspiration'. The fresh flowers or leaves were also used to destroy or drive away fleas, and in Europe during the medieval period for strewing floors.

Other names for the Ox-Eye include Dog Daisy, White Weed, White Daisy, Field Daisy, Dun Daisy, Moon Daisy, Maudlin Daisy, Great Ox-Eye, Goldens, Gowan Horsegowan, Maudlinwort and Marguerite The plant's specific name of *leucanthemum* simply means white, referring to its flowers and is derived from the Greek word *leucoma*

Infusions are still prescribed by herbalist for their antispasmodic, diuretic and tonic principles, mainly in the treatment of asthma

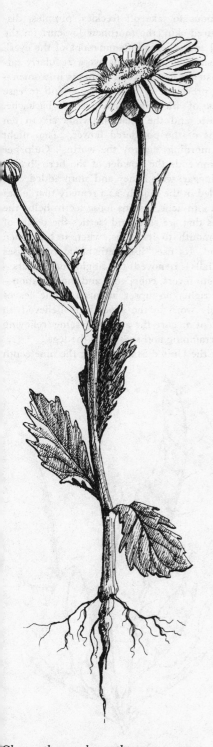

Chrysanthemum leucanthemum

whooping-cough and nervous excitability (although large doses can cause sickness) and as an external lotion for applying to ulcers and sores. The leaves have an acid, tingling taste and the flowers are bitter. In Italy the young leaves are occasionally eaten in salads.

The Tansy (*C. vulgare*, syn. *Tanacetum vulgare*), like the previous species, is native to most of Europe (including Britain) and parts of Asia. It grows in pastures, grassy verges, waste and similar places. The stiff, erect stems grow to 1m/3ft high, and bear finely divided feathery leaves, while from June onwards dense clusters of flat-topped, small button-like yellow flowers appear. Although native to the regions above, this was yet another plant taken to New World by the early settlers, where it soon naturalized itself.

The herb's familiar name of Tansy is believed to be derived from the Greek word *athanasia*, meaning immortality, referring either to the flowers, which are long-lasting and when dried tend to retain a natural appearance, or perhaps to the plant's ancient use 'for preserving the bodies of the dead from corruption'. A late example of the latter is provided by Samuel Sewell, the New England Puritan, who recalls that the body of a friend of his was kept for some time by being packed in Tansy leaves. The herb was commonly used at this time, both in America and Europe 'to keep flies from corpses', and to 'drive bugs and vermin away'.

Of its medicinal uses during the early part of the Middle Ages little is known for certain. It was one of the plants mentioned as grown in the herb garden of Charlemagne the Great, at the end of the eighth century, and also in the Swiss monastery of St Gall, a Benedictine establishment, which was then rapidly becoming renowned as a centre of learning.

In England some time after the Norman Conquest, it became a regular custom to 'eat of Tansy pudding on an Easter Sunday', Turner later explaining: 'It was well divised of Phisicianes of old tyme that after Easter men should use tanseyes to drive away the wyndenes yt they have gotten all the lent before with eatyng of fish, peasen, beanes and diverse kynds of wynde making herbes.'

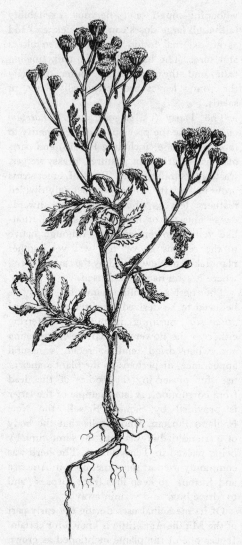

Chrysanthemum vulgare

Coles in 1656 was of the opinion people ate Tansy at Easter 'as a wholesome antidote to the salt fish consumed during Lent', which counteracted any ill effects of the 'moist and cold constitution of winter . . .' Others firmly believed it was eaten in spring 'to avoid the summer sickness'.

Of its numerous medicinal uses Turner observes the herb was used as a face wash by 'our women in Englande and some men that be sunne burnt and would be fayre.' The distilled water applied was regarded as

'virtuous to take off freckles, pimples, discoloured skin, the morphew [a scurf on the face] and relieves inflammations of the eyes'. Infusions or decoctions were regularly administered for 'nervous thoughts in women – as a preventer of miscarriage – and to ease aches of the joints all over – backache, rupture and the sciatica,' while six to ten grains of the powdered flower, taken night and morning 'destroy the worms'. Culpeper recommends the powder of the herb 'boiled in vinegar, with honey and alum added, and gargled in the mouth' as a remedy that 'eases the tooth-ache, fastens loose teeth, helps the gums that are sore' and 'settles the palate of the mouth to its place, when it has fallen down'. Its use 'dissolveth blood by bruises and falls – removeth the singing of the ears – helpeth fevers, colic, gout and the digestion – and rights an upset stomach.' The leaves simply worn in the shoes were believed 'to prevent or cure the ague' the same 'relieving the cramping and spasms of the legs'.

In the United States during the nineteenth

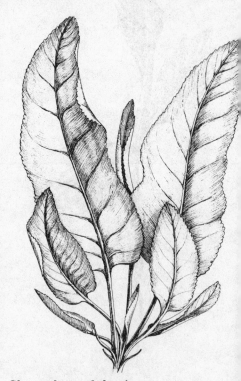

Chrysanthemum balsamita

ntury cold infusions prescribed in small
ɔses were 'found useful in convalescence
ɔm exhausting diseases, dyspepsia, hysteria
ɪd jaundice. The warm infusion is dia-
ɪoretic and emmenagogue. It bears a good
putation in suppressed menstruation, but
ɪould only be used when the suppression is
ɪe to morbid causes.'

Tansy roots mixed with certain chemicals
ɪoduce a green dye (which is still used in
inland), the leaves a greenish-yellow and the
ɪwers a gold or orange-tan. The dye from
ɪe leaves was often used to colour cakes and
ɪns.

Infusions of this bitter aromatic herb are
ɪll given for their anthelmintic, emmena-
ɪgue, stimulant and tonic principles, mainly
ɪ promoting perspiration to sweat out colds,
ɪills and influenza, and in hepatic, bilious,
ɪphritic and female complaints. It is said to
ɪlp prevent miscarriage and to ease swollen
ɪd varicose veins, although it should never
ɪ taken in excess for it can act as an irritant.
ɪfusions are also administered for expelling
ɪorms in animals and children.

In the United States, the bruised leaves are
ɪmetimes applied as a household remedy for
ɪeating rheumatism and bruises.

As a culinary herb the leaves of the Tansy
ɪe still added in small amounts for flavouring
ɪkes, puddings, omelettes, stews and other
ɪshes.

Its other common names include Buttons,
ɪtter Buttons, Bachelor's Buttons, Ginger,
ɪrsley Fern, Scented Fern and Cheese.

The Costmary (*C. balsamita*, syn. *Tana-
tum balsamita* or *Balsamita vulgaris*), which
ɪ supposed to be native to the Orient but is
ɪw found widely naturalized in southern
ɪurope and western Asia, was yet another
ɪmiliar member of the Chrysanthemum
ɪnus to become well-known to the people of
ɪurope, especially during the sixteenth and
ɪventeenth centuries. This aromatic peren-
ɪial has bluntly toothed, oblong or oval leaves
ɪd somewhat woody flowering stems about
ɪn/3ft. high, bearing loose clusters of
ɪllowish button-like flowers in summer.

The commonest name of this plant, Cost-
ɪary, has evolved over the years from the
ɪreek word *kostos*, or the Latin *costus*, an

aromatic Oriental herb with a spicy flavour,
the 'Mary' being added during the medieval
period in honour of the Virgin Mother, to
whom the species was dedicated in several
European countries. Indeed the herb had
become so popular that during the sixteenth
century crops were specially cultivated in
Spain for export. At about this period the
plant was introduced to England and grown
mainly for the sake of its leaves, which were
added to salads and used in cooking. It
became known there by several other names,
for instance Goose Tongue referred to the
shape of the leaves, Bible-Leaf because its
leaves were used as bookmarks in churches,
and Alecost as it was added for flavour to a
variety of alcoholic brews.

Elizabethan writers inform us that the
leaves were employed 'to sweeten floors and
closets by strewing' and often dried and mixed
with lavender to perfume linens and cupboards. Of its medicinal uses, it 'cleanseth
inwardly which is foul – openeth obstructions
and dissolveth putrefactions of their evil
effects – and will strengthen the inward
parts'.

By the middle of the seventeenth century it
had become one of the commonest of English
herbs. Culpeper prescribed it for agues, liver
complaints, ulcers and to rid children of
worms. Ointments of it were also used
throughout Europe 'for the bruisings in the
skin – hot veins and painful sinews – running
scab – the itch – scorching of gunpowder
blasts – and for body lice – scabies and crabs'.
After Culpeper's time the use of Costmary in
medicine declined, although it was still
officially listed in the *British Pharmacopoeia*
until 1788, and often given for dysentery.
Bryant writes in 1783: 'It is a pity it is not
continued, as from its sensible qualities it
seems superior to many aromatic plants now
in credit.'

Today the leaves and dried flowers however can be employed in the kitchen and
included sparingly in salads, pot-pourri and
in meat and vegetable stews; it goes quite well
with chicken and veal. The fresh or dried
leaves make a pleasant-tasting tea, formerly
prescribed for its astringent and antiseptic
effects.

The roots from crops commercially grown are nowadays included as an ingredient in very expensive perfumes, having a fragrance similar to that of lemon, chrysanthemum and mint.

The somewhat fleshy leaves of the Corn Marigold (*C. segetum*), which is native to the cornfields and arable lands of most of Europe and the British Isles, were formerly used in the home to produce a good yellow dye. This erect, greyish looking annual, 20–60cm/

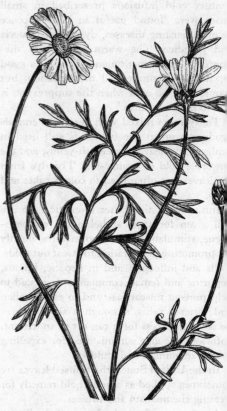

Chrysanthemum cinerariaefolium

7–23in. high, produces its bright golden yellow daisy-like flower heads on solitary stalks, from about June to the end of the summer, and is one of the species from which the popular annual Chrysanthemums of the ornamental garden have been raised.

The important insecticide known as Pyrethrum powder is obtained from the dried powdered flowers of the Dalmatian Pyrethrum (*C. cinerariaefolium*) native principally to the Dalmatian Coast, although grown in other countries such as Japan. Three other species possess similar properties, the Persian Insect Flower, (*C. marschallii*), the Persian Pellitory (*C. roseum*) and *C. carneum*.

The botanical name of this genus, Chrysanthemum, is derived from the Greek *chrysos*, meaning gold, and *anthemon*, flower.

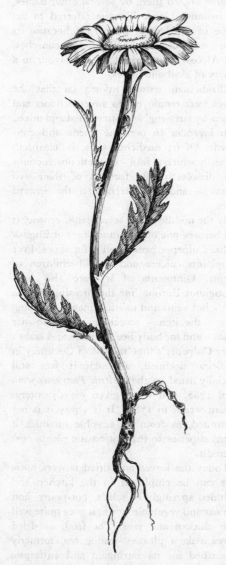

Chrysanthemum segetum

ICHORIUM

ompositae, the Daisy family

hicory, Endive

nly four species belong to this genus of shy rooted biennial or perennial flowering erbs common to much of Europe and Asia, d only two were used in medicine. The ost important was the Chicory (*C. intybus*) stiff, toughly stemmed perennial 30–120cm/ –47in. high, having spreading upright ranches and lance shaped, somewhat variable aves, and bearing from June to September, ong the stems at the base of the leaves, most unstalked flowers ranging in twos and rees and consisting of bright blue ray

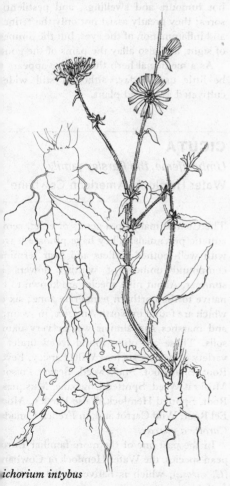

ichorium intybus

florets only. Native to most of Europe (except Iceland) and much of western Asia, including central Russia, it is found in waste ground, by the borders of fields and by tracks and road-sides, mostly on gravel or limestone soils. It is known in many other countries having been introduced as a commercial crop, for example, North and South America, eastern Asia, South Africa, New Zealand and Australia.

The generic name of this herb, *Cichorium*, from which the word Chicory is derived, appears to date from before the birth of Christ, when it was listed by the Greeks as *kichora* or *kichoreia*. Variations of these were known both to the ancient Egyptian and Arabian physicians, to the latter as *chicouryeh* and later on as *chicourey*.

Whatever its origins this plant was certainly known to the Romans who ate the roots as a vegetable, as mentioned by Horace, Virgil and Pliny, or added them to their salads, while Galen informs us that, medicinally, it was the friend of the liver. The bruised leaves were applied as a poultice to ease swellings and inflamed eyes, besides being taken internally for their tonic and digestive effects, often in the latter case by boiling the root in broth.

During the medieval period, it was regarded as a cleansing plant and was regularly prescribed as a diuretic, laxative and tonic, especially 'as a strengthener of weak and feeble stomachs'. Tusser, in 1573, regarded it as a useful remedy for the ague and used it with the Endive. Culpeper also thought: 'The water is effectual also for sore eyes that are inflamed' and 'for nurses' breasts that are pained by the abundance of milk'. This 'fine, cleansing, jovial plant' as Parkinson called it, was also prescribed inwardly 'for swoonings and passions of the heart – loss of appetite – gout – dropsy – the ache – heat and headaches in children – and for helping the liver and blood.' Externally applied it 'allays swellings and inflammations – wheals, ugly pushes, spots and pimples' as well 'as pestiforous sores and St Anthony's Fire' if applied with vinegar. During the reign of Charles II of England the water distilled from the flowers formed one of the ingredients which, with violet flowers, were made into the English

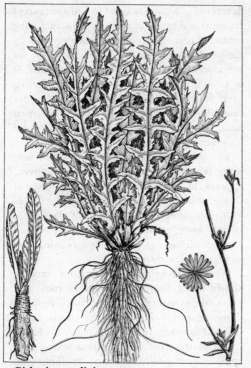

Cichorium endivia

confection known as 'Violet Plates'.

The roots are still prescribed for their tonic, laxative and diuretic principles. These are usually decocted and taken freely to relieve jaundice, liver troubles, gout and rheumatic complaints. The Syrup of Succory makes an excellent laxative for children.

Several highly developed varieties of this species are grown in gardens or are commercially cultivated nowadays for the sake of their tap roots. These are dried, roasted and ground down, and substituted or blended with coffee. The shoots or young leaves when blanched are often included in salads or cooked as a vegetable dish.

The root of a similar species, the Common or Garden Endive (*C. endivia*), is also added to coffee mixtures or grown as a salad plant. This somewhat glaucous annual or biennial is native to southern Asia, although widely cultivated in various leaf forms in many other countries, as in southern Europe, where it is sometimes found naturalized.

As Culpeper recorded: 'Common garden

Endive bears a longer and larger leaf tha[n] succory, and abides but one year, quick[ly] running up to stalk and seed, and the[n] perishing. It has blue flowers, and the seed so much like that succory, that it is hard [to] distinguish it.' As a 'fine cooling cleansir[g] plant' he prescribed 'the decoction of th[e] leaves, or the juice, or the distilled water – [to] cool the excessive heat of the liver an[d] stomach – the hot fits of agues, and all oth[er] inflammations' and to cool 'the heat an[d] sharpness of the urine, and the excoriation of the urinary parts'. Culpeper regarded th[e] seed as having 'the same properties, thoug[h] rather more powerful' and as 'available f[or] faintings, swoonings and the passions of th[e] heart'. Outwardly applied 'they serve [to] temper the sharp humours of fretting ulcer[s] hot tumours and swellings, and pestilenti[al] sores; they greatly assist not only the redne[ss] and inflammation of the eyes, but the dimne[ss] of sight, and also allay the pains of the gout[.]'

As a medicinal herb the Endive appears [to] be little used today, although still widel[y] cultivated as a salad plant.

CICUTA
Umbelliferae, the Parsley family
Water Hemlock, American Cowbane

The Cicutas make up a genus of erect, sem[i]-aquatic perennials. They have pinnate leave[s] with well-toothed leaflets and bear termin[al] compound umbels of whitish flowers i[n] summer. About nine species are known to b[e] native to the northern temperate zone; six [of] which are found in North America, in swamp[s] and marshes and similar wet or very dam[p] soils. These are often found listed under [a] variety of names, such as Wild Parsley, Feve[r] Root, Snakeroot, Snakeweed, Beaver Poiso[n,] Muskrat Weed, Spotted Cowbane, Musquas[h] Root, Spotted Hemlock, False Parsley, Moc[k] Eel Root, Wild Carrot and, in French Canad[a,] *Carotte à moreau*.

In the past one of the more familiar Euro[-]pean species, the Water Hemlock or Cowban[e] (*C. virosa*), which is native to the norther[n] and central parts of that region, although now widely naturalized elsewhere, as in the British Isles and North America, was frequently used as a poison. This virulent herb is found in or near the fresh water of ditches, ponds and marshes, where its stout, hollow branching stems reach 1½m/5ft high, sometimes more, and bear in July and August, rather large, long-stalked umbels of pure white flowers.

The extracted juice from the hollow parsnip or dahlia-like tubers of this species

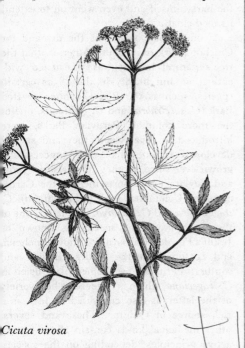

Cicuta virosa

provided the poison, but to be completely effective it had to be used while fresh. Within a short time the victim would complain of stomach pains, followed by 'a terrible retching sickness' generally accompanied 'with the grinding of the teeth – violent hiccough – uncontrollable and powerful urination – with delirium – convulsions and dreadful seizure to watch,' the spine sometimes curving backwards in the form of a bowstring, the 'blood running from the ears'. Death if it came would result 'from asphyxia'. Not all the fatalities recorded as caused by this plant were the result of intended poisonings, for the roots have often been mistakenly eaten as

parsnips. Nevertheless, poisonous as the Water Hemlock is, chemists nowadays extract a volatile alkaloid known as Cicutine from its roots, and this when properly used is very helpful in relieving epilepsy, convulsions and psychosis.

The American Cowbane or Cowbean (*C. maculata*), often known as the Spotted Water Hemlock, occurs mainly to the east of the Rocky Mountains, and is one of the most poisonous plants found in the United States, having caused the deaths of many children and adults who, as with the previous species, dug up the roots believing them to be parsnips or artichokes and therefore edible. Unfortunately, at certain times of the year just one mouthful of the root can severely poison or kill. Grazing cattle are often affected by eating the young shoots as they appear in spring. Poisonous as it is, the American Cowbane was formerly prescribed for sick and nervous headaches, but is seldom used nowadays. The alkaloid Cicutine previously mentioned is also present in this plant, as it is in the Western Water Hemlock (*C. douglasi*), found from Alaska south to California.

For obvious reasons, herbalists rarely if ever prescribe any of the Cicuta genus.

CIMICIFUGA
Ranunculaceae, the Buttercup family
Black Cohosh

Most of the Cimicifugas are hardy herbaceous perennials, native to North America, China and Japan. They grow from 1–1½m/3–5ft high, producing in late summer long graceful spikes of white or whitish flowers.

The generic name of these herbs, Cimicifuga, is derived from the Latin *cimex*, a bug, and *fugo* or *fugere*, to flee or drive away, referring to the insecticidal properties found in the leaves of some of the species, although only one, the Black Cohosh or Black Snake Root (*C. racemosa*, syn. *Actaea racemosa* or *Macrotys actaeoides*), appears to have been widely prescribed in medicine. This tall leafy perennial is native to North America, where it is found in woods and shady hillsides, in both Canada and the United States, bearing from May to August slender feathery racemes of white flowers 30–90cm/11–35in. long.

Only the hard, black knotty roots or rhizomes of this species were used in medicine, from which a resinous, bitter tasting substance known as Cimicifugin or Macrotin was obtained. This was successfully used 'in cholera, periodical convulsions, fits, epilepsy, nervous excitability, asthma, delirium tremens and many spasmodic affections, and in consumption, cough, acute rheumatism, neuralgia and scrofula.' It was also 'very valuable in amenorrhoea, dysmenorrhoea and other menstrual and uterine affections.' The 'saturated tincture of the root' was valued as an 'embrocation in all cases of inflammation of the nerves, tic douloureux, crick in the back or sides, rheumatism, old ulcers, etc.,' and 'as a way of inducing perspiration' besides being 'good for the whooping-cough – as an antidote against poison'. One of the herb's more common names, that of Black Snake Root, refers to its use in snakebites, and is so-called to distinguish it from the Common or Virginian Snake Root (*Aristolochia serpentaria*). Fluid extracts or tinctures of the root were occasionally administered 'as very useful in palpitations of the heart, and cardiac affections generally'.

The rhizomes are still valued and prescribed in various forms for their astringent, alterative, diuretic and emmenagogue effects. Overdoses or large doses cause feelings of nausea.

The herb's other common names include Rattle Root, Squaw Root, Rattle Weed and Bugbane.

CINCHONA
Rubiaceae, the Madder family
Jesuit's Bark, Peruvian Bark

The Cinchonas make up a fairly large genus of evergreen shrubs and trees, about 70 species of which are native to the Andes of South America, Colombia and Peru. They have opposite entire leaves, and bear panicles of fragrant usually whitish-pink to purplish coloured flowers, followed by numerous winged seeds.

The Incas are believed to have used several of these species in the treatment of fevers, long before they came to the attention of the Western world in the early 1640s, when it was taken to Spain by the Jesuits. They used infusions of the bark as a cure for malarial fevers, hence the name Jesuit's Bark. One of the first Cinchona species to be raised in England was grown at Upton in Essex by Dr John Fothergill (1712–80) who prescribed the bark himself and even went on to extend its medicinal use.

At one period, such was the demand for Cinchona bark from South America, that the tree's natural habitat was threatened with extinction, but luckily in the 1850s certain species, such as the Red Cinchona or Red Bark (*C. succirubra*) and *C. officinalis*, one of the more common Peruvian Barks, were introduced to Java, where they and several developed varieties have been successfully grown ever since, as they have also in India and Ceylon. Other sorts include the Carthagena or Colombian Bark (*C. lancifolia*). *C. condaminea* and *C. calisaya*. The latter, one of the more important species, is known as Jesuit's Powder, Calisaya or Yellow Cinchona, and is found in the Andes, Bolivia and southern Peru. A closely allied plant listed as *C. ledgeriana*, which is believed to be a variety of the latter, is also cultivated in Java as a rich source of Quinine. These and several other medicinal kinds contain about twenty active principles, depending on the species, the most familiar of which is Quinine and this is mainly prescribed in tropical countries as a febrifuge in malaria. Other important constituents include Cinchonine, Cinchonidine, Quinidine, Quinamine, Hydroquinine, Hydrocinchonidine and Homocinchonidine.

During the late nineteenth century thirteen species provided the Cinchona bark of commerce, although only four were recognized in the *Pharmacopoeia* of the United States, and these were prescribed there, as they were in Britain and Europe, for their 'tonic, antiperiodic astringent' and 'eminent febrifuge effects'. As 'a topically (or externally) antiseptic' it was 'of much value when

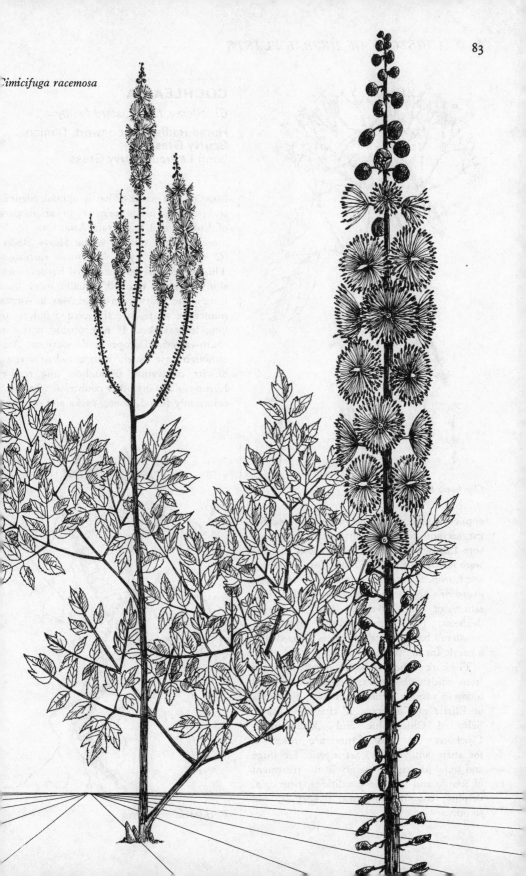

Cimicifuga racemosa

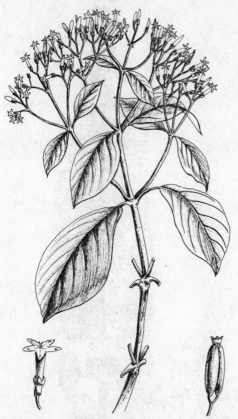

Cinchona lancifolia

applied to gangrenous ulcerations, or used for gargles and washes in erysipelas, ulcerated sore throat and mouth . . .' Liquid extracts were sometimes used in both North America and Europe as a cure for drunkenness, although overdoses produced headaches, vertigo, irritation of the intestines and sometimes deafness. The Victorians also added the powdered bark to tooth powders or used it as a gargle for the throat.

The bark of the Cinchonas, mostly obtained from cultivated species, is still widely used today in various forms, as in pills, Tinctures or Elixirs of Cinchona, Elixirs of Calisaya, Salts of Cinchonine and Cinchonidine, Cinchona wine. Most of these are prescribed for their antiperiodic, astringent, febrifuge and tonic principles, mainly in the treatment of febrile and typhoid conditions, neuralgia, debility, coughs, influenza, dyspepsia, and so on.

COCHLEARIA

Cruciferae, the Mustard family

Horse Radish, Spoonwort, Danish Scurvy Grass, Long Leaved Scurvy Grass

Most of this genus of hardy annual, biennial and perennial herbs are native to various parts of Europe and temperate Asia. One of the more familiar species is the Horse Radish (*C. armoracia*, syn. *Armoracia rusticana*). This robust, hairless perennial has large and shiny, slightly toothed, usually wavy basal leaves, and bears from about May to August numerous white, sweetly scented flowers on long leafy spikes. It is probably native to south-eastern Europe and western Asia, although now widely naturalized as a result of its cultivation throughout the rest of Europe and many other countries, where it is commonly found among rocks and on waste

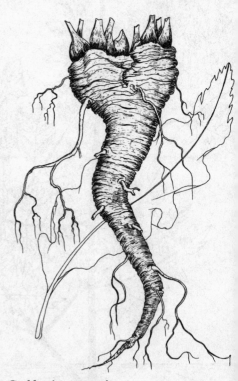

Cochlearia armoracia

ground and similar waste places.

Pliny is believed to have recommended this particular plant for its medicinal uses under the name of Amoracia, a word of uncertain meaning. It is also possible that it is the Wild Radish of the Greeks, listed as *Raphanos agrios* in the *Great Herbal*. Gerard described it in 1597 as *Raphanus rusticanus*, and this is the name used in the London *Pharmacopias* of the eighteenth century. The more familiar botanical name of *C. armoracia* was previously used by Culpeper – the Latin *cochleare* or *coclear*, meaning spoon, refers to the shape of the genera's leaves – although since his time the plant has been reclassified as *Armoracia rusticana*. The most common current name of Horse Radish is probably derived from the Latin *radix*, meaning root, with the prefix 'horse' indicating that this species is the coarser growing kind, thus distinguishing it from the edible Radish (*Raphanus sativus*). Its other names have included Wild or Mountain Radish, Great Raifort and Red Cole.

Of its known medical uses Gerard tells us as a condiment the root was pounded 'with a little vinegar put thereto' which was 'commonly used among the Germans for sauce to eate fish with and such like meates as we do mustarde'. A custom to which Parkinson in the 1640s also refers.

As an internal medicine, the root was regarded as a very strong diuretic, and the majority of the apothecaries and physicians of the medieval period prescribed it for 'relieving the stone and gravel – the dropsy – sciatica – and the pains of the gout' and, like Boerhaave, for the scurvy when little or no fever was present. Coles agreed with Culpeper in saying: 'Of all things given to children for worms, horseradish is not the least, for it soon killeth and expelleth them.' The bruised root was also applied direct to chilblains, facial neuralgia and various paralytic complaints. Taken infused in wine, the root 'readily promotes the perspiration,' while 'the syrup relieves the cough of the influenza – whooping cough – and the hoarseness'.

The root is still prescribed infused or in syrups, for its diaphoretic, diuretic and stimulant principles, as in dropsy, and is an

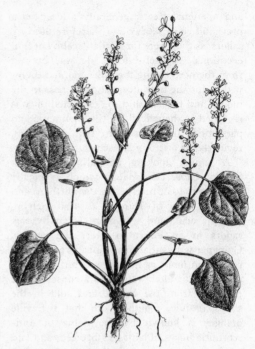

Cochlearia officinalis

excellent stimulant for the digestive organs.

The leaves of several other Cochlearia species were formerly prescribed in medicine. One such was the Spoonwort or Scurvy Grass (*C. officinalis*), a small hairless biennial or perennial, having erect or spreading branched stems up to 50cm/19in. tall, with fleshy, long-stalked heart- or kidney-shaped leaves, and bearing in summer terminal racemes of numerous white flowers. It is mostly found in the northern and western parts of Europe, where it grows on cliffs and banks by the sea, on salt marshes and similar maritime districts, and occasionally inland on mountain sides, in wettish stony or sandy soils.

Culpeper writes of it: 'The root is made of many white strings, which stick deeply into the mud, wherein it chiefly delights, yet it will abide in the more upland and drier ground, and tastes brackish there, but not as much as where it feeds upon the salt water.'

The fresh leaves of this species have a very pungent odour and a bitter taste, and were prescribed for their antiscorbutic, diuretic and aperient effects, generally infused as a preventative of scurvy and therefore used by sailors, as they were for similar 'scabby or foul eruptions'. A useful tonic ale was brewed from the herb, while the 'juice gargled therewith helps the foul ulcers and soreness in the mouth and throat', and the extracted oil was regarded as 'beneficial for the rheumatic and paralytic.' Infusions can still be taken, regularly, as a strong antiscorbutic.

A similar looking annual, the Danish Scurvy Grass (*C. danica*) which is mostly found in the salt marshes in the northern and western parts of Europe, is also rich in ascorbic acid, and was often eaten by sick sailors in an effort to avert the scurvy. Culpeper writes that this plant: 'Is a powerful remedy in moist asthma, or scorbutic rheumatism. A distilled water and a conserve, are prepared from the leaves, and sold in the shops, its juice together with that of Seville oranges is known by the name of antiscorbutic juices. The leaves bruised, and laid to the face, or any other part, takes away spots, freckles and sun-burns; but those of delicate complexions cannot bear the application without injuring them.' Other names for this species include Early Scurvy Grass and Ivy-Leaved Scurvy Grass.

The Long Leaved or Sea Scurvy Grass (*C. anglica*) is found on the muddy shores in much of north-west Europe. Culpeper tells us: 'This kind is used along with the others as antiscorbutics ... but abounding more in saline, it may be used to good purposes as a diuretic.'

COLCHICUM
Liliacea, the Lily family
Meadow Saffron

The Colchicums make up a genus of about 30 species of hardy bulbous flowering plants, most of which are native to parts of Europe, Asia, North Africa, Iran, India and the Himalayas. Of these only one, the Meadow Saffron (*C. autumnale*), was used to any extent in medicine. This hairless perennial, native to the damp meadows of much of

Europe, has shiny green, lance-shaped leaves 12–30cm/4–11in. long, and in the autumn, after the leaves have died down, bears solitary rosy-purple or white crocus-like flowers on weak stalks.

The active parts of this herb consist of the fleshy bulb resembling that of a tulip, and the seed, both having been employed for centuries as a poison. These were powdered down and added to alcoholic drinks, which were then administered to the victims. Dioscorides warned of its poisoning effects, while Theophrastus, the Greek philosopher-

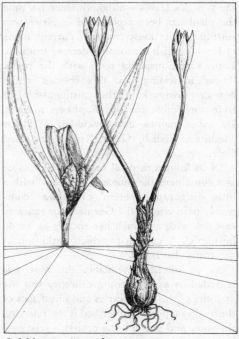

Colchicum autumnale

scientist, records that it was occasionally taken in small amounts by slaves, when they were upset or offended simply to make themselves ill.

The botanical name of the genus, Colchicum, is derived from the Greek *Kolchis* or the Latin *Colchis*, an ancient district in Asia Minor, the home of Medea the sorceress where, according to legend, the bulbs first grew, having sprung from the drops spilt by Medea as she was brewing a liquor.

This vegetable arsenic, as it was often called, was frequently used in Europe and the

Mediterranean region in the medieval period, to dispose of unwanted people Turner warned the English of its dangers when he wrote, in 1563, 'much of it is stercke poyson, and will strongell a man and kill him in the space of one day.' And strangle it would. The first symptoms normally appeared after several hours 'by fire in the throat and mouth' with 'a terrible unquenchable thirst and frequent sickness' lasting a day, followed by 'anguishing colic and bloody diarrhoea', with the central nervous system gradually becoming paralyzed, the unfortunate victim finding it extremely difficult even to breathe, often resulting in 'a tormenting death within two days'. Having enumerated its fearful symptoms, Culpeper asserted that it was, when properly prepared, 'a safe but powerful medicine'.

Deadly as the Meadow Saffron was, the bitter whitish juice from its corms had long been valued as a remedy for the gout, and is believed to have been first used by the ancient Egyptians over 4,000 years ago. James I, King of England (1603–25), was obliged to partake of the herb having been prescribed it by Sir Theode Mayerne, his physician, who mixed small portions of the root with the powder of unburied skulls, which at that period were often included in cures. Anton Freiherr von Stoerck (1731–1803) managed to work out the proper extract and started using it in 1763 as a specific for gout taken in wine, thus eliminating most of the previous hit and miss methods.

The Colchicum was also cultivated in the United States during the eighteenth and nineteenth centuries, much as it was in Europe, for its sedative, cathartic and diuretic principles, which were put to good use in 'gouty rheumatisms, dropsy, and palpitations of the heart'.

An alkaloid known as Colchicine is nowadays extracted from the roots and seed of the herb and this is given in pill form in the treatment of gout and other rheumatic complaints.

It has since been discovered that Colchicine, a very powerful drug well able to withstand boiling, drying and storage, will upset the normal processes of cell division in plants and is now used in experimental genetic work, as a means of creating new forms and species.

COLLINSONIA
Labiatea, the Mint family
Stone Root

This strongly scented North American Mint, the Stone Root (*C. canadensis*), is native to the moist woods from Canada to Carolina, its four-sided stems reaching 30–120cm/11–47in. high, having large, coarsely serrate-ovate leaves, and bearing greenish-yellow flowers from about July to September.

In nineteenth-century medicine, the whole of this pungent and spicy herb was prescribed for its antispasmodic, astringent, diaphoretic, diuretic and stomach-tonic effects, although its chief virtues were regarded as 'laying concentrated in the roots' – a knobby, greyish-brown rhizome, which with its

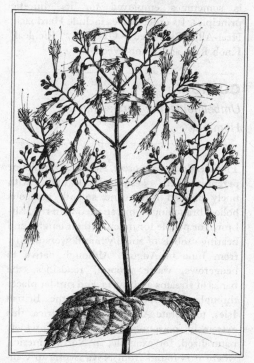

Collinsonia canadensis

numerous brittle rootlets was only administered when fresh. These were employed 'with
good effect in chronic catarrh of the bladder –
whites – weakness of the stomach – and for
the disorders of the urinary organs'. Its use
was believed to 'exert a strong influence over
the mucous tissues' and 'is a very fair stimulant, and a gentle tonic and diuretic'. The
active principle of the herb, known as
Collinsonin after Peter Collinson its dis-
coverer, was classed as a 'very valuable
remedy for haemorrhoids and all other
diseases of the rectum'. The average dose was
from about two to five grains.

The leaves were also applied externally in
fomentations and poultices to 'bruises,
wounds, blows, sprains, contusions, cuts,
ulcers and sores, etc.'

Herbalists still prescribe the roots, mostly
in liquid extracts or tinctures, in the treatment
of haemorrhoids, bladder complaints and as a
general diuretic.

Two of the plant's more familiar names,
Horsebalm and Horseweed, refer to its use in
North American veterinary practice, where it
is sometimes employed for its diuretic
principles. Its other names include Hardback,
Heal-All, Richweed, Ox-Balm, Richleaf,
Knob Root and Knob Weed.

CONIUM
Umbelliferae, the Parsley family
Hemlock

The Hemlock is an erect, slender, biennial or
perennial herb ½–2½m/1½–8ft high, with
finely divided leaves and smooth glaucous
hollow branching stems, spotted with reddish-
brown or purple for much of their length, and
bearing umbels of small white flowers mainly
from June to August. Although native to
hedgerows, waste ground, roadsides, the
banks of streams and rivers, and similar places
throughout Europe, including the British
Isles, temperate Asia and North Africa, this
extremely poisonous herb is now widely
naturalized, for example, in North America,
where it is found from Nova Scotia to California, and in Chile, and occasionally in other
South American countries.

The ancient Roman name for the Poison
Hemlock was Cicuta, a Latin word used
throughout the medieval period until, probably in 1541, it was transferred by Gesner and
other authorities to the Water Hemlock
(*Cicuta virosa*) a related plant also of the
Umbelliferae family. In 1737 Linnaeus, to
avoid confusion, allocated this particular
Hemlock the botanical name of *Conium
maculatum*. This new generic name of Conium
itself was derived from the Greek *koneion* or
konas, to spin or whirl, referring to the
disastrous effects on the body should any part

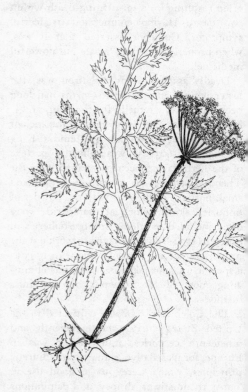

Conium maculatum

of the plant be eaten for it causes, even in
small amounts, 'a terrible vertigo' possibly
followed by death. Maculatum, the herb's
specific name, means spotted or speckled, and
alludes to the purplish mottling of the stems,
said to represent the brand of Cain, put there
after he had committed murder. The commonest name, Hemlock, has been used

probably since the Anglo-Saxon period, when it was known as *Hemlic* or *Hymelic*, which is possibly derived from *hoem* or *healm*, meaning straw, and *leac*, a leek or plant, referring perhaps to the dry and hollow stems that are left after the herb has flowered. Its other names include Common Hemlock, Poison Parsley, Conium, Spotted Hemlock, Herb Bennet, Spotted Corobane, Musquash Root, Beaver Poisoner, Kex and Kecksies.

Although the Hemlock has been used since ancient times as a medicinal herb, it was also administered, especially by the Greeks, as a very reliable poison. Its juice is also believed to have been one of the main ingredients of the Hemlock cup' which according to Plato was given to the philosopher Socrates 'from the hands of the State'. Numerous other people have since died, having accidently eaten the fruits as anise, or the long fleshy tap root as parsnip. The poisonous constituents are said to be less strong in the root, although the whole of the plant, even in small amounts, is capable of killing. Within a few minutes the unfortunate victim's sight would fade or blur, his mouth would tingle or burn, followed by sickness, vertigo, convulsions and diarrhoea, with paralysis of the central nervous system, the whole of the body from the feet up going stiff and cold, with death, should it come, occurring from respiratory failure. During the whole of this process the victim's mind was said to remain unaffected.

Such a poisonous plant had to be administered very carefully when it came to be used in medicine. During the medieval period it was only taken for 'the bite of mad dogge' when its bitter juice was mixed with Betony and Fennel seed, which was not only applied to the place, but mixed with wine and drunk, such was the fear of rabies. Later on the juice was occasionally administered as a last resort, as an antidote for strychnine and other virulent poisons.

The Hemlock could however be safely used externally in poultices and ointments to risings, hard or otherwise – inflammations – indolent tumours – tumults and swellings – wheals – pushes – creeping ulcers – pains of the joints all over – scrofulous affections' and to St Anthony's Fire'. The monks and other religious sects of the fifteenth and sixteenth centuries also made use of the roasted root for relieving the pains of gout and applied it not only to the painful part affected, the foot, but to their hands and wrists. In the 1760s, it began to be used by Stoerck, both externally and internally as a cure for cancerous ulcers.

The juice of the Hemlock *Succus conii*, is still valued by chemists as it contains several alkaloids, one of which is Coniine. This is extracted from the leaves and young shoots, just as the fruits begin to form, generally towards the end of June, and is prescribed under strict medical supervision in tinctures and extracts for its sedative, anodyne and antispasmodic effects, in such illnesses as asthma, epilepsy, whooping cough, angina, chorea and stomach pains. Overdoses produce narcotic poisoning with paralysis and loss of speech.

CONVALLARIA
Liliaceae, the Lily family
Lily of the Valley

This small hardy herbaceous perennial, the Lily of the Valley (*C. majalis*), with usually two broad, long stalked leaves 8–20cm/3–7in. tall, is found in the wild throughout Europe, including the British Isles, Soviet Russia, north east Asia and North America. It grows locally in shady woods and thickets, generally in damp, but well-drained sandy loam or limestone humus rich soils. Its creeping rhizomes and underground stems produce from April to June one-sided racemes of small pure white bell-shaped pendulous flowers, followed by green berries turning red.

The generic name of the herb, Convallaria, is derived from an older name, *Lillium convallium*, thus Lily of the Valleys. Majalis, its present-day specific name, alludes to May, its main flowering period. Due to the whiteness of the flowers, it was formerly associated in several European countries with the Virgin Mary, which led to another common name, Our Lady's Tears. Long before this, in the fourth-century *Herbarium of Apuleius*, it was known as Glovewort and used in the care of the hands. Apuleius also informs us that the plant was found by Apollo and given by him to Aesclepias, the Greek physician or leech.

Gerard, perhaps quoting Joachim Camerarius of Nurenburg, recommended: 'The floures of May Lillies put into a glasse, and set in a hill of ants, close stopped for the space of a moneth, and then taken out, therein you shall find a liquor that appeaseth the paine and griefe of the gout, being outwardly applied; which is commended to be most excellent.' Besides this rather unusual remedy Gerard recommends: 'The flowers of the Valley Lillie distilled with wine, and drunke the quantitie of a spoonefull' to 'restore speech unto those that have the dumb palsie and that are falne into the Apoplexie ...' He adds: 'The water aforesaid doth strengthen the memory that is weakened and diminished; it helpeth also the inflammations of the eies, being dropped thereinto.' Matthiolus observed that the Lily of the Valley strengthened the heart and combated spasms and palpitations, while the Russian peasants gave it in the treatment of dropsy resulting from heart complaints.

For relieving the headache or pains of the migraine, a few of the flowers dipped in wine and eaten was said to be very effective, and these when powdered were added as a major ingredient to 'errhines and cephalic snuffs'.

The whole herb is still used for its important cardiac tonic and diuretic principles mostly in tinctures and fluid extracts and to a lesser degree infused, especially in cardiac debility, dropsy, valvular heart disease and other closely related illnesses. In action it resembles the Foxglove (Digitalis), although rather less powerful than that plant and therefore safer to administer internally. Nevertheless all parts of the herb are listed as potentially poisonous and its indiscriminate use in fairly large amounts can cause a heart attack. The main symptoms of its poisoning effects are a very slow pulse, cold clammy skin, dizziness, severe pains of the stomach and intestines, with vomiting, purging and diarrhoea, followed by delirium, and if the dose was large enough finally coma and death. The active constituents are a group of cardiac glucosides.

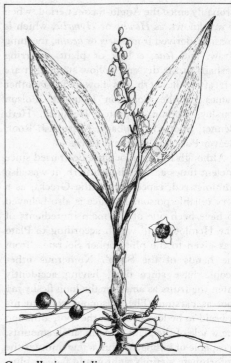

Convallaria majalis

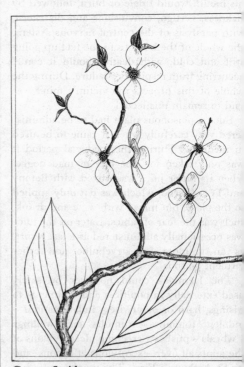

Cornus florida

Even so in parts of Germany a delicious wine is made from the flowers mixed with raisins. A green to yellow dye can be extracted from the leaves, the colour depending largely on the season when gathered.

The plant's other common names include Mugget, May Lily, Male Lily, Lily Convalle, Lily Constancy, Liroconfancie, Jacob's Tears and Ladder to Heaven.

CORNUS
Cornaceae, the Dogwood family
Flowering Dogwood, Common Dogwood, Red Osier

About 50 species of Dogwood are native to the northern hemisphere, the greater number consisting of hardy, deciduous, rarely evergreen trees and shrubs, some with showy bark, variegated or highly coloured leaves, or attractive flowers.

Of the 18 species that occur wild in the United States, mostly to the east of the Rocky Mountains, one or two were and still are included in herbal medicine. The most important, which is also one of the more showy American kinds, is the Flowering Dogwood or Cornel (*C. florida*) of the eastern and central parts of the United States, a slow growing tree or large shrub 3–10m/9–32ft high, with opposite oval leaves, which bears in April and May a mass of flowers surrounded by pinkish-white or rose-red bracts followed by red berries.

The active part of this particular Cornus, known as Cornine, is found in the rough brownish bark, or the root bark, which on its removal from the tree was first dried and then soaked in water to extract its healing virtues which, with the seed, were first used by the American Indians in the treatment of fevers. It was later employed as a substitute for the Peruvian Bark and was prescribed 'when the foreign remedy is not to be obtained, or when it fails, or where it cannot be administered.' For this and for 'general body exhaustion' decoctions were prescribed taken in wine-glassful doses. The species' 'best virtues' were however 'exerted in the shape of an ointment'.

This was regarded as 'detergent in all inflammatory conditions, destructive to morbid growths, and at variance with diseased nutrition. It stimulates granulations, increases the reparative process, induces circulation of healthy blood to the parts, removes effete matter, vitalizes the tissues, and speedily removes pain from the diseased parts.'

Liquid extracts or the dried powdered bark infused are still prescribed for their tonic, astringent and slightly stimulant principles in the treatment of exhaustion and fever, and for relieving headache.

The very hard, closely grained wood, which is also known as American Boxwood, American Dogwood, Dog Tree, Flowering Cornel and Green Ozier is used in the making of shuttles for the textile trade.

The botanical name of this family, Cornus,

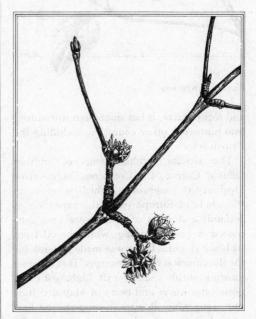

Cornus mas

actually refers to the durability of the wood, and is derived from *cornu*, a horn. Similarly in the Cornelian Cherry (*C. mas*) a deciduous shrub or small tree which reaches 2–6m/6–19ft high, and produces small umbels of yellow flowers in early March before the leaves appear. Although native to central and south east Europe, where it grows in woods, hedges

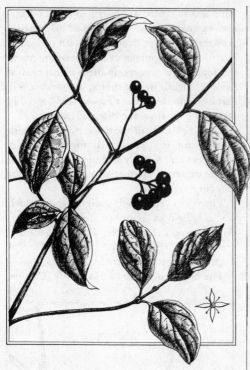

Cornus sanguinea

and rocky places, it has since been introduced into numerous other countries, including the British Isles.

The slender reddish twigs of another familiar Cornus, the Common Dogwood or Dogberry (*C. sanguinea*), which is native to the whole of Europe (with the exception of Iceland) and parts of Asia, were once employed in basket making, while the oil from its black globular fruits was made into ink for the illumination of manuscripts. It is an erect growing shrub 1–4m/3–13ft high, with opposite oval leaves and bears in May and June numerous white flowers in long-stalked flat-topped clusters. In the past the juice of the herb was regarded as a cure for hydrophobia. Diseased and mangy dogs were sometimes washed in decoctions of it, thus Hound's Tree, another common name. Its oil is nowadays added to soaps.

In North America the Red Osier or Silky Cornel (*C. sericea*) was substituted for the Flowering Dogwood, the first species described, and is mostly found in the eastern part

of the United States in wet ground. It reaches a height of about 1–4m/3–13ft, producing in June and July abundant greenish-yellow flowers in small but attractive clusters, followed by blue berries. As with the Flowering Dogwood, the dull purplish and somewhat warty bark of the species was the part prescribed, and this together with the root bark was classed as astringent, bitter and tonic, and administered infused 'for disease of the womb – to check the vomitings of pregancy – and is of service in typhoid fever and the dropsy'. It is still used in the treatment of dyspepsia and diarrhoea and is sometimes found listed as Rose Willow, Red Willow, Blueberry, Swamp Dogwood and Female Dogwood. During the Victorian period its powdered bark was added to a range of tooth powders, as a whitener of teeth and preserver of the gums.

The insipid scarlet fruits of the Bunchberry or Dwarf Cornel (*C. canadensis*, syn. *Chamaepericlymenum canadense*), a low growing shrub, indigenous to the woods of much of North America, were at one time eaten by the

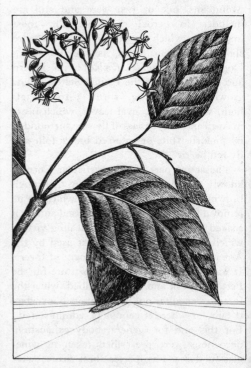

Cornus sericea

Indians there as a nutritious food; they are still added to puddings. The red berries of another species bearing the name Dwarf Cornel (*C. suecica*) were also eaten as a food by the Indians of North America and at one time in Scotland and other parts of Europe as a tonic for the appetite under the name of Lus-a-chraois – Plant of Gluttony. This little creeping arctic or alpine perennial grows from 6–20cm/2–7in. tall and is found on the moors and heaths and on the mountains in northern and arctic Europe, Asia and America.

Other species known to have been used in herbal medicine include the Round-Leaved Dogwood (*C. circinata*) from the eastern part of the United States and the Kizziljiek or Redwood (*C. mascula*) from Asia Minor. The astringent fruits of the latter have been used in cholera and are still given for bowel complaints, and the flowers for diarrhoea. The red stain from this plant makes the dye used for the fez.

CROTON
Euphorbiaceae, the Spurge family
Cascarilla, Croton Seed

This very large genus of Euphorbiaceous plants, many of which possess fairly important medicinal properties, are native for the most part to a wide range of tropical countries.

The dried bark of one of the more familiar kinds, the Cascarilla (*C. eleuteria*, syn. *Clutea eleuteria*), a small tree, with alternate, lanceolate-ovate leaves, and producing small white flowers in March and April, found its way into the markets of Europe during the seventeenth century, where it was used in medicine for its aromatic, stimulant and tonic principles.

The natural habitat of this species is referred to in *eleuteria* its specific name, alluding to Eleuthera near Providence, one of the islands of the Bahamas, while Croton the genic name is derived from the Greek *kroton*, meaning a tick, supposedly referring to the appearance of the seeds of the various species.

On the world's markets this hard aromatic

brownish-yellow bark, which was exported from Nassau, was seen as short-quilled compact pieces, perhaps 5cm/2in. in length, often covered with fine lichen (*Verrucaria albissima*). These were powdered down, infused and taken in small amounts as a bitter tonic 'for dyspepsia – flatulence – intermittent fevers – dysentery and diarrhoea' as 'an expectorant in chronic bronchitis', and as valuable 'in convalescence from acute diseases – debility – and nocturnal pollutions'. It was

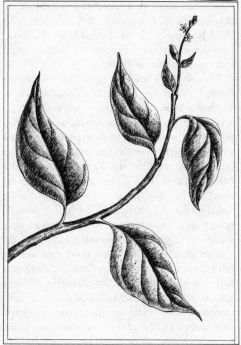

Croton eleuteria

frequently combined with Cinchona to arrest vomiting caused by the use of that bark, or was used as a substitute. It is still used in medicine in the form of Tinctura Cascarillae and Infusion Cascarillae. The powdered bark appears to have been added from time to time to tobaccos as a flavouring. It gives off a fragrant smell when burnt, although in fairly large amounts this caused sickness and giddiness. Other names for the species include Sweet Wood Bark, Sweet Bark, Bahama Cascarilla, Elatheria, Aromatic Quinquina, False Quinquina and Cortex Thuris.

In the West Indies a useful black dye is

extracted from the Cascarilla, while infusions of the leaves taken as a tea are regarded as good for the stomach.

An almost identical Mexican tree, the Copalche Bark (*C. pseudochina*, syn. *C. niveus*), was prescribed for much the same as above. A second species from that region, the Mexican Dragon's Blood or Sangre de Drago (*C. drago*) is still valued there for its vulnery and astringent effects. The bark of the Argentinian tree *Pogonopos febrifugus*, which is sometimes used as a Cinchona substitute, is also known in commerce as Cascarilla. The Wild Rosemary (*C. cascarilla*) from the West Indies was formerly believed to be the actual source of Cascarilla Bark.

The oil from another species, the Croton Seed, Tiglium or Klotzsch (*C. tiglium*, syn. *Tiglium officinale*) was prescribed, generally as a last resort, as a very powerful and forceful purgative, which rarely if ever failed. This was obtained from a small tree or shrub indigenous to India, the East Indies and the Malabar Coast, which has alternate, petiolate-ovate leaves, and bears yellowish flowers in erect terminal racemes, followed by smooth filbert sized fruits or capsules, each containing three seeds, generally of a mottled appearance.

The expressed oil from these seeds contains a substance known as Crotonic Acid and this was prescribed for its cathartic, irritant and rubefacient effects. As a cathartic administered in very small doses, it acted extremely quickly, often in less than an hour, although only slightly larger amounts are recorded as having caused violent sickness, severe pains and on occasions a violent death. In many cases it was taken mixed with Castor Oil. It is still given today in the treatment of constipation, generally in the much safer form of a capsule or pill. Externally applied as a liniment with olive oil, it produces inflammation of the skin with pustular eruption and was used for its counter-irritating and vesicatory effects 'in relieving the gout – rheumatism – neuralgia' and so on. The 'Liniment of Croton Oil' for obvious reasons is rarely used nowadays. At one time a single drop of this oil, placed on the tongue was administered to those 'in a coma – stupor – or in a sluggish lethargic torpor'. It was said to

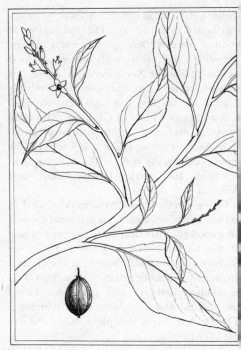

Croton tiglium

be very effective.

Other species known to have been formerly used in herbal medicine include *Croton micans*, *C. sanguifolius* and *C. hibiscifolius*.

CYCLAMEN
Primulaceae, the Primula family
Sowbread

The Cyclamens belong to a small family of bulbous plants. They have heart-shaped leaves, white spotted or mottled along the veins, and (according to the species) white, pale-pink, rose-red or reddish to plum-coloured flowers with reflexed petals. Their generic name of Cyclamen is derived from the Greek word *kyklaminos*, with *kyklos*, meaning circular, referring perhaps to the spirally arranged leafstalks of some kinds.

Of the known Cyclamen species employed in medieval medicine, all are native to various parts of southern Europe, where they are found in woods, thickets and other bushy places. One of their commonest uses at that time was in the treatment of ear disease, the individual leaves supposedly resembling the human ear. For this reason Paracelsus, the Swiss physician, prescribed the plant for this during the sixteenth century.

In Britain, the corms of these plants were known medicinally long before they were actually cultivated there. Turner, in 1551, tells us he had not seen Cyclamen or Sowbread growing in England. By 1597 Gerard possessed at least two species, the Ivy-Leafed Cyclamen (*C. hederifolium* syn. *C. neapolitanum* or *C. europaeum*), the sort usually prescribed at that time in medicine, which was found wild in France, Switzerland, Italy, Yugoslavia, Albania, Greece and Turkey, and *Cyclamen coum* from the Turkish island of Cos. About thirty years later Parkinson was cultivating about ten different sorts.

In England the corms were principally used to assist women in childbirth and at first were thought to be very potent indeed. Turner writes: 'it is perillous for weomen with chylde to go over this roote' a warning

Gerard later heeded for he fenced his in with sticks, fearing that if a pregnant woman should unknowingly walk over the top, she would immediately miscarry. The juice of the corm was also added to ointments and applied as a salve or poultice to indolent ulcers, and used as a wash during the all too frequent smallpox epidemics.

At the present time the Cyclamens appear to be little prescribed in herbalism, while one or two of the species are even regarded as having a poisonous nature, containing the glucoside known as Cyclamin. In homoeopathic medicine the fresh roots in the form of a tincture are applied externally to the region of the bowels for its purging effects.

DAEMOMOROPS
Palmaceae, the Palm family
Dragon's Blood Palm

Most of the species belonging to this genus of climbing Palms, have ornamental leaves, long flexible stems, bearing pointed berries about the size of a cherry, and are native to the warmer regions of the world, including India, Sumatra, Malaya and Penang.

The medicinal part of the plant was obtained from the berries of certain species, which as they ripen become covered in a reddish, rather brittle, resinous substance, formerly used by the natives for its astringent principles. The resin itself was usually separated from the fruits by placing them in a bag or sack and subjecting them to a vigorous beating, after which they were shaken out and sorted. The resin was then heated until plastic and moulded into balls or sticks for export. This end product, still found on the world's markets, generally wrapped in leaves, is known in its various forms as Stick, Lump, Reed, Tear, Drop or Saucer Dragon's Blood and is nowadays employed as a colouring agent in pharmacy, the arts, and in varnishes, stains, toothpastes, plasters and tinctures. It is also used to stain marble red and is applied in a solution to the heated stone; the hotter the stone the deeper the colour penetrates.

As an astringent medicine the resin was

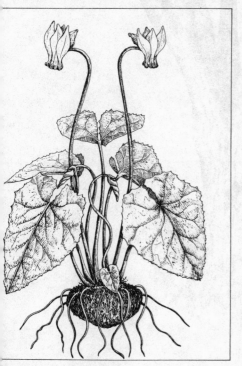

Cyclamen hederifolium

Daemomorops draco

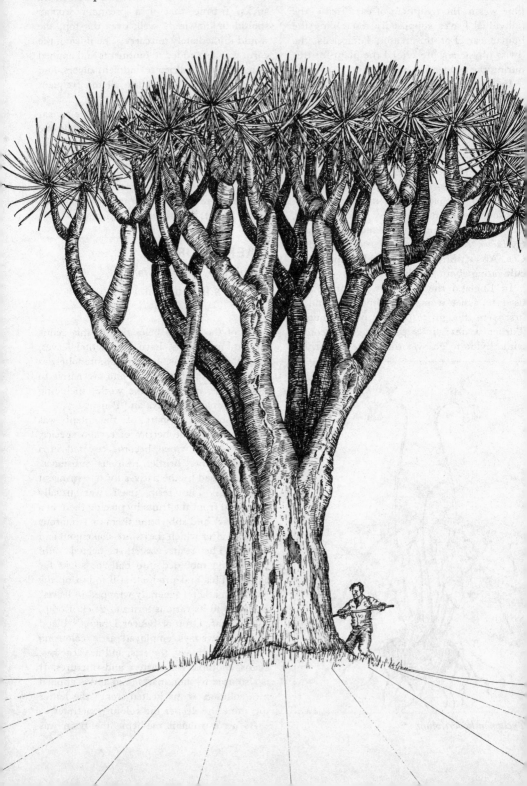

administered in doses of ten to thirty grains in the treatment of dysentery and diarrhoea, and occasionally when mixed with other ingredients as a cure for syphilis, although at present it is rarely if ever internally prescribed. It is sometimes added as an ingredient to external plasters, for which it was popularly used during the nineteenth century.

The principal species prescribed in medicine was the Dragon's Blood Palm or Blume (*D. draco*, formerly *Calamus draco*) from Malaya, Sumatra and the East Indies, sometimes found listed as Draconis Resina or Sanguis Draconis. Other species used in that region include *Daemomorops didynophyllos*, *D. propinquus* and *D. micrancanthus*. The resin from two other plants known to have been employed as astringents in native medicine include *D. draconcellus* from Borneo and the Socrotrine Dragon's Blood (*D. cinnabari*). The latter is still exported from Bombay and Zanzibar, sometimes under the name of Zanzibar Drop and this is used for some of the purposes given above.

DAPHNE

Thymelaeaceae, the Daphne family
Mezereon Spurge, Spurge Laurel, Mediterranean Mezereon

The Daphnes consist of about 40 species of toughly barked evergreen or deciduous trees, many with fragrant flowers and a low habit of growth. They are native to Europe including the alpine regions, and Asia, through to China and Japan.

Their botanical name Daphne, commemorates the nymph of that name, the daughter of the river god, who according to Greek legend prayed for help when running from Apollo in an effort to escape his advances, and as a result was transformed into this sacred tree.

The most common species, often known during the medieval period as the Mezereon Spurge, (*D. mezereum*) is an erect, little branched deciduous shrub ½–1m/1½–3ft high. It bears purplish-pink or rarely white flowers, borne in dense lateral clusters before the short-stalked alternate lanceolate leaves ap-

pear, followed by fleshy scarlet ovoid berries. Formerly it had several uses in medicine. Native to the woods of much of Europe, including the British Isles, western Asia and Siberia, it is generally found in chalky or limestone soils, but is now, having escaped from cultivation, naturalized in both Canada and the United States.

According to Culpeper: 'A decoction made of a dram of the bark of the root in three pints of water, till one pint is wasted, and this quantity taken in the course of a day, for a considerable time together, has been found very efficacious in resolving and dispersing venereal swellings and excrescences. The bark of the root, or the inner bark of the branches, is to be used, but it requires caution in the administration, and must only be given to people of robust constitutions, and very sparingly even to those; for if given too large a dose, or to a weakly person it will cause bloody stools and vomiting; it is good in dropsy and other stubborn disorders. A light infusion is the best mode of giving it.'

Although extremely poisonous – it often proved fatal to children in the past – the Russian peasantry used to prescribe thirty berries as a body purge, while the French regarded fifteen as a fatal dose. In Britain fifteen berries eaten between them are known to have killed six pigs. The Russians also used the bark for treating diseases of their horses hoofs. In Germany a tincture of the berries was occasionally given for relieving neuralgia, and in other European countries, including England, for 'relieving scrofulous diseases – inward pains – chronic rheumatism – snakebite – syphilis – and various other skin diseases', while a piece of the root 'chewed in the mouth readily relieves the toothache.' The latter remedy can result in excessive pain, and the juice simply applied to the skin often causes blistering.

The powdered bark, the root and rootbark are still prescribed in herbalism, either decocted or as liquid extracts, for their alterative, diuretic and stimulant principles, mainly in rheumatism. Larger doses than recommended will act as an irritant poison, causing vomiting and violent purging. It is sometimes applied in the form of a lotion to

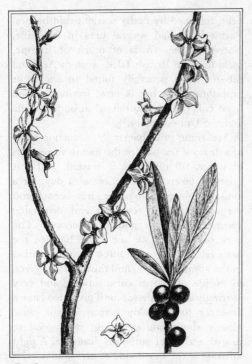

Daphne mezereum

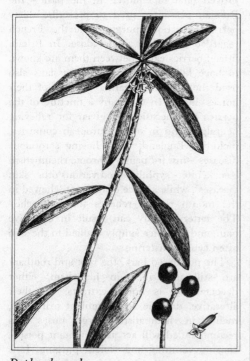

Daphne laureola

indolent ulcers, although this causes redness and blistering.

Other names for this species include Spurge Olive, Dwarf Laurel, Flowering Spurge, Kellerhals, Wild Pepper and Mezzereon. The latter, one of its commonest names, is a Middle Latin word derived from the Arabian or Persian *mazariyun*.

The Spurge Laurel or Evergreen Laurel (*D. laureola*) is neither a Spurge nor a Laurel, but a small evergreen shrub ½–1m/ 1½–3ft high, with dark glossy-green, broad and leathery, lanceolate leaves, and which bears from February to April, lateral clusters of small drooping greenish-yellow flowers, followed by black and fleshy egg shaped berries. It is native to much of Europe including Britain, where it is found in open woods, especially those with chalky soil.

The caustic bark of this shrub was sold on the markets as Mezereon Bark, and was at one time listed in the official medicine of several countries, including Britain and the United States. Its uses were similar to those of Mezereon Spurge. The leaves have been used as an emmenagogue, although they often caused vomiting and purging. The leaves and root were also taken as 'a means to procure abortions'.

The Mediterranean Mezereon, Garland Flower or Spurge Flax (*D. gnidium*), a native of the bushy places and uncultivated ground of that region, is an erect little branched evergreen shrub ½–2m/1½–6½ft high, having numerous, glaucous, leathery, linear-lance shaped leaves and bearing clusters of small sweetly scented flowers, brownish outside and white within, followed by red or black fleshy berries. The leaves were on occasions substituted for both the species listed above. Alternatively, it was used for the cleansing of wounds and at one time was listed in the official medicine of the United States and in the *British Pharmacopoeia*. In France, where the bark is still used in herbal medicine, it is known as *Sainbois* or *Garou*.

Other species prescribed for their vesicant and stimulant effects, or as substitutes for those already mentioned, include *Daphne alpina* from the Alps, *D. pontica* from Asia Minor, *D. tartonaira* and *D. thymeloea*.

DATURA
Solanaceae, the Nightshade family
Thornapple, Metel, Tolguacha

About 25 or so species make up this genus of annual or shrubby perennial flowering plants, which are native chiefly to tropical America, Peru, Mexico, southern Europe, India and parts of Asia.

The most familiar species of all, the Thorn-

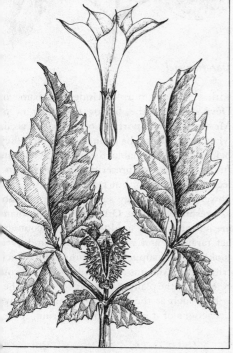

Datura stramonium

apple (*D. stramonium*), although its native country is unknown, has naturalized itself throughout the temperate regions, including the whole of Europe, Asia and North America, where it is most common, having sown itself from seed in waste places and on rubbish dumps. This coarse growing, hairless branching annual 40–100cm/15–39in. tall, has lobed or sharp-toothed broadly-oval leaves and bears white or purplish funnel shaped flowers from about July to the autumn. These are followed by spiny egg-shaped fruits, hence

Thornapple the common name, which as they ripen split into four, revealing many wrinkled black kidney-shaped seeds inside.

The use of this particular species in medicine dates back to an early period in Indian and Russian history, when the seeds were ground down, mixed with water and used by cheats and thieves to drug and stupefy their victims before robbing them. The same concoction was employed by the 'thugs', members of an ancient Indian religious organization, who robbed and murdered in the service of Kali, the goddess of Destruction. At the same time the seeds were prescribed in that country to relieve a wide range of complaints from epilepsy to hysteria and in heart disease. The generic name of Datura is also referred to in some early Sanskrit writings as *dhustura* or *dhatura*. In China this and various other species were prescribed under the name of *man-to-lo* for diseases of the feet, as well as for their sedative effects. In ancient Greece the priests of Apollo at Delphi took small amounts of the leaves themselves for added inspiration when making prophecies. Avicenna, the eleventh-century Arabian physician, who valued this plant in medicine, tells us that its 'nut' or seed, brought about intoxication.

In Europe the seed of the Thornapple became well-known as an easily administered poison during the Renaissance. When taken with the leaves of Henbane (*Hyoscyamus niger*) it brought on a form of 'Black Madness' causing the victim hallucinations, intoxication and mental derangement.

Gerard recorded that the 'Thornie Apple' was first seen in Britain when he received some seed 'of the right honourable the Lord Edward Zouch; which he brought from Constantinople ... The juice of Thornapples boiled with hog's grease to the form of an unguent or salve, cures all inflammations whatsoever, all manner or burnings and scaldings as well of fire, water, boiling lead, gunpouder, as that which comes by lightening and that in very short time ...' It was also believed that should anyone be foolish enough to sleep under the leaves of one of these fetid smelling plants, it would kill him.

The common Thornapple became well-known in North America as Jimson Weed, a contraction of Jamestown Weed, where a number of soldiers and settlers had been poisoned after eating its leaves. Another American name, Fireweed, originated in Virginia during the seventeenth century, because the plant was one of the first to spring up after a fire. By the nineteenth century the herb was prescribed throughout most of that region for its anodyne, antispasmodic and narcotic effects, in 'mania – convulsions – twitch – epilepsy – gastritis – delirium tremens – enteritis – neuralgia – rheumatism – and period pains'. The dried leaves were also smoked there, as in Britain and the rest of Europe, for 'spasmodic asthma and coughs' or was given in the form of a tea, although fatalities were occasionally recorded due to its improper use. Its poisoning effects are said to be similar to the Deadly Night-shade (*Atropa belladonna*) with intense pain, dilation of the eyes, very unpleasant hallucinations and maniacal delirium. The active constituents are a combination of Scopolamine, Hyoscyamine and Atropine. The leaves contain from 0.2 to 0.5 per cent of these alkaloids, depending on the climatic conditions during the growing season.

The leaves and seed, mostly obtained from cultivated plants, are still employed in the medicine of many countries, and are prescribed for the three basic principles mentioned above. Tinctures or Extracts of Stramonium are added to bronchial medicines and other preparations such as asthma powder, while the dried leaves are included in special cigarettes, which are smoked for asthma and bronchial complaints.

The seeds of *Datura metel*, a plant found in India and other tropical countries, were given by prostitutes to their clients, who, when well sedated, were easy to rob.

The Tolguacha or Toloache (*D. meteloides*), a Datura native to the south-western parts of the United States, once had a wide range of medicinal uses, especially for relieving pain in the setting of broken bones, and even amputations. A shrubby perennial with grayish leaves and slender forking stems 60–90cm/23–35in. high, it bears in late autumn, white trumpet-shaped flowers, tinged

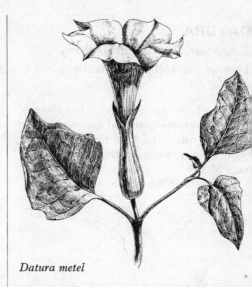

Datura metel

with violet and purple. Under the name of Devil's Weed, the brujos or sorcerers of Mexico ate small portions of its root or seeds when they wanted hallucinations, which they believed would enable them to foretell the future. They also prescribed the stems and leaves in medicine, but reserved the fragrant flowers for previously selected victims, who, as a result, went mad. Other American Indians are known to have used this plant to counter-act tarantula and rattlesnake bites and even took it for its supposed immunity. One such tribe, the Mahuna of southern California referred to the plant as *Qui-qui-sa-waal*. Other tribes, such as the Yokut and Luiseno, gave decoctions of it in the form of a drink, some-

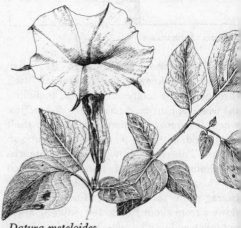

Datura meteloides

times over a period of several days, when initiating adolescent boys into manhood, while the Yaqui Indians of northern Mexico extracted the juice from the root, mixed it with water, to bring on convulsions, visual distortion and colourful hallucinations, a very dangerous procedure sometimes resulting in amnesia or death. The Algonquins of north-eastern America also prescribed the species under the name of Wysocean.

Several other species had their uses. The Inca priests gave *Datura inoxia* in fairly large amounts to deaden feeling in the sick before performing painful operations. No doubt the Hyoscyamine and Scopolamine contained within the plant caused the patient to fall into a trance-like state, resulting in a very deep sleep, or even death-like coma.

Besides the common Thornapple described above, at least seven other Daturas are known to grow in the Andean region of South America, namely *Datura arborea*, *D. suaveolens*, *D. aurea*, *D. candida*, *D. dolichocarpa*, *D. sanguinea* and *D. vulcanicola*. All of these have been added from time to time, generally in the form of the powdered seed, to a wide selection of beverages and drinks, mainly to bring on narcosis with the usual visual and hallucinatory effects during the waking periods, which in many cases was supposed to help the taker predict the future and to communicate with the spirits of the dead. Two or three of these plants are of a shrubby perennial nature and are sometimes cultivated in gardens as ornamentals. The most popular are *Datura arborea*, with white flowers and reaching 3m/9ft in height, *D. suaveolens* (syn. *D. knightii*) growing to 4m/13ft and with white flowers, both of which are known as Angel's Trumpets and *D. sanguinea*, about 3m/9ft tall with reddish or sometimes orange yellow flowers tinged with green.

The Chibchals of Colombia went even further with these plants and administered decoctions of *Datura aurea* to the wives, servants, and slaves of men who had just died and buried them with the deceased. The Jivaro, an Indian tribe from eastern Ecuador, are still said to give decoctions of Datura seed as a form of punishment to their children when they misbehave, and also take it as a way of allowing their ancestors to visit them through the hallucinations.

Several of the above species are still used in medicine, including one or two not mentioned, such as the Chinese Datura (*D. ferox*) which is employed in homoeopathy; *D. fastuosa* from tropical India, one of the more toxic varieties, and *D. quercifolia* from Mexico.

DELPHINIUM
Ranunculaceae, the Buttercup family
Stavesacre, Field Larkspur, Larkspur

The Delphiniums are hardy, branching, annual or herbaceous perennials of varying heights up to 2m/6ft, bearing bluish flowers in erect spike-like clusters, mainly from May to August. The original species from which the present-day hybrids and numerous varieties are descended are native mainly to Siberia, Syria, China and India.

Their generic name, Delphinium, is derived from the old Greek word *delphinion*, with *delphis* or *delphin* meaning dolphin. Gerard says this is because 'the floures, and especially before they be perfected, have a certaine shew and liknesse of those Dolphins . . .'

One of the species native to southern Europe and Asia Minor, the Stavesacre or Staves-Acre (*D. staphisagria*), is known to have been employed by both the Greeks and Romans as an external medicine, as mentioned by Dioscorides, while Pliny described its use as a parasiticide, which gave rise to Louse-wort and Licebane, two more common names. This is a stout elegant, upright, hairy annual, or robust biennial, has broad palmate leaves, bears long spikes of bluish-grey flowers from about May to August and is generally found in waste or stony places, reaching about 1m/ 3ft high. In England it was Turner who first wrote of it, telling us in 1551: 'I never saw it growing out of Italy but only in gardines.' Culpeper also observed it was: 'A native of warm countries, but grows in gardines' and 'flowers in July'.

In medicine only the seed was used and then with the utmost caution, generally being prescribed in the form of a powder in

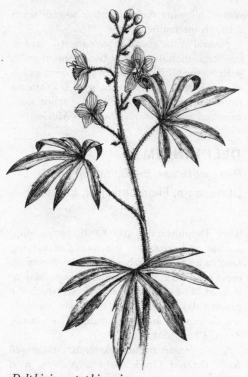

Delphinium staphisagria

'gargarisms for relieving toothache and masticatories', although this was occasionally taken internally in small doses 'against rheumatic and venereal disorders', and 'in dropsy', which frequently 'caused vomiting and bloody purging'. Coarsely powdered, the seed was regarded as a reliable household remedy for 'strewing' on children's hair 'to kill domestic vermin'. The same decocted and applied to 'the itch' was said to be very effective.

The seeds, which have a bitter tingling taste, contain a poisonous constituent known as Delphinine and this is added to lotions, washes and ointments for its vermin destroying properties. It has been prescribed on occasions to arrest the convulsions caused by strychnine, a rather dubious procedure, for Delphinine itself causes the pulse to slow, with paralysis of the spinal cord often causing death by asphyxia.

In 1572, Tusser tells us of another species, *Delphinium consolida*, the Field Larkspur,

which became the parent of the taller branching sorts of Larkspur commonly grown in gardens. This slender rooted annual has spreading branches 40–60cm/15–23in. high, with sessile alternate leaves, and spikes of bright bluish-purple flowers. Although native to Europe, where it was used as a wound herb, it soon became naturalized in the United States on its introduction there, growing freely in woods and fields.

In the United States of the nineteenth century, the whole of the plant was prescribed for its 'acid principles', which were mainly employed as an insecticide. At one period the leaves and flowers were used by the army as 'an external application to kill body lice', while 'the water or juice distilled from the flowers' was said to be good for the eyes. Tinctures of the seeds were also administered 'as a cure for asthma – the colic of purging – as an antidote to poisoning – and as a specific for cholera morbus'. As a wound herb, one of the plant's more ancient uses, the juice of the leaves was applied direct and this is referred

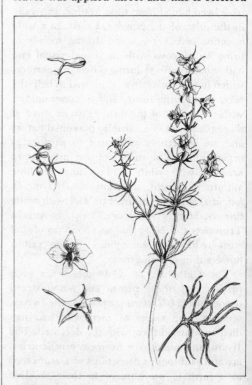

Delphinium consolida

to in *consolida* its specific name, meaning to consolidate. The same was recommended 'to stay the bleedings of the piles'. Its other common names include Larks Heel, Lark's Claw, Lark's Toe and Knight's Spur.

The seed is still used in the form of a tincture as a parasiticide and insecticide for destroying body lice and nits and sometimes in spasmodic asthma and dropsy.

Another kind of annual Larkspur, *Delphinium ajacis*, was introduced to Britain from southern Europe in about 1573, deriving its specific name *ajacis* from Ajax the Greek

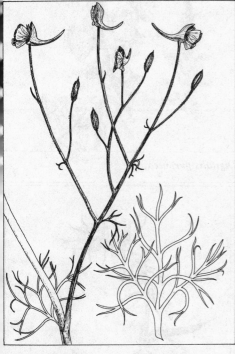

Delphinium ajacis

hero of the Trojan war. According to legend the plant supposedly sprang from his blood. Thirty years later this had become a common English 'weed of the cornfield', a pretty plant with feathery leaves, ½–1m/1½–3ft high, bearing deep blue, occasionally pink or white flowers in long loose spikes. On its introduction to North America it soon became widely naturalized in the eastern parts of the United States where it is sometimes known as Rocket Larkspur. Gerard, however, called it the

Wild Larkspur, thus keeping it distinct from the garden Larkspur (*D. consolida*). As a medicinal herb it was prescribed or substituted mostly during the sixteenth and seventeenth centuries for some of the illnesses listed above.

The effects of the Larkspur's poison are similar to those of the Monkshood (*Aconitum napellus*). Smaller doses cause severe irritation of the stomach, violent purging, with death if it comes, occurring from asphyxia or a heart attack. The poisonous constituents of the Larkspurs consists of a group of complicated alkaloids used sometimes by chemists. These are not affected by drying or storing.

DIGITALIS
Schrophulariaceae, the Figwort family
Foxglove, Yellow Foxglove

These stately, erect, biennial and perennial herbs are native to Europe and parts of west and central Asia.

One of the more familiar species, the Common Foxglove (*D. purpurea*), a tall unbranching biennial ½–1½m/1½–5ft high, with most of its leaves confined to a basal rosette, is native to much of western and central Europe, including the British Isles. It is generally found in shady places, in open woods and on heaths, especially in acid soils. The long tapering spikes of bell or thimble shaped, drooping, bright mottled pinkish purple spotted flowers are borne from about May to September. This now grows in many other countries, including the United States, where it is believed to have been introduced to New England by the late 1750s.

The Anglo-Saxons referred to this and the other species of the genus as *foxes glofa* probably meaning the glove of the fox, or as *foxes gleow*, *gleow* likening these plants to an arch of bells, a contemporary musical instrument. In England these names appear to have evolved to Folksglove by the reign of Edward III (1327–77) and in time to Foxglove. The botanical name of Digitalis was allocated to the genus in 1542 by Fuch the German herbalist and is derived from the Latin *digitus*, meaning finger, referring to the shape of the flowers, as does the German name of *Fingerhut*, a finger hat or thimble. The specific *purpurea* simply means purple, the dominant colour of the flowers, hence Purple Foxglove, another common name. Others include Dead Man's Bells, Witches Thimbles, Fairy Thimbles, Gloves of Our Lady, Bloody Fingers, Floppy Dock, King Elwand, Foxbell and Flowster-Docken.

Of its early medicinal uses little is recorded. In Ireland the ancient Druids are known to have valued it, as did the thirteenth-century Physicians of Myddvai in Wales, who applied the leaves as an external medicine. Dodoens in 1544 administered it internally boiled in wine as an expectorant, a remedy which poisoned many people.

Parkinson recommended the bruised herb or the expressed juice in the form of an ointment for scrofulous swellings and the bruised leaves for 'cleansing old sores and ulcers'. As Culpeper noted: 'The herb is familiarly and frequently used by the Italians to heal any fresh or green wound, the leaves being bruised and bound thereon; and the juice thereof is also used in old sores, to cleanse, dry and heal them . . . The decoction hereof made up with sugar or honey, is available to cleanse and purge the body both upwards and downwards, sometimes of tough phlegm and clammy humours, and to open obstructions of the liver and spleen.' For the falling sickness (epilepsy) Culpeper prescribed two handfuls of the decocted herb 'with four ounces of polypody in ale', which he says had been found by late experience 'to cure divers of the falling sickness, that have been troubled with it above twenty years'.

The herb was first included in the *London Pharmacopoeia* of 1650, although it appears to have been little prescribed in the treatment of heart disease at that time. This very important use was first brought to the attention of the medical profession by William Withering, a Birmingham physician, late in the eighteenth century. He had started to use the plant as a diuretic in 1775 after learning that the leaves were employed as a rather unreliable cure for dropsy in parts of Yorkshire. He spent ten years finding out what the active

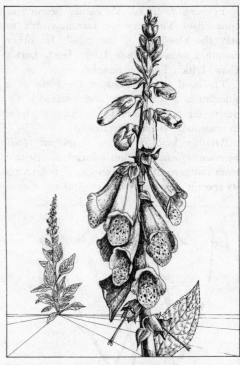

Digitalis purpurea

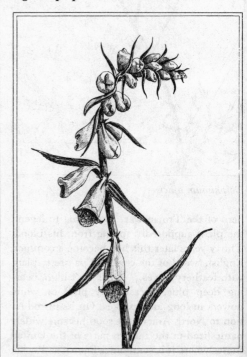

Digitalis grandiflora

part was, together with the accurate dose, finally using the blade of the leaf after discarding the midrib and leaf-stalk. His book *An Account of the Foxglove and Some of its Medicinal Uses* was published in 1785.

The powdered leaves of the Foxglove became the source of the drug Digitalis, a mixture of cardiac glycosides, which are now administered by doctors, mostly in tinctures, fluid extracts and infusions, or in tablet form, for their cardiac tonic, sedative and diuretic principles, as heart stimulants and in dropsy, especially when the latter is connected with heart trouble. The use of the drug also reduces the tremendous swellings in the legs and ankles.

If not properly prescribed by a physician this herb is best left well alone, owing to the cumulative effect of the poison. Many people have died through eating its bitter leaves; it takes only a few to cause paralysis and death from a heart attack. Digitalis is sometimes used as an antidote for Aconite poisoning and for this is usually injected.

A second European species is the Yellow or the Large Yellow Foxglove (*D. grandiflora*, syn. *D. ambigua*), an erect perennial 40–100cm/15–39in. tall, with glandular stems, which bear large creamy yellow flowers from June to September. It is found among rocks and in forest clearings in the mountains, and the lance-shaped leaves were collected and used for their medicinal uses, more or less as the species above.

DRIMYS

Magnoliaceae, (or Winteraceae) the Magnolia family

Winter's Bark, White Cinnamon

The Drimys are a small genus of handsome evergreen trees or shrubs, native mainly to South America, Australia and Tasmania.

Of these the species principally prescribed in medicine was the Winter's Bark (*D. winteri*), an evergreen spreading tree or large bush 10–12m/32–39ft high, having leaves 5–20cm/5–7in. long, fragrant when bruised, and aromatic ivory-white flowers in large loose clusters. In its natural habitat this species is found in Chile and Brazil and south to the Straits of Magellan, although sometimes grown in other countries as an ornamental for the frost-free flower garden.

The tree's common name of Winter's Bark dates from 1597 and is so named in honour of Captain Winter, the commander of the *Elizabeth* under Sir Francis Drake who, on the return voyage from the Straits of Magellan, used its pungent tasting bark as a spice and medicine to relieve his crew of scurvy. The bark is believed to have been previously administered in that region by the native people as a stimulant, aromatic and as a tonic

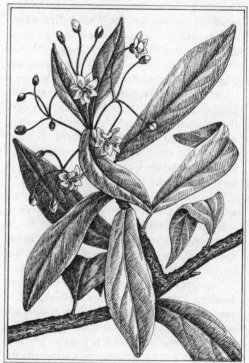

Drimys winteri

in certain stomach complaints, such as flatulence and indigestion. Its other names include Winter's Cinnamon, Wintera Aromatica, Wintera and True Winter's Bark.

The bark of a second species, *Drimys chilensis*, from Chile, was sometimes substituted for that of the above, and very occasionally *Drimys aromatica*, from Victoria and Tasmania in Australia. The latter has smaller leaves and bears its whitish flowers in small clusters and grows in the form of a rather dense bush.

Their generic name is derived from *drimys*, meaning acrid, referring to the biting taste of the bark, which appears to be little used nowadays probably due to its scarcity, although it is still recommended in the treatment of indigestion, colic, flatulence, etc. In South America an infusion of the powdered bark is still prescribed for relieving diarrhoea.

As the above species became harder to obtain, so they were gradually replaced in medicine by the False Winter's Bark (*Cinnamodendron corticosum*), known also as Red Canella or Mountain Cinnamon, a shrubby tree from Jamaica and the West Indies, where it is cultivated and prescribed for the same diseases as the True Winter's Bark.

The whitish bark of the White Cinnamon (*Canella alba*) was often passed off as Winter's Bark. This erect tree reaching about 15m/49ft high, is branched only at the top and has dark shiny alternate laurel-like leaves, bearing small clusters of violet coloured flowers, followed by greenish oblong berries, turning to blue and finally glossy black. It is found in the Bahamas, the West Indies and Florida.

The commonest name of this shrubby aromatic tree, White Cinnamon, was given to it by the Spaniards on their arrival in South America, for they believed it to be an actual species of the Cinnamomum genus. They introduced its pale orange-brown bark into Europe under that name and it reached England around 1600. The flowers, which rarely open to the full, are collected, carefully dried and added to warm water to give off a musk-like fragrance which is used for perfuming rooms and to remove unpleasant odours. The shredded bark is added to tobacco.

The powdered bark of the White Cinnamon was formerly prescribed for the same diseases as the Winter's Bark, and occasionally with Aloes as a purgative. It is still employed as a condiment and as an aromatic bitter for stomach complaints, and having a clove and cinnamon odour is sometimes mixed with other medicines. Its other names include West Indian Wild Cinnamon, Wild Cinnamon, White Wood and Canellae Cortex.

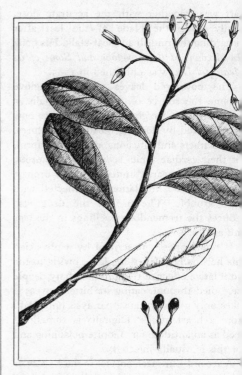

Canella alba

DROSERA
Droseraceae, the Sundew family
Common Sundew, Great Sundew, Longleaved Sundew

About 100 species of this insect-catching genus of perennial herbs are known and these are native mainly to Australia, Europe including Britain, South Africa and North America. Throughout this range they are found in peat bogs and damp heaths, often in sphagnum moss, their leaves usually forming a basal rosette near the soil, the latter varying in shape depending on the species. From the centre of these leaves rises a slender naked stalk, bearing small star-like, white, pink or crimson flowers, in loose one-sided terminal clusters, normally opening in the sunshine. The upper surfaces of the leaves are covered with sensitive glandular hairs and a sticky glistening honey-like substance that is attrac

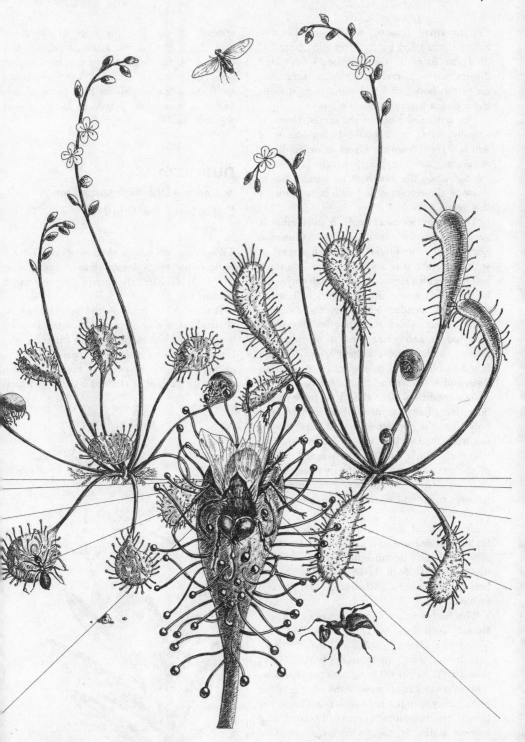

Drosera rotundifolia (left) and *Drosera anglica* (right)

tive to small insects, which on alighting become entangled by it. After the insect has died the hairs of the leaf bend over and downwards to secrete a digestive substance on to the body, and the plant then absorbs the proteins from the insect's body.

The botanical name of the genus, Drosera, actually refers to this viscid dew-like fluid and is derived from the Greek *droseros*, dewy, or *drosos*, dew or juice, which is usually exuded when the sun is at its height, hence Sundew the common and collective name of this genus.

The main species used in medicine is generally known today as the Common Sundew (*D. rotundifolia*), a smallish perennial, with flattened rosettes of stalked roundish yellow-greenish leaves, covered with sticky red hairs, which bears in summer small white flowers on slender leafless stems 5–12cm/ 2–4in. high. Although native to the bogs, peat moors and damp heaths of much of Europe, including the British Isles, it is also found in North and South America, Russian Asia, India, China and South Africa.

As a medicinal herb the bitter juice of the flowering plant was prescribed infused, not only for the 'spasmodic and dryness of tickling coughs' but as 'a preventative of whooping cough' and for 'the wasting disease of the consumptive'. The fresh juice, which contains citric and malic acid, was applied to 'remove corns and warts' and occasionally 'to curdle milk'.

The infused herb, tinctures, solid and liquid extracts are still prescribed for their anti-asthmatic, demulcent and expectorant principles, mainly in the treatment of chronic bronchitis, coughs, whooping cough and asthma.

The herb's other common names include Roundleaved Sundew, Dew Plant, Red Rot, Youthwort, Herba Rosellae and Rosa Solis.

Culpeper also made use of the Great Sundew (*D. anglica*) listing it as the Sundew. This is a similar species to the above, often hybridizing with it, although having narrower leaves, tapering into the usually erect and hairless stalks. It, too, is native to most of Europe including the British Isles. The leaves were prescribed much as for the previous species, as was also the juice of the stem.

A third species, the Longleaved Sundew (*D. intermedia*) which is native to the peat bogs of most of Europe, was sometimes substituted in medicine for both of the above, and this was often listed, as is the Great Sundew, as *Drosera longifolia*.

DUBOISIA
Solanaceae, the Nightshade family
Corkwood Tree, Pituri

This genus of tallish shrubs or small trees indigenous to Australia was named after F. N. A. Dubois, the French botanist who died in 1812.

Before the arrival of the white man in Australia, the aborigine tribes of the interior made use of the inodorous but bitter tasting leaves of the Duboisias as a type of narcotic, calling it *Pituri*. These were moistened with water, then rolled or chewed into quids which

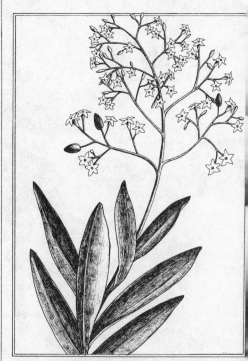

Duboisia myoporoides

ere then taken for the stimulating effect, mainly to ward off hunger and fatigue. One species known to have been used this way was the Corkwood Tree (*D. myoporoides*), a labrous looking shrubby bush or small tree bearing whitish flowers in axillary clusters which is found mainly in New South Wales, Queensland and New Caledonia. The leaves of this particular plant have since been found to contain several alkaloids, including Scopolamine, which in small doses causes excitement then hallucinations, depending on the amount consumed, although larger doses have severely poisoned and even killed at times. The aborigines of the interior still use its leaves as an easy means of capturing game, by simply poisoning the water holes where the animals drink.

As a medicinal herb the leaves were prescribed for their sedative, hypnotic and mydriatic principles, while one of the alkaloids Sulphate of Duboisia was occasionally substituted for Atropine. A tincture of it is still used in homoeopathic medicine for paralysis and in the treatment of some eye infections.

The leaves of a second Australian 'Pituri' (*D. hopwoodi*), a similar but smaller species, were also chewed by the aborigines, again for their narcotic effects. This shrubby plant contains a bitter tasting alkaloid known as Piturine, which is supposed to be similar if not identical to Nicotine.

EQUISETUM

Equisetaceae, the Horsetail family
Field Horsetail, Dutch Rush

About 25 species of this distinctive flowerless genus are known, and the majority of these are native to the northern temperate regions, where they thrive in damp and watery places, specially in acid soils. The different sorts consist mainly of a perennial rootstock, from which grow tall leafless, hollow jointed annual stems, which develop at regular intervals smaller scale-like branches arranged in whorls, these replacing the leaves. Repro-

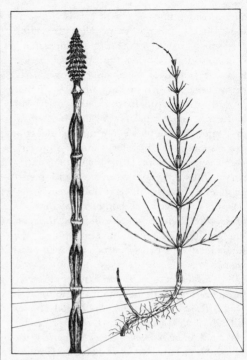

Equisetum arvense

duction is by means of the creeping roots, or by dispersal of minute spores, borne at the top of the fertile stems.

The general appearance of these plants has been likened to the tail of a horse, and is referred to in Equisetum the generic name. This is believed to have been used by Pliny and is derived from the Latin *equus*, a horse, and *seta*, a bristle. Several of the common collective names refer to much the same thing, such as Mare's Tail, Cat's Tail and Horsetail.

The species mostly used in medicine was the Field or Corn Horsetail (*E. arvense*) which is native to most of Europe, including the British Isles, and as its specific name suggests, it is often found growing in fields, as well as in meadows, gardens and on railway embankments, where it tends to be invasive, its pale brown unbranched fertile stems appearing in early spring, before the rough green sterile ones.

The use of this species dates back at least to the time of the Romans, who applied the bruised leaves to bleedings, at the same time adding the young shoots to salads for their tonic effects, the poorer people even eating the green parts as a rather unpalatable vegetable dish. During the medieval period it was regarded as a valuable wound herb, being 'very powerful to stay bleedings, either inward or outward.' It would also 'stay laxes or fluxes – cure ruptures in children – heal foul and inward ulcers – running ulcers – excoriation of the bladder – gut and entrails – and help the stone, dropsy and the stranguary'. Outwardly applied in a warm fomentation or compress 'it eases inflammations – pustules – the scab – and other such eruptions of the skin' including, according to Culpeper, 'the swelling heat and inflammation of the fundament or privy parts, in men and women.'

Several other species are known to have been prescribed in medicine including the Dutch Rush (*E. hyemale*), the Wood Horsetail (*E. sylvaticum*), the Great or River Horsetail (*E. maximum*, syn. *E. fluviatile*), the Marsh Horsetail (*E. palustre*) and the Smooth Horsetail (*E. limosum*). Most of the species have since been found to contain an extremely high content of silica, especially *E. hyemale*. This simple plant consists of a stiff, rough, dark evergreen stem up to 60cm/23in. or more in height. Gerard informs us that bunches of it were sold for polishing metal, for which it was exported from Holland to England under the name of Dutch Rush. He also says it was used for scouring pewter, hence Pewterwort, another common name. It was also used by fletchers and combmakers to polish their work and by milk-maids to cleanse their pails, thus Scouring Rush. Other names applying to one or more of the species include Shavegrass, Bottlebrush and Paddock Pipes.

The sterile stems of the Field Horsetail are still given for their diuretic and astringent principles, mainly in liquid or fluid extracts, decoctions or teas, in dropsy and kidney complaints, gravel, cystitis, ulcers of the urinary tract, haemorrhages and for soothing disordered bladders. Decoctions applied as a wash will help stop wounds from bleeding and ease inflammations, swellings and various skin eruptions.

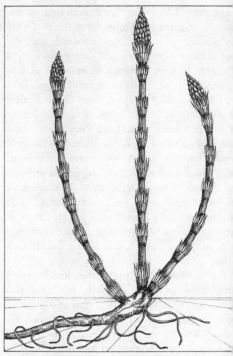

Equisetum hyemale

ERIGERON
Compositae, the Daisy family
Fleabane

Most of the Erigerons are hardy herbaceou plants, native principally to the norther temperate regions, including north-wes America, eastern Europe and the Himalayas

One of the more common North America species, the Fleabane (*E. canadense* sy *Conyza canadensis*), an annual 'weed' native t Canada and the northern and middle States was formerly prescribed in herbal medicin for its astringent, diuretic and tonic effects This stiff, erect and leafy plant, which i found in fields, meadows, by roadsides an similar places, has a bristly unbranched ster 1½–2m/5–6½ft high, with lance-shaped leave and bears numerous greenish-white or yel lowish flowers, with yellow disk florets in lon lax branching clusters, from about June t September.

When the early settlers in North America discovered that the whole of this plant could be used in medicine, some seed was dispatched back to Europe, where, in 1640, Parkinson mentions it as an American species that was not then found growing wild in England.

Culpeper certainly knew of the American species and listed it as Simson, Canada Fleabane or Flea-Wort, the last two names being derived 'because the seeds are so like fleas'. He tells us: 'The juice of this, as well as the sweet Fleabane or Erigeron Acre, is an excellent pectoral; but being unpleasant is not often used; however, if the decoction or infusion be sweetened with capilary or syrup of Maidenhair, it may be used with success in consumptive cases.'

In Canada and the United States the whole of the plant was prescribed during the nineteenth century 'as useful in gravel, diabetes, dropsy, and many kidney diseases' and 'can also be employed in diarrhoea, dysentery, etc.' The volatile Oil of Erigeron, which resembles Oil of Turpentine in action, was also frequently prescribed.

Herbalists still prescribe infusions of this rather astringent plant in the treatment of gravel and kidney disease, for tonsillitis, ulcers and inflammation of the throat.

The Fleabane's other names include Prideweed, Butter Weed, Colt's Tail and Horse Weed. The plant's generic name, Erigeron, is derived from the Greek *eri*, early, and *geron*, old man, literally meaning old man, alluding to the worn-out appearance of several of this species even when in flower.

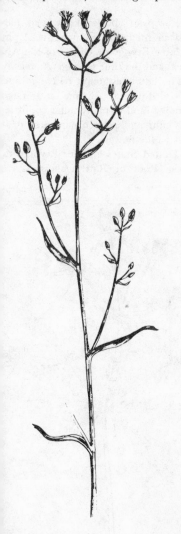

Erigeron canadense

ERYNGIUM

Umbelliferae, the Parsley family
Sea Holly, Field Eryngo,
Buttonsnake Root

The Eryngiums make up a large genus of spiny perennial flowering plants, with broad grayish-blue leaves and light blue flowers, native mainly to North and South America, Europe and parts of Asia.

The principle species used in medieval herbal medicine was the Sea Holly (*E. maritimum*), often known as the Sea Hulver or Sea Holm, a stiff branched, spiny perennial 30–60cm/11–23in. high, having stalkless, glaucous, spiny-toothed holly-like leaves, bearing from June to September light blue thistle-like flowers; a fairly common plant in most of Europe, including the British Isles, where it is usually found, as its specific name suggests, by the sea, mostly in sand and on shingle beaches.

The parts generally prescribed in medicine were the long white aromatic roots, which were also valued as a form of tonic and

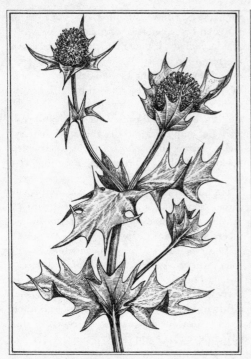

Eryngium maritimum

Eryngo, and possessing more or less the sam
medicinal properties.

The eating of the roots as an aphrodisiac o
'restorative' seems to have been very popula
during the sixteenth century when they wer
candied and sold as 'kissing comfits'.

The roots of both the species mentione
above are still prescribed for their diaphoretic
diuretic, expectorant and stimulant prin
ciples, mainly in bladder diseases, uterin
irritation and as a restorative. These can b
decocted and taken freely in wineglassfu
doses. The flowering tops are said to be ver
nutritious.

Other European species known to hav
been used in medicine include the Alpin
Queen, Alpine Eryngo or Queen of the Alp
(*E. alpinum*) and the Blue Eryngo (*E. amethy
stinum*). The latter, although native to suc
countries as Bulgaria, Albania and Yugo
slavia, is now found in many other countrie
where it is cultivated as an ornamental for i
bright violet-blue flowers.

In the United States another Eryngo, th
Buttonsnake Root or Rattlesnake's Maste

stomachic by the Anglo-Saxons. Traditionally,
the best time to lift them was in the early
autumn, from plants up to two years old.
These were believed to possess many virtues.
and were used during the medieval period
throughout Europe 'to ease cramps and convulsions – expel the stone – remove obstructions of liver and spleen – impostumes in the
ear – relieve the yellow jaundice – dropsy –
colics coming of wind – to provoke urine
– ease melancholy of the heart – and to help
in the quartan and quotidian agues'. Dr
Thomas Muffel (1553–1604) recommended
the root with sugar for giving to people
'withered and consumed with age'.

Gerard also cultivated the Field Eryngo
(*E. campestre*), a pale yellowish-green, spiny-
leaved, densely branched perennial, less thick
set than the previous species, bearing small
pale blue or whitish-green flowers surrounded
by long narrow bracts, which is native to
much of Europe, except the north. In the
wild this plant is found in dry grassland, on
grassy banks and in stony places, the roots of
both species being sold on the markets as

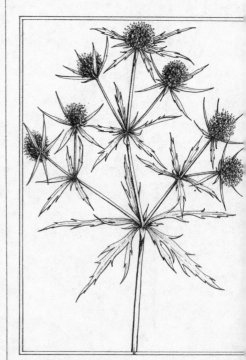

Eryngium campestre

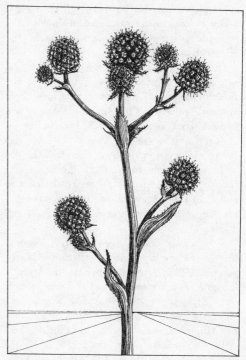

(*E. aquaticum*), was once widely administered for its diaphoretic, diuretic, expectorant and stimulant principles and in large doses as an emetic. This perennial is indigenous to the swamps and low wettish soils from Virginia to Texas, where it grows from 30–150cm/ 11–59in. high. It has long narrow taper-pointed leaves and bears in summer inconspicuous pale or whitish flowers.

During the late nineteenth century, the use of its root was regarded as an 'aphrodisiac, exciting venereal desires' and 'a strengthener of the procreative organs' besides being 'very useful in dropsy, nephritic and calculous affections'. It was also recommended for haemorrhoids, venereal disease, insect and snake bites.

The dried and fresh roots are still employed in homoeopathic medicine in the form of a tincture.

ERYTHRONIUM
Liliaceae, the Lily family
Dog's Tooth Violet, Adder's Tongue

Eryngium aquaticum

Although generally known as Dog's Tooth Violets, this genus of dwarf growing bulbous plants belongs to the Lily family. The majority are native to North America, have attractive broadly-oval shaped greenish leaves, curiously mottled with reddish brown, purple and occasionally white, and bear solitary drooping flowers on stems 10–30cm/3–11in. high.

Only one species, the common Dog's Tooth Violet (*E. dens-canis*), is known to have been prescribed in the medicine of medieval Europe, and this is indigenous to parts of the Mediterranean region and south-east Europe, where it is found in meadows, heaths and woods. Its generic name of Erythronium (Gr. *erythronion*) is derived from the Latin *erythos*, meaning red, which refers to the elegant drooping flowers of this species which appear from April to May, while Dog's Tooth refers, as does its specific name, to the yellowish-white pointed bulbs, which Culpeper tells us are 'full of a slimy pulp'. These were formerly eaten in several of the Mediter-

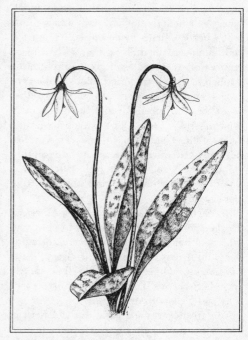

Erythronium dens-canis

ranean countries in the treatment of worms, and may have been introduced to England for this purpose during the latter part of the sixteenth century.

Only the fresh gathered bulbs were classed as suitable for inclusion in prescriptions 'for they dry very ill and generally lose their vertues entirely'. The expressed juice was administered internally 'for the worm in children' and to 'speedily ease the pains of the belly which are produced thereby'. If the child was unable to stomach the juice, the bulbs were boiled in milk to lessen their bitter taste. It was regarded as a very powerful remedy with small doses taking quick effect.

Another species of Dog's Tooth Violet was discovered by the early settlers in North America. This became known as the Adder's Tongue (*E. americanum*) and is found in rich open ground, or in thin moist woods and along the banks of streams from Nova Scotia to Minnesota and south to Florida and Arkansas. Each plant produces a single drooping yellow flower in April or May. Unlike the European kind, the leaves of this species were found to be more active than the roots and were prescribed in various medicines 'as emetic, emollient and antiscorbutic when fresh; nutritive when dried'. The fresh root simmered in milk or the fresh bruised leaves were regarded as of great help 'if often applied in a poultice' to scrofulous tumours or ulcers, which was generally taken together 'with the free internal use of the infusions in wineglassful doses.' The sweetish tasting juice of the plant infused in cider was also administered during the nineteenth century 'in dropsy – for relieving the hiccough – vomiting – hematemesis, and bleeding from the lower bowels'.

In their turn, the bulbs of the American Dog's Tooth were exported to England where, although known, they were not cultivated until 1665, the year of the Great Plague of London. Other names for this species include Serpent's Tongue, Fawn Lily, Trout Lily and Yellow Snowdrop.

The fresh leaves and corm of the American Dog's Tooth Violet are only occasionally used nowadays, usually in the form of a poultice

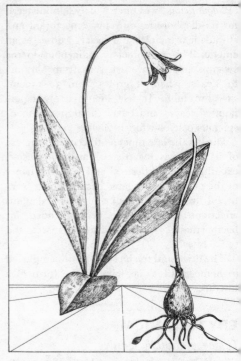

Erythronium americanum

for applying to swellings and tumours, etc. The European species does not appear to be prescribed at all.

ERYTHROPHLOEUM
Leguminosae, the Pea family
Sassy Bark

This large and spreading African tree, the Sassy or Saucy Bark (*E. guineense*), is native to the Sudan, Nyasaland and the west coast of Africa. The hard bark of the trunk and branches form the medicinal part, which is sometimes found on the world's markets in small and flat or slightly curved warty-looking pieces, the thickness and length depending on where taken from the tree.

In the past this inodorous but very acrid bark, that varies in colour from grey to brownish-red, was used by the West African natives in their trials by ordeal and in sorcery and witchcraft rites. Internal use causes constriction of the throat and gullet, accomanied by a prickling feeling and numbness. Overdoses cause violent headache, stricture of the brow, severe vomiting, followed by coma and death.

The principle poisonous constituent, known as Erythrophleine, has a similar effect on the body as Digitalis and from this was derived Erythrophleic acid and Manzconine, the latter a volatile alkaloid. These have been employed from time to time in various forms, as an uncertain remedy for treating mitral disease of the heart, in dropsy, which unfortunately upsets the stomach, and as an application to the cornea to bring about relief for failing eyesight. The powder alone causes violent sneezing.

The infused bark is still given in several countries for its astringent, laxative and narcotic effects, as in diarrhoea, dysentery, passive haemorrhage, etc.

The tree's other names include Mancona Bark, Doom Bark, Ordeal Bark, Nkasa, Casca Bark, Red Water Bark and Cortex Erythrophlei.

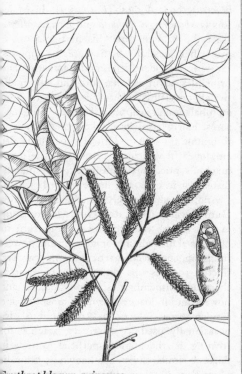

Erythrophloeum guineense

EUCALYPTUS
Myrtaceae, the Myrtle family
Blue Gum, Kino Eucalyptus

There are over 300 species of Eucalyptus, a genus of quick growing evergreen trees with leathery leaves containing a fragrant volatile oil, and native chiefly to Australia and Tasmania, where they are generally known as Gums, Ironbarks or Stringybarks. Some species thrive in moist soils, others in regions subject to drought. Others, again, develop into very large timber-bearing trees, while many of the smaller kinds are planted in warmer countries as ornamentals in gardens and parks.

About 25 or so of the species are valued for the oils they contain, which in commerce are divided into three basic groups: the medicinal, the industrial and the aromatic.

The medicinal kind was formerly derived from the leaves and shoots of the Blue Gum or Stringy Bark (*E. globulus*) from Tasmania. This tall graceful tree, which may reach 55m/180ft in height, has dark shiny sickle-shaped leaves, glaucous when young, and bears single or two to three almost stalkless whitish flowers about 4cm/1½in. across, followed by waxy button-like fruits.

One of the first Europeans to realize the potential of this species was the German botanist and explorer Baron Ferdinand von Müller, the Director of the Melbourne Botanical Gardens from 1857 to 1873. He suggested that the aromatic oil from its leaves resembled Cajaput Oil (*Melaleuca leucadendron*) and might be of use as a disinfectant in marshy districts subject to fever. As a result, seed was planted in Algiers. It thrived, but the expected antiseptic fragrance of the leaves was exceeded by the action of the roots, which appeared to consume vast amounts of water. Within five or six years the marshy, unhealthy region had dried out, and with no water to breed in, the malaria-carrying mosquitoes quickly faded away. As a result, the Fever Tree, as it became known, was extensively planted in other tropical, sub-tropical and temperate regions in an effort to

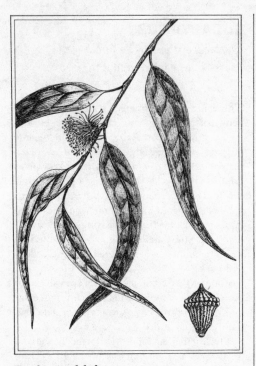

Eucalyptus globulus

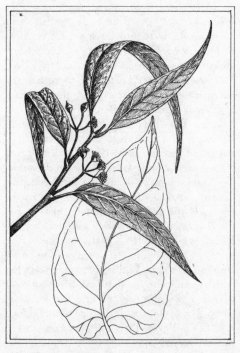

Eucalyptus rostrata

dry out swamps and marshes, thus ridding large areas of malaria and yellow fever.

In Australia, the leaves of the Blue Gum became, and still are, widely used as a household remedy in the treatment of many diseases and minor complaints, where at the first sign of any sickness, decoctions would be kept simmering as a fumigant on the stove twenty-four hours a day. In Britain and Europe during the late nineteenth century the oil of the leaves, which is powerfully antiseptic and composed mainly of Euca lyptol, was given for fevers and febrile conditions, pulmonary tuberculosis and was applied or inhaled for relieving asthma, bron 'chitis, sorethroat, croup, whooping-cough scarlet-fever and even diptheria and typhoid The dried leaves were also smoked like cigarettes for asthma, while the oil in the form of an aperitif was taken as a digestive.

Although the oil used in medicine is still obtained in part from this particular Blue Gum, several other species with a more pleasant aroma are used nowadays. Among these are the Silver Malee Shrub (*E. poly bractea*), the Gully Ash (*E. smithii*), the Male Box (*E. bakeri*), *E. dumosa* and *E. australiana*

At the present time this particular oil is prescribed generally in tinctures or vapours for its antiseptic, antispasmodic and stimulant principles, as in asthma, sore and spasmodic throat complaints, where it is mostly taken as an inhalant and is applied direct to ulcers and sores. Fairly large doses taken internally tend to irritate the kidneys. Eucalyptus Oil is also employed in veterinary practice in the treat ment of septicaemia, parasitic skin complaints distemper in dogs and influenza in horses.

Another valuable tree, the Kino Eucalyptus Gum Eucalyptus or Red Gum (*E. rostrata*) exudes a dark reddish-brown gum from its bark, used in medicine for its tonic and power ful astringent effects, particularly in powders tinctures and syrups, for complaints affecting the mucous membranes of the stomach and bowels, and in lozenge form for tonsillitis and similar throat infections. Red Gum is also occasionally used in veterinary practice for treating diarrhoea and superficial wounds in dogs. A similar substance known as Gum or Gum Kino is obtained from the dried juice of the Bastard Teak (*Pterocarpus marsupium*) of the Leguminosae Order, from Ceylon and the Indian Peninsula, and is similarly prescribed.

Several species of Eucalyptus, including *E. globulus* and *E. resinifera*, yield what is known as Botany Bay Kino, a dark reddish-brown resin obtained by making incisions in the trunk and when dried this is administered as an astringent.

Certain other kinds are valued for their perfumed oil, such as the Citron-Scented Gum (*E. citriodora*), the Paddy River Box (*E. mac-arthurii*), the Lemon Scented Ironbark (*E. staigeriana*), *E. sturtiana* which smells of apples, while *E. odorata* is used in the making of soap. Some species like the White Top Peppermint (*E. radiata*) and the Peppermint Gum (*E. dives*) yield oils which, as their common names suggest, taste of peppermint.

In the mining industry the oils from some species, including that of *E. dives* and *E. amygdalina*, are used for separating zinc salts from those of lead, while the very hard, durable wood of others is employed in ship-building and heavy construction.

The botanical name of this genus, Eucalyptus, is derived from the Greek *eu*, meaning good or well, and *kaluptos*, covered, thus well-covered, referring to the cap-like calyx that covers the unopened flowers.

EUPHORBIA
Euphorbiaceae, the Spurge family
Gum Thistle, Sun Spurge, Caper Spurge, Large Flowering Spurge

---

This large genus consists of well over 1000 species of annual and perennial herbs, shrubs and trees, native to the temperate and tropical regions of the world. The majority contain a milky and powerfully acrid and very poisonous juice or sap, hence Milkwort their collective and common name. According to Pliny, the generic name, Euphorbia, a Latin word derived from the Greek *euphorbion*, commemorates Euphorbus the physician of King Juba II of Mauritania, who is reputed to have first used the juices of these plants in medicine.

One of the perennial species, the Gum Thistle (*E. resinifera* syn. *E. officinarum*) from Morocco and the Atlas mountains, a leafless cactus-like plant up to 1m/3ft or just over in height, with fleshy quadrangular stems and small bright yellow flowers, was known to both Dioscorides and Pliny. Its active medicinal part, the juice, was procured by cutting the stems and then allowing them to bleed. After the sap had dried in the sun into a waxy yellowish or brownish substance it was collected in leather bags and powdered down. This end product, a very acrid highly inflammable latex or resin, was extremely violent in its effects, and even its dust caused severe inflammation of the nostrils. Even so,

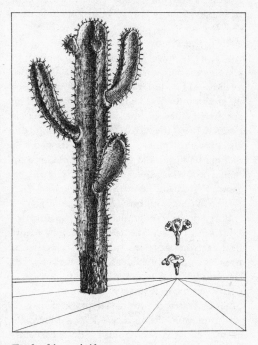

Euphorbia resinifera

powerful as it was, the ancient herbalists prescribed it as a drastic form of purgative and as a vesicant to raise blistering on the skin. It was also used at one time throughout much of Europe in the treatment of dropsy, and when mixed with the beetle known as Spanish Fly (*Cantharis vesicatoria*) as 'a blistering plaister for gout', or with other substances was snuffed as an errhine for relieving chronic complaints of 'the eyes, ears and the brain'.

It is rarely prescribed nowadays because of the deaths its use is known to have caused. The resinous gum is still employed in commerce, being added to paints used for preserving the bottom of ships and as an anti-fouling composition for the same.

Other names for the species include Poisonous Gum Thistle, Darkmous, Dergmuse, Euphorbium Bush and Gum Euphorbium.

The Sun Spurge (*E. helioscopia*), a hairless usually unbranched annual 10–50cm/4–19in. tall, with finely toothed oval leaves and bearing broad umbels of flowers with yellowish bracts from about April to November, was formerly used as a 'certain body purge', and is usually found in cultivated soils and waste ground throughout the whole of Europe, including the British Isles, parts of Asia and North Africa, and is now naturalized elsewhere. In the past its juice was popularly applied to warts and corns, and as a 'cure' for sore eyelids. The latter remedy often causes inflammation and intolerable pain. The specific name of the herb, *helioscopia* is derived from the Greek *helios*, meaning sun, and *skopein*, to look, referring to its habit of turning its flowers to the sun. Other common names for this species include Churnstaff Seven Sisters and Wart Spurge.

The Wood Spurge (*E. amygdaloides*), a robust, downy perennial up to 80cm/31in. tall, with lanceolate leaves, bears yellow flowers from April to July, and is native to the woods and thickets of Europe, except for the north. Its juice was also applied as a corrosive to corns and warts, although its use often ulcerated the flesh. The bark of its root was sometimes administered as a febrifuge, as was the Cypress Spurge (*E. cyparissias*) which again is indigenous to the woodlands and hedgerows of Europe (except the north) and western Asia. The erect stems 20–50cm/7–19in. high, and small unstalked linear leaves and yellow flowers of this species rise from long creeping rhizomes. Pliny referred to this species as *cyparissias*, now its specific name, to indicate Cyprus, which he believed to be its country of origin. In parts of France its juice is still prescribed as a forceful purgative although it can act as a violent poison, not only to humans but also sheep.

The juice of an Australian Spurge (*E. drummondii*) often kills cattle and sheep, while that of *E. cremocarpus* was formerly used by the aborigines to poison fish in pools. The Irish Spurge (*E. hyberna*), or as Culpeper called it the Knotty Rooted Spurge, was used for a similar purpose in Ireland, where some bruised leaves were placed in a basket, which was simply let down into the water, a very effective method for killing fish downstream. The juice was often included in so-called cures for syphilis before the use of mercury, and as a 'reliable' purgative.

Other species prescribed as purgatives in both Europe and the Mediterranean region include the Purple Spurge (*E. peplis*), the Spiny Spurge (*E. spinosa*), *E. apois* and *E. aleppica*, while the Petty Spurge (*E. peplus*) together with the Marsh Spurge (*E. palustris*) were regarded as 'hopeful cures in hydrophobia'. Culpeper tells us that the Petty Spurge 'is a strong Cathartic, working violently by vomit and stool, but is very offensive to the stomach and bowels by reason of its sharp corrosive quality, and therefore ought to be used with caution.'

The young fruits of another European species, the Caper Spurge (*E. lathyris*), have from time to time been pickled as a substitute for Capers, a very dangerous and potentially poisonous procedure. This robust hairless biennial is found in both waste and cultivated soils, where it reaches 1m/3ft high or more, having narrow opposite leaves, producing after its flowers, smooth, three sided hairless fruits 8–20mm/¼–¾in. across. From these was and still is extracted a colourless, inodorous, but very poisonous oil, known as 'Oil of Euphorbia' which when taken produces violent purgative effects besides severely irritating the mucous membrane of the intestinal canal. In France between ten and fifteen seeds on their own are still taken for their powerful laxative effects. The juice of the leaves are also vesicant and produce blisters if applied to the skin and will even remove body hair.

Other species known to have been prescribed as emetics and purgatives include *E. portulacoides*, *E. laurifolia*, *E. papillosa* all from South America, and *E. buxifolia* from

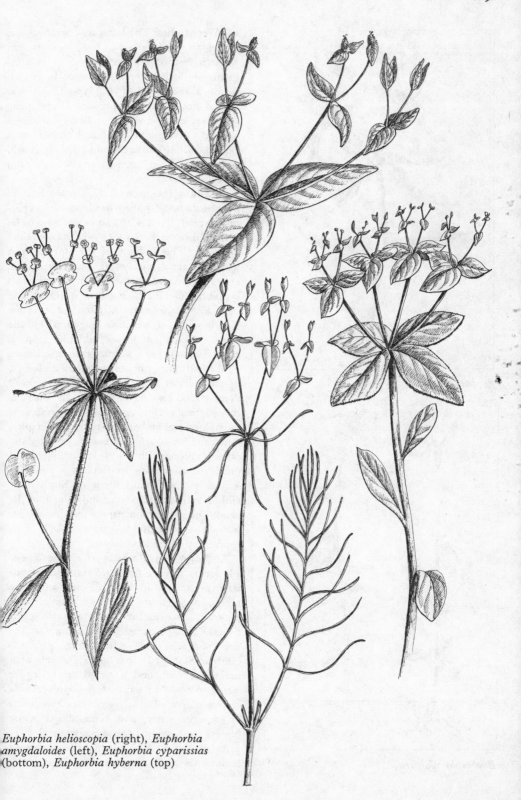

Euphorbia helioscopia (right), *Euphorbia amygdaloides* (left), *Euphorbia cyparissias* (bottom), *Euphorbia hyberna* (top)

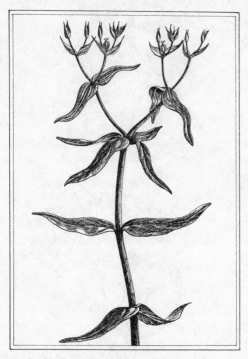

Euphorbia lathyris

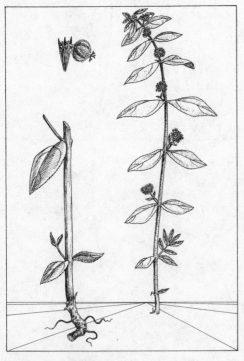

Euphorbia pilulifera

the West Indies. The latter was prescribed as a purgative in Java and in India as a vesicant when it formed a major ingredient of ointments applied to syphilitic sores. In central America the juice of *E. hypericifolia* was valued for its astringent principles in relieving dysentery and diarrhoea, and was sometimes applied to the eyes even though this at times caused partial blindness and pain. It is still prescribed as an astringent, although of a narcotic nature.

In Brazil the juice of *E. linearis* and *E. heterodoxa* was 'applied to ulcers of a syphilitic nature'. That of the latter was said to be able 'to dissolve both cancerous and syphilitic growths'. The Indians of the interior also used the acrid juice of *E. cotinifolia* as an arrow poison. Other sorts used as antisyphilitics include *E. canescens* in Spain, and both *E. parviflora* and *E. pilulifera* in India. The last named, which is known as Asthma Weed, is common to several other tropical countries, and has a slender cylindrical stem with bristly hairs, opposite lanceolate leaves, in the axils of which appear the very small dense round clusters of flowers. In Australia this particular Spurge was much prescribed for its pectoral and antispasmodic principles, especially for coughs, chronic bronchitis and other pulmonary disorders. It is still used for much the same thing in decoctions, tinctures and as a 'Compound Elixir of Euphorbia', and for relieving hay-fever and catarrh of the head. Other common names for this species include Queensland Asthma Weed, Pillbearing Spurge and Catshair.

A North American species, the Large Flowering Spurge (*E. corollata*), was popularly prescribed in that region during the nineteenth century for its 'emetic, diaphoretic, expectorant and epispastic principles'. This perennial plant is found in the dry woods and fields of both Canada and the United States. It has a large yellowish branching root, and a round erect slender stem 30–60cm/11–23in. high, with sessile oblong-obovate leaves, sometimes smooth at other times hairy, and bears showy white flowers from about June to September.

As an 'efficacious' emetic, the powdered bark of the root was prescribed in doses of

en to twenty grains, and 'As an expectorant
t is administered three grains at a time, mixed
vith honey, molasses or sugar; as a cathartic,
rom four to ten grains are required . . . It is
egarded as one of the best remedies ever
liscovered for the dropsy.' Nevertheless the
terb appears to be little used nowadays
)ecause of its irritating and potentially
)oisonous effects. Its other names include
3looming Spurge, Milk Weed, Wild Apple,
3owman's Root, Purging Root, Emetic Root,
Hippo Root and White Purslane. The juice
)f this particular plant, together with that of
everal others, was used by the American
ndians to dissolve warts and similar growths
n the skin. They also administered the juice
)f E. prostata, from the south-western parts
)f the United States, as an antidote for the
)ites of rattlesnakes and spiders. The juice of
he root obtained from an Indian species, E.
igularia, a tree held sacred to the goddess of
erpents, was prescribed for much the same
:hing and was both applied and taken
nternally.

Many other Spurges have been employed

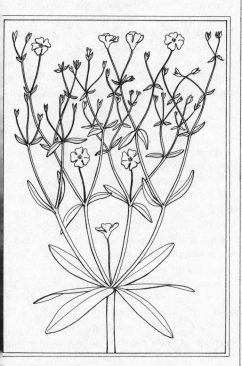

Euphorbia corollata

from time to time in herbal medicine including the Mountain Snow (*E. marginata*), *E.
iata* and *E. humistrata* from North America,
the Leafy Spurge (*E. esula*), the Sea Spurge
(*E. paralias*) and the Dwarf Spurge (*E. exigau*)
from various parts of Europe, and *E. tetra-
gona* and *E. antiguorum* of the African coast.

FOENICULUM
Umbelliferae, the Parsley family
Fennel, Florence Fennel, Carosella

Only one species of Foeniculum is listed by
botanists, the Common or Garden Fennel
(*F. vulgare*, syn. *F. officinale* or *Anethum
foeniculum*). This hairless, strong-smelling,
graceful, glaucous perennial ½–1½m/1½–5ft
high, has much divided dark green feathery
leaves, and bears from July to September
flat umbels of yellow flowers. It is believed
to be native to southern Europe, where it is
found in waste and cultivated soils, especially
in the Mediterranean regions of France and
Italy, although it is now widely naturalized in
the rest of Europe, as in Britain, where it is
mostly found near the sea, and parts of
temperate Asia.

From this species over the centuries,
certain distinct forms have been developed,
such as Finnochio, known also as the Sweet
or Florence Fennel (sometimes listed as *F.
vulgare dulce*, or as *F. dulce*), and the Carosella, known as the Italian or Sicilian Fennel
(listed as *F. vulgare piperitum*, or as *F.
piperitum*), both of which are grown as
vegetables in parts of southern Europe.

The use of the common type, or Wild
Fennel as it is sometimes known, dates back
to the ancient Egyptians, the Greeks and the
Romans, all adding its aromatic fruits and the
more succulent shoots to their dishes. Pliny,
writing of its medicinal uses, tells us it was
employed for twenty-two remedies alone and
goes on to say that when serpents had cast
their skins, they then rubbed against the
plant to sharpen their sight. Perhaps because
of this observation, the juice of the herb was
taken to improve the human eyesight;
cataracts were supposedly removed simply by

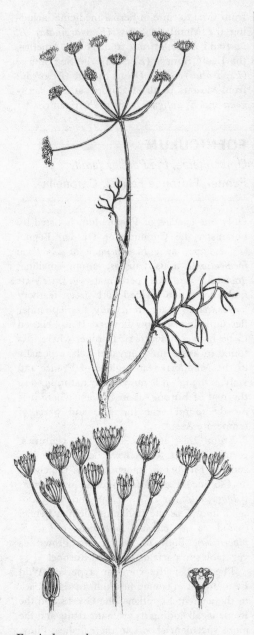

Foeniculum vulgare

The generic name of the Fennel, Foeniculum, is derived from *foenum* a Latin word meaning hay, to which its smell is believed to have been compared, and this seems to have evolved by the Anglo-Saxon period into *finol* or *fenol*, and in time to Fenkel, another of its common names. The Romans certainly liked the smell of the Fennel, and laid the herb under their bread when baking, for added fragrance, while the soldiers mixed the seed in with their regular meals, thus assuring themselves of fighting strength and courage. The early Greeks while training for the Olympic Games ate the seed as a valuable health-giving food and to help control their weight.

By the medieval period the use of Fennel had become entwined with witchcraft and superstition, when sprays of it were used with certain other herbs, such as St John's Wort (*Hypericum*), as a protection against evil forces, being regularly hung inside houses and churches or above doors to protect those inside against the devil, while the seed was placed in keyholes to bar the passage of any inquisitive ghost. In 1281 the household of King Edward I of England is known to have been consuming the seed at the rate of 8½ to 10lbs per month. Around this time, too, the poorer peasants ate the seed when hungry to make themselves feel full and to keep up their strength, while fat people ate it in the hope of becoming thin.

Culpeper writes: 'The seed boiled in wine and drunk, is good for those that are bit with serpents, or have eat poisonous herbs or mushrooms.' In his day, the seed, the leaves and the roots were made up into several medicinal forms, which were taken 'as good for the breaking of wind – to provoke urine – to break and ease the pain of the stone – stay the hiccough – allay the heat and loathings of the stomach, and the gripings therof – open obstructions of the liver, gall and spleen – and to ease the painful and windy swellings of the spleen – as also in gout and cramps'. Culpeper also recommended 'The leaves or seed, boiled in barley water and drunk' as 'good for nurses, to increase their milk, and make it more wholesome for the child'.

Parkinson writes of its great use 'to trimme

eating its root, while the blind ate the whole plant in the faint hope of restoring some vision. At the same time the Chinese and Hindu people regarded Fennel as a potent herb for neutralizing snakebites and scorpion stings.

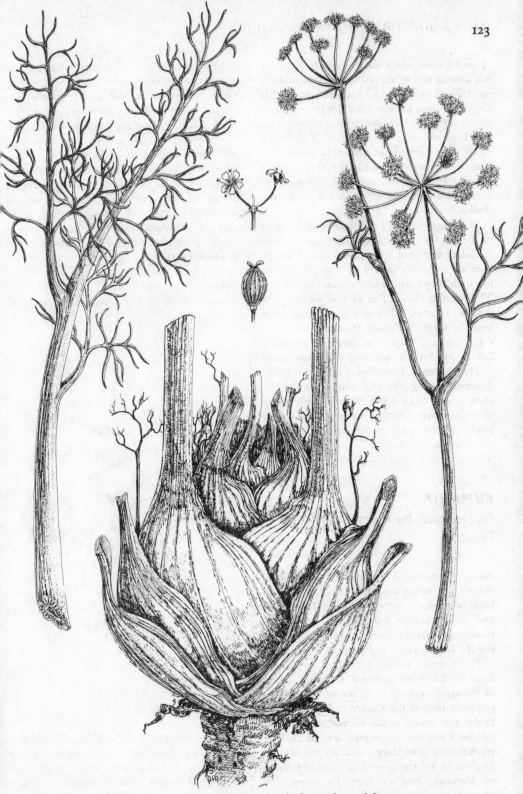

Foeniculum vulgare dulce

up and strowe upon fish, as also to boyle or put among fish of divers sorts, Cowcumbers pickled and other fruits,' and that 'the seed is also much used to be put into Pippen pies and divers other such baked fruits, as also into bread, to give it a better relish.' The young stems were sometimes added to salads, although Stevenson, in the *Gentleman Gardener's Director* of 1796, warns to 'take care of the green worm that is often met with in the Stalkes.'

The fruits of the Fennel are still used in medicine for their aromatic, carminative, stimulant and stomachic principles, although they are generally added to other medicines for their flavouring and carminative effects. The volatile Oil of Fennel has similar properties to that of Dill, and when diluted down into the form of Fennel Water, is added to Gripe Water, which is given to teething babies and infants suffering from flatulence.

The Common Fennel was introduced into America during the eighteenth century by some priests from Spain, where it still grows in the vicinity of their missions. It was later grown commercially in the United States by the Shakers.

FUMARIA
Papaveraceae, the Poppy family
Fumitory

About 35 species of Fumaria are known, the majority of which are rather floppy, delicate hairless annuals, with finely divided leaves and small tubular red to pink or whitish flowers. It is native mainly to Europe, including the British Isles, and parts of Asia.

The generic name, Fumaria, is derived from the Latin *fumus terrae*, meaning smoke of the earth, and refers either to their smell, probably that of the Common Fumitory, or to the appearance of the foliage, which early on dewy summer mornings was likened to smoke rising from the ground. By the Middle English period the word had become *fumeter* or *fumytere*, and in time Fumitory, the present-day collective and common name.

From the time of the Anglo-Saxons onwards the use of some of this genus became much entwined in witchcraft and superstition, when the leaves were burned for their smoke, which was firmly believed to possess the power to expel and to protect against evil spirits and spells. The principal species employed for such purposes, the Common Fumitory (*F. officinalis*), is a variable, straggling or climbing, branched annual 40–70cm/15–27in. tall, bearing slender racemes of dense-stalked, numerous, crimson-tipped purplish flowers, from about April to September. It is found in cultivated soils and waste places throughout most of Europe and western Asia, and is now naturalized elsewhere, as in North America, South Africa and Australia.

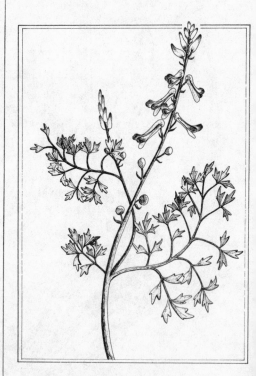

Fumaria officinalis

In the past the juice from the leaves of this species was decocted or distilled and added to syrups and essences. These were then prescribed 'to open obstructions of liver and spleen – procure an abundance of urine – to help the gout and yellow jaundice – drive forth the plague and pestilence – to clarify the blood of saltish and choleric humours, the cause of leprosy, scabs, tetters, itchings, scurvy – and eruptive breakings out and similar scorbutic affections of the skin'. The distilled water alone 'gargled often therewith' with a little water and honey of roses added, 'helps heal sores of the mouth and throat', while the dried herb in a powder, including the seed 'taken for some time together' is 'effectual for morbidness and melancholia'. Culpeper writes: 'The juice dropped into the eyes, clears the sight, and takes away redness and other defects in them . . . The juice of the Fumitory and docks mingled with vinegar, and the places gently washed or wet therewith, cures all sorts of scabs, pimples, blotches, wheals, and pushes which rise on the face or hands, or any other part of the body.' John Hill in the 1750s wrote: 'Some smoke the dried leaves in the manner of tobacco for disorders of the head with success.'

In North America, during the late nineteenth century, the fresh green leaves were prescribed for their tonic principles. The flowers and tops were also taken 'macerated in wine' in 'dyspepsia, with partial good effect'.

Infusions or liquid extracts of the herb are still prescribed, for their aperient, diuretic and slightly tonic principles, mainly for stomach and liver complaints, or in the treatment of skin diseases. The flowers were once used to make a yellow dye for wool.

Several other species known to have been prescribed in the herbal medicine of Europe include Small or Small Flowered Fumitory (*F. parviflora*), Climbing Fumitory (*F. claviculata*), Ramping Fumitory (*F. capreolata*), Wall Fumitory (*F. muralis*) and Narrow-Leaved Fumitory (*F. spicula*).

A number of North American species were also used, one of the most important being the rather bitter tasting and more powerful American or Indian Fumitory (*F. indica*). Others from that region include Spongy Flowered Fumitory (*F. fungosa*), Glaucous Fumitory (*F. sempervirens*) and Naked Stalked Fumitory (*F. cucullaria*).

GENTIANA

Gentianaceae, the Gentian family

Yellow Gentian, Field Gentian, Marsh Gentian, Cross Leaved Gentian, Marsh Felwort, Five-Flowered Gentian, American Gentian, Sampson Snake Weed

The Gentians make up an extensive group of annual, biennial and perennial flowering plants from many parts of the world.

Their botanical name, Gentian, refers to Gentius, the King of Illyria (180–167 B.C.) who is reputed, according to both Pliny and Dioscorides, to have discovered their ability to suppress the symptoms of fevers. Their use probably dates back at least a thousand years before this, one species having been recorded on a papyrus in a tomb at Thebes.

One of the commonest species used in the medicine of medieval Europe was the Yellow or Great Yellow Gentian (*G. lutea*), a stout, handsome hairless perennial ½–2m/1½–6½ft high, having large oval-pointed strongly ribbed leaves, and bearing whorled spikes of yellow star-shaped flowers from about June to August. It is native to the woods, meadows and damp places of central and southern Europe.

The large and bitter tasting roots of this plant provided the medicinal portion and these were prescribed for 'hysteria – female weakness – debility – agues – griping pains in the side – yellow jaundice – dyspepsia – tough phlegms – scabs – itches – fretting sores – ulcers – intermittents – scrofula – as a strengthener of the stomach – restorer of the appetite – comforter of the heart – breaker of stone' and 'as an admirable remedy to kill the worms'. Gerard certainly used the herb in England.

He also grew the Gentianella, which was generally known as the Little Felwort (*G. acaulis*), a smaller plant often forming mats of rich, glossy green leaves on the ground, spread by underground shoots, and bearing in May and June beautiful blue trumpet-shaped flowers. This possessed similar medicinal properties to the previous plant and was

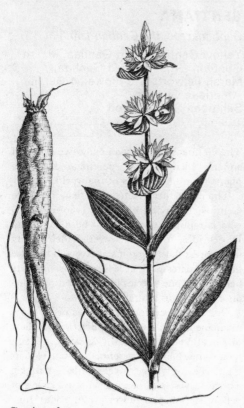

Gentiana lutea

prescribed for similar complaints.

The root of three other European species were freely and indiscriminately mixed with both the above; the Brown or Hungarian Gentian (*G. pannonica*) with its brownish-purple flowers spotted with purple black, the Purple Gentian (*G. purpurea*) with purple-red flowers, yellowish at their base and often striped and spotted with green, and the Spotted Gentian (*G. punctata*) with large pale yellow, purple spotted flowers.

Gerard also cultivated the Field Gentian (*G. campestris*, syn. *Gentianella campestris*), the Marsh Gentian (*G. pneumonanthe*) and the Cross or Cross-Leaved Gentian (*G. cruciata*). Of these, the Field Gentian is an erect, branched, annual or biennial 10–30cm/4–12in. high, which is found in pastures and grassy places in much of Europe, including the British Isles. It produces in August and September terminal clusters of dull purple,

or, on rare occasions, white flowers. At one time this was a much sought after plant, especially in Sweden, where it was employed in brewing in place of the hop. The Marsh Gentian, a rather rare plant, also grows in Britain, as it does in bogs, marshes and wet heaths in most of Europe. An erect, un-branched leafy stemmed perennial 30–50cm/ 4–19in. high, it bears a cluster of bright blue trumpet-shaped flowers, streaked with green from about July to October. Gerard tells us that 'the later physicians hold it to be effectual against pestilential diseases and the bitings and stingings of venemous beasts.' It was sometimes referred to as the Calathian Violet. The third species, the Cross-Leaved Gentian, a robust broad-leaved, leafy perennial up to 50cm/19in. tall, produces its dull blue flowers in dense terminal axillary clusters, from about June to September, and is native to south-eastern and central Europe. During the late medieval period, the root of this plant was regarded as possessing power-ful medicinal virtues, and at one time were considered a cure for rabies. A tincture of the root is still used in homoeopathic medicine in the treatment of hoarseness and sore throat.

Other species known to have been pres-cribed in the herbal medicine of Europe and the British Isles, include the Felwort, Bald-money or Autumn Gentian (*G. amarella*, syn. *Gentianella amarella*), the Vernal or Spring Gentian (*G. verna*) and the Milkweed or Willow Gentian (*G. asclepiadea*). Culpeper said that the Gentian 'helps agues of all sorts, and the yellow jaundice: as also the bots in cattle: when kine are bitten on the udder by any venomous beast, stroke the place with the decoction of any of these, and it will instantly heal it.'

Culpeper also made use of the Marsh Felwort (*Swertia perennis*), a closely related plant. This erect unbranched and hairless perennial 20–60cm/7–23in. tall, has pale greenish lance-shaped leaves, and bears from July to September terminal clusters of dark violet-purple flowers. It grows in marshes and boggy meadows in the mountains of southern Europe, although now naturalized elsewhere. He mentioned it as 'a very good stomachic', adding that 'The country people use it as an

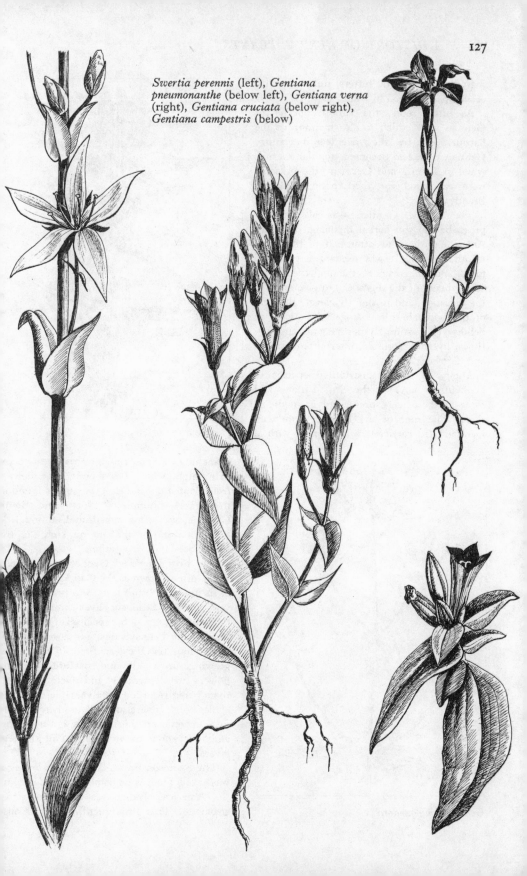

Swertia perennis (left), *Gentiana pneumonanthe* (below left), *Gentiana verna* (right), *Gentiana cruciata* (below right), *Gentiana campestris* (below)

ingredient in making bitters, mixing it with orange peel steeped in wine.'

As bitter roots, the various species of Gentian were added to ales to improve the flavour, and by the seventeenth century Gentian Wine had become a popular aperitif, while in Austria and Germany the peasants were renowned for their potent Gentian Brandy.

The Yellow Gentian was also widely prescribed in the herbal medicine of North America during the latter half of the nineteenth century. It was used as a powerful tonic and improver of the appetite, as a strengthener of the digestion, to give force to the digestion, and to slightly elevate the heat of the body, besides being 'very useful in debility, exhaustion, dyspepsia, gout, amenorrhoea, hysteria, scrofula, intermittent worms and diarrhoea'.

About 40 widely distributed species of Gentian are native to the United States and some of these were prescribed in medicine there. The root of the Blue or American Gentian (*G. catesbei*), a perennial with a

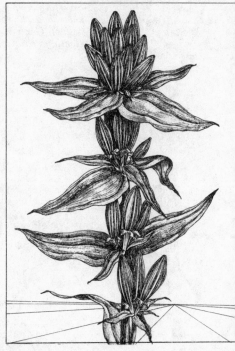

Gentiana andrewsii

branching root and rough stems up to 30cm 11in. high, which bears large blue flowers from September to December and is found in the grassy swamps of North and South Carolina, was often substituted, although 'a little inferior' for the foreign kind, 'in the same doses and preparations'.

The Five Flowered Gentian (*G. quinqueflora*), often known as the Gall Weed because of its intensely bitter taste, was prescribed 'as very useful in headache, liver complaints and the jaundice, etc.' This species is found from Vermont to Pennsylvania 'and a variety of it throughout the Western States', both types growing in woods and pastures, bearing flowers in September and October, their roots being regarded 'as a valuable tonic and cholagogue'. These are still used in tincture form in homoeopathic medicine as a stomachic and tonic, and in the treatment of intermittent fevers.

The Sampson Snake Weed (*G. ochroleuca*) was at one time, as its name suggests, used by the American Indians as an antidote for snakebite. This little plant, which is also

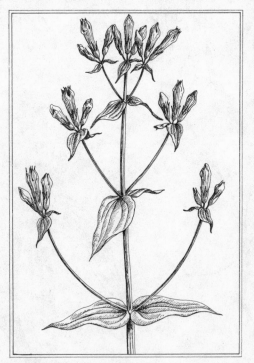

Gentiana quinqueflora

known as the Yellowish-White Gentian, the Straw-Coloured Gentian or Marsh Gentian, is found in Canada and occasionally in the southern States, where it produces its straw-coloured flowers in September and October. Although the root was classed as the official part the leaves were sometimes used, both for their anthelmintic, astringent, bitter and tonic principles, mainly in 'dyspepsia, intermittent dysentery, and all diseases of periodicity'.

Other species providing American gentian root included *Gentiana andrewsii*, *G. puberula* and *G. saponaria*.

The roots of many of the Gentian species are still prescribed in medicine as a bitter vegetable tonic in general debility, weakness of the digestive organs, lack of appetite etc.

The old English name of Bitterwort, once used in reference to several of the species, alludes to the intensely bitter roots of this genus, as does Felwort, *fel* being the ancient word for gall.

GERANIUM

Geraniaceae, the Geranium family

Herb Robert, Dove's Foot, Cut Leaved Cranesbill, American Cranesbill

About 150 species of true Geraniums or Cranesbills are known, the majority of which are native to the northern temperate zones. They have deeply cut and sometimes fern-like leaves, and bear rather strongly scented flowers which vary in colour from whitish-pink to red, purple and occasionally almost to black. They are not to be confused with the cultivated 'Geraniums', which are really Pelargoniums.

The botanical name of the genus, Geranium, is believed to have been used by Dioscorides, and is derived from the Greek *geranion* or *geranos*, meaning crane, referring to the seed pods that were likened to the beak of that bird; hence Cranesbill, their collective name, which distinguishes them from the Heron's Bill of the Erodium genus, a closely related group of plants of the Geraniaceae Order, and so-called because of their long-beaked fruits.

Of the 39 species of true Geranium native to Europe, the one chiefly used in medicine during the medieval period was the Fox Geranium or Herb Robert (*G. robertianum*), a variable and strong smelling, sparsely haired, annual or biennial 10–50cm/4–19in. high, with deeply cut ferny leaves, frequently reddish stems, which bears pinkish or rarely white flowers from about April onwards. It is found by the edges of open woods, hedges, in rocks and shingle, and on walls, in most of Europe, temperate Asia and North Africa, although now naturalized in many other regions of the world, including both North and South America.

As a medicinal herb the whole of this plant was prescribed for relieving 'inflammations of the eyeballs – of the conjunctiva – ulcers of the tonsils, throat and mouth – diarrhoea – retention of milk in the breasts – bleedings of wounds – irritation of the skin – facial neuralgia – haemorrhage of the private parts

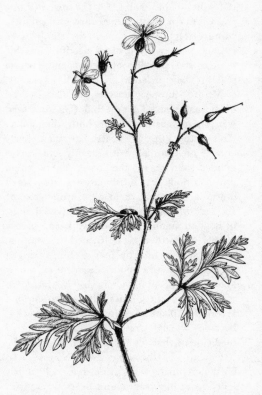

Geranium robertianum

in women – torpor – and to help the diabetic.'
(In the latter, its use has since been found to
reduce the sugar level of the blood.)

During the seventeenth century Culpeper
'commended' it 'against the stone, and to
stay blood, where or however flowing', and
writes that 'it speedily heals all green wounds,
and is effectual in old ulcers in the privy parts,
or elsewhere.' Its juice is still regarded by
herbalists as possessing valuable styptic
properties.

The Dove's Foot Cranesbill (G. molle) had
several varied uses and is a common, often
prostrate, branched downy annual, found
throughout Europe and parts of Asia, in
fields and in waste and similar places. It has
rounded lobed leaves and bears smallish pink
or rosy-purple flowers from about April to
September.

Of its medicinal uses Gerard observes:
'The herbe and roots dried, beaten into most
fine pouder, and given halfe a spoonfull
fasting, and the like quantitie to bedwards in
red wine, or old claret, for the space of one
and twenty daies together, cure miraculously
ruptures or burstings . . . if the ruptures be
in aged persons, it shall be needfull to adde
thereto the powder of red snailes (those
without shels) dried in an oven . . .'

A third European species, the Cut Leaved
or Jagged Leaved Cranesbill (G. dissectum)
was often substituted for both the above.
This rather untidy coarse growing hairy
annual or biennial, with deeply cut leaves
divided almost to the base, bears small
purplish-pink or whitish flowers from April
onwards. It is native to all Europe (except
Iceland) where it is found in cultivated soils,
in hedges, among rocks, on walls and grassy
places. Gerard also cultivated an annual
species sent to him by Jean Robin, listing it
as 'Geranium nondum descriptum,' now
known as the Shining Cranesbill (G. lucidum).

The American Cranesbill (G. maculatum),
a common plant of eastern North America,
became widely prescribed in the herbal
medicine of that region especially during the
latter part of the nineteenth century. An
erect perennial 30–60cm/11–23in. tall, it has
hairy spreading leaves, and bears from April
to June, usually pale to rosy purple flowers.

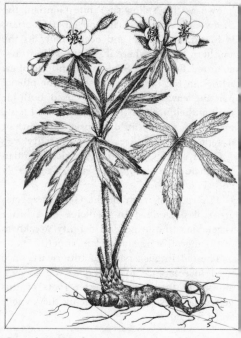

Geranium maculatum

It generally grows in open woodland and
meadows, mostly from Newfoundland south
to Georgia and Missouri.

The thick rough knotty roots of this species
were employed for their 'powerful astringent
principles' as in 'the second stage of dysentery,
diarrhoea and cholera infantum' often 'in
infusion with milk'.

Professor O. Phelps Brown recommended
that because of its 'freedom from any nauseous
or unpleasant qualities, it is well adapted to
infants and persons with fastidious stomachs.'

The active part of the root, known as
Geranin, is still prescribed by herbalists, in
liquid extracts or infusions, for its astringent,
styptic and tonic principles, mainly for
relieving piles, internal bleeding, as an
injection for leucorrhoea and excessive
menstruation and occasionally as a gargle.

Other common names for the American
Cranesbill include Dove's Foot, Crowfoot,
Alum Root, Alum Bloom, Shameface, Old
Maid's Nightcap, Wild Geranium, Wild
Cranesbill, Spotted Cranesbill, Stork's Bill
and Spotted Geranium.

GEUM

Rosaceae, the Rose family

Wood Avens, Water Avens,
Throat Root

The Wood Avens (*G. urbanum*), or Avens as
it is called, was highly esteemed throughout
most of Europe, including the British Isles.
An erect little branched perennial up to
90cm/23in. tall, with pinnate leaves, it bears
yellow flowers in June or July, and is native
to Europe, North Africa and western Asia,
where it is found in woods, hedges and in
similar shady or damp situations.

During the medieval period, the upper
leaves of the Avens, with their three leaflets,
together with the flowers, with their five
golden-coloured petals, were symbolically
associated with the Holy Trinity and the
Five Wounds of Christ on the Cross. As the
devil was believed to become powerless if he
dared approach it the roots were dug up and
put in church and house, to protect those
inside. As a further preventative measure, the
flowers and leaves were carved or painted on
the walls within the churches, where they are
occasionally found today.

Other names for the Wood Avens include
Colewort, Herb Bennet or Bennet, while
urbanum, its specific name, is derived from the
Latin *urbanus*, meaning town or city dweller,
for that was where the species was once found.

In herbal medicine, the roots of the plant
were 'valued principally as an aid to digestion',
for which they were prescribed by Paracelsus,
for catarrhs of the stomach and intestines.
This use is referred to in Geum, the generic
name, which is derived from the Greek
genein, to taste, or *geuo*, meaning agreeable
fragrance. To obtain this 'delicate flavour and
taste' the roots were dug up in the spring,
steeped in wine and taken regularly to
'helpeth digestion – warmeth a cold stomach
and open obstructions of the liver and spleen'.
The juice of the fresh root, or the powder of
the dried root in a decoction was said to have
the same effect, and was taken 'for the
diseases of the chest and breast – pains and
stitches in the side – inward fluxes – other

burstens and ruptures – wind colics – and the
spitting of blood caused by falls'. For diarrhoea the dried stringy roots were 'beat to
powder' and this taken in wine 'binds the
body and belly and stops all the torments
thereof'. Used outwardly, body wounds could
'be bathed therewith a decoction', while the
same 'taketh away spots or marks in the face
being washed therewith'. According to
Culpeper: 'It is very safe; you need have no
dose prescribed; and is very fit to be kept in
everybody's house.'

Teas or infusions of the dried herb or root
are still given by herbalists as a tonic, in cases
of dyspepsia, general debility, body weakness
and as an astringent for relaxed throats. The
aromatic roots are also used to flavour gin.

A second member of this family, the Water
Avens (*G. rivale*), was employed in the herbal
medicine of North America, in more or less
the same manner as the Wood Avens was in
Europe, for treating a range of stomach
complaints. This erect, hairy, little branched
perennial grows from 20–60cm/7–23in. high,
has a woody root, and produces drooping bell-
shaped flowers of yellowish-purple or red. It
is found from Newfoundland to New Jersey

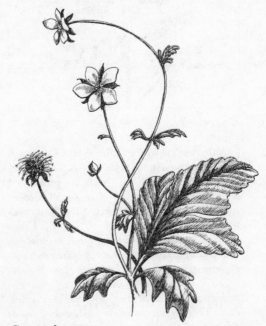

Geum urbanum

and west to Alberta and Colorado, in marshes, wet fields and similar places in dampish soil, as is suggested in *rivale*, meaning riverside, its specific name.

This particular species, which is often known as the Purple Avens or Chocolate Root, appears to have been prescribed more in medicine in the United States than it was in Europe and Russian Asia, where it is also found as a common plant, but whose apothecaries apparently preferred the Wood Avens.

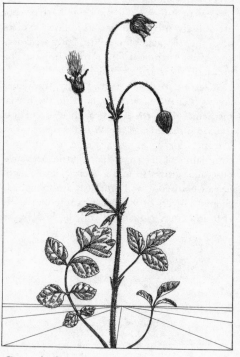

Geum rivale

Although the whole of the Water Avens was considered in America as 'containing medicinal properties' the part normally prescribed was the aromatic root, which was classed as tonic and astringent, 'its virtues being extracted by alcohol or boiling water'. These were administered during the nineteenth century 'in passive and chronic hemorrhages – chronic diarrhoea and dysentery – leucorrhoea – dyspepsia – pulmonary affections – and congestions of the abdominal viscera, etc.' The herb's name of Chocolate Root refers not only to the colour of its root, but to

its use in the making of a beverage once used as a substitute for cocoa. Its other names include Indian Chocolate, Water Flower, Cure-All, Nodding Avens and Drooping Avens.

A third species of Geum, the Throat Root or White Avens (*G. virginianum*) which is common only to the United States, was often prescribed in American medicine for the same purpose as the Water Avens. This perennial plant has a small crooked root, with stems 60–90cm/23–35in. high, and produces its small white flowers from about June to August.

Both the Water Avens and the Throat Root are still sometimes prescribed in American herbal medicine for their tonic and astringent effects, as in dyspepsia and similar stomach disorders, passive haemorrhage and diarrhoea.

GLECHOMA
Labiatae, the Mint family
Ground Ivy

Only one species of this small genus appears to have been employed in herbal medicine, the Ground Ivy (*G. hederacea*, syn. *Nepeta glechoma*). This hairy, aromatic perennial with prostrate rooting stems and long-stalked kidney shaped leaves, bears whorls of two lipped bluish-purple flowers mainly from March to June, but sometimes flowers throughout the year. Although native to most of Europe, including the British Isles, where it is found in meadows, ditches, hedge banks and shady places, the Ground Ivy is also common from Russia through China to Japan, as it is in Canada and the United States, having become widely naturalized there.

In the past this often carpet forming plant was listed as *Nepeta glechoma*, a close relation of the Catmint, with Glechoma derived from the Greek word *glechon*, mint or thyme. Hederacea, its present specific name means ivy-like, and probably refers to the shape of its leaves and to its creeping habit, which was likened to that of the Common Ivy (*Hedera helix*), thus Ground Ivy, the Glechoma's common name.

At one time, and especially in Britain during the middle and latter part of the medieval period, the herb's bitter-tasting evergreen leaves were valued as an ingredient when brewing with grain, to clarify, improve the flavour and to give the brew 'keeping strength'. One of the plant's more common names, Gill-go or Gill-creep-by-the-Ground, refers to this use, the word Gill coming from the French *guiller*, meaning to ferment ale.

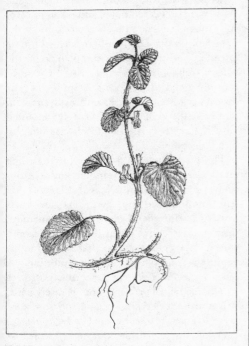

Glechoma hederacea

As ale houses were frequently known as gill houses, and gill also meant girl or sweetheart, the plant came to be known in some areas as Hedgemaids or Haymaids. Its other names include Turnhoof, Tun Hoof, Alehoof, Cat's Foot, Gill-over-the-Ground, Creeping Jenney, Gill-go-by-the-Hedge, Robin-run-in-the-Hedge, and in North America as Creeping Charlie.

As a medicinal herb the Ground Ivy had various uses. Prescribed for its astringent, diuretic and stimulant principles, it 'acted on the bladder and kidneys – would cure digestive troubles – ease the griping pains of the wind and choleric humours of the belly and spleen – openeth the stoppings of the liver and gall – provoketh abundant urine – womens courses – relieve fever – sciatica – gout – the gout of the hands, feet and knees – coughs and colds' and was regarded as a singular herb 'for inward wounds – exulcerated lungs or other parts' and as an excellent wash 'for the running scab – sores and ulcers in the privy parts'. Gerard writes: 'Ground-Ivy is commended against the humming noyse and ringing sound of the eares, being put into them, and for them that are hard of hearing.' Strong decoctions of the leaves in wine with a little honey added 'if gargled therewith eases the sore mouth or throat', while the leaves in a simple poultice 'helpeth green wounds, being bruised and bound thereto' and which 'stays the spreadings and eatings of cancers – cleanses fistulas and ulcers – the itch, wheals, and similar breakings out in the skin'. Gerard goes on to write: 'Ground-Ivy, Celandine and Daisies, of each a like quantitie, stamped and strained and a little sugar and rose water put thereto, and dropped with a feather into the eies, taketh away all manner of inflammation, spots, webs, itch, smarting, or any grief whatsoever in the eyes, yea although the sight were nigh hand gone.' A similar prescription was used for horses and cattle with eye trouble.

In the United States during the nineteenth century, the Ground Ivy was administered 'in diseases of the lungs and kidneys, asthma, jaundice, hypochondria, and monomania'. Infusions were regarded as 'very beneficial in lead-colic, and painters who make use of it are seldom, if ever, troubled with that affection.' Furthermore: 'The fresh juice snuffed up the nose often cures the most inveterate headache.'

Herbalists still prescribe the aromatic bitterish leaves for their astringent, diuretic and tonic effects, mainly infused in the form of a tea, in the treatment of coughs, kidney diseases, indigestion, nervous headache and occasionally as a lotion for tired and sore eyes. It can be combined with Chamomile Flowers or Yarrow, as a poultice for abscesses and whitlows.

At one time the trailing stems were made

into wreaths for the dead, and were given to horses as a vermifuge. There are occasional reports of cattle having been poisoned by eating the herb, but usually they tend to avoid it because of its bitter taste. Bees, on the other hand, like the flowers.

Several old English recipes recommend the Ground Ivy for inclusion in home-made jams, and that the young spring leaves be added to soups, gruels and other vegetable dishes.

GRATIOLA

Scrophulariaceae, the Figwort family
Hedge-Hyssop

The majority of the species belonging to this genus are native to Europe, parts of Asia, and to both North and South America. Several have been used in herbal medicine throughout the world, one of the better known of these being the Hedge-Hyssop or Gratiole (*G. officinalis*). This hairless perennial 20–60cm/7–23in. tall has quadrangular stems and

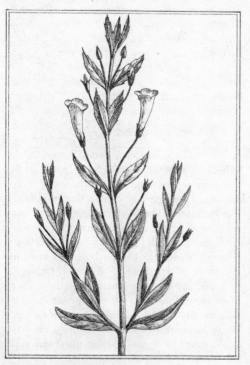

Gratiola officinalis

numerous opposite lance-shaped leaves, and bears from May to October solitary pinkish-white flowers on long stalks in the axils of the upper leaves. It is native to the wet meadows, marshes and similar watery places of most of Europe, except for the north.

The generic name of this herb, Gratiola, is derived from the Latin *gratia*, meaning grace, referring to the healing properties of this and of several other species.

The inodorous, but very bitter tasting brownish-yellow rhizomes were the parts generally prescribed in official medicine, and these were powdered down and taken in carefully measured amounts, sometimes under the name of Gratia Dei, 'in scrofula – chronic affections of the liver – complaints of the spleen – and for producing urine.' Culpeper recommended it as 'very helpful for the dropsy, gout and sciatica; outwardly used in ointment they kill worms, the belly anointed with it; and are excellent to cleanse old and filthy ulcers'.

The plant contains two very bitter tasting glycosides known as Gratiolin and Gratiosolin. Infusions of the powdered roots are still administered by herbalists for their cathartic, diuretic and emetic principles, mainly in infections of the liver, jaundice and spleen. Larger doses than prescribed induce vomiting followed by violent purging. A second species, *Gratiola peruviane*, possesses similar medicinal properties but is rarely used.

A third species known as *Gratiola amara* (syn. *Herpestis amara* or *Curanga amara*) contains the glycoside Curanjiin, which is prescribed in the East Indies under the name of Curanja, for its tonic and febrifuge effects.

HELLEBORUS

Ranunculaceae, the Buttercup family
Christmas Rose, Stinking Hellebore, Green Hellebore

christ tide (1629)

About 11 species of this extremely poisonous genus of erect, hardy, evergreen or deciduous perennials are native to southern Europe and Asia, the majority producing their flowers in

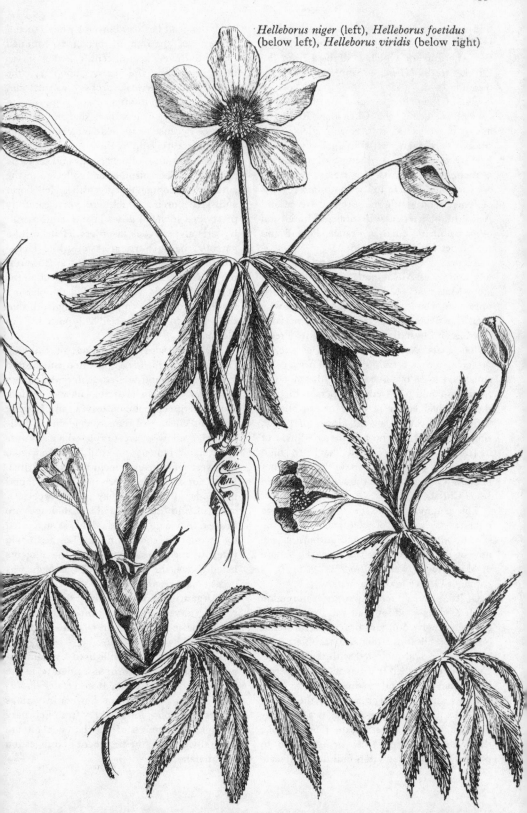

Helleborus niger (left), *Helleborus foetidus* (below left), *Helleborus viridis* (below right)

mid-winter or early spring. Their rather virulent nature is referred to in Helleborus, the generic name which is derived from the Greek words *helein*, to injure, and *bora*, meaning food.

One of the principal species to be used in ancient medicine, the Christmas Rose (*H. niger*), a handsome low growing plant, with smooth dark evergreen shining leaves, bears from December to April single white flowers 3–10cm/1–4in. across on stems 15–30cm/ 6–11in. high. Native to the mountain regions of central and southern Europe, Greece and Asia Minor, it is now naturalized in several other countries, such as France, Poland and the Soviet Union.

According to Pliny, this particular species was known as Melampode, and was named after Melampus, a Greek shepherd turned physician, who lived about 1400 B.C. and who used the plant in the treatment of nervous diseases and hysteria, after noticing its effects on his goats. As it was regarded as such a powerful herb, a certain amount of prayer and ritual had to be observed before the root and rhizomes could be lifted. The person digging them up had either to chew on, or shortly before have eaten, several cloves of garlic, simply to ward off the poisonous effluvia of its roots. Gerard recorded that: 'In high Dutch it is called Christ's herbe, and that because it floureth about the birth of our Lord Jesus Christ.'

The common name of Black Hellebore refers to the colour of its roots, as does the specific *niger*, although some authorities are now of the opinion that the Black Hellebore of the Greeks was *Helleborus officinalis*, a native of Greece and Asia Minor.

Of its 'Virtues' Gerard wrote: 'A purgation of Hellebor is good for mad and furious men, for melancholy, dull and heavie persons, and briefly for all those that are troubled with black choler, and molested with melancholy.' Culpeper prescribed the root as 'very effective in quartan agues and madness' and to 'help falling sickness, the leprosy, both the yellow and black jaundice, the gout, sciatica and convulsions. Used as a pessary, the roots provoke the terms exceedingly; also being beaten to powder, and strewed upon foul ulcers, it eats

away the dead flesh and instantly heals them.' The use of the root in medicine continued well into the eighteenth century, when it was prescribed for 'the palsy, apoplexy, the insane and hysterical, dropsy, worms and amenorrhoea', but after that it appears to have been more or less discarded in domestic practice because of its toxic effects.

Chemists still employ the blackish rhizomes for their diuretic, emmenagogue and cathartic principles. The rhizomes are collected in the autumn and contain two glycosides Helleborin and Helleborein, which are very carefully prescribed in small doses in the treatment of hysteria and nervous disorders. Helleborin, a narcotic, has a burning taste, while Helleborein is sweetish. The latter, a powerful purgative, has a similar poisoning effect on the heart as Digitalis. At one period the demand for these roots was so great in England, that they had to be especially imported from Germany.

The Setterwort, Bear's Foot or Stinking Hellebore (*H. foetidus*) was often substituted for the above, and is a stout, foetid, hairless perennial 30–80cm/11–31in. tall, having dark green evergreen palmate leaves, and bearing drooping clusters of numerous globular, bell-shaped, yellow-green purple-edged flowers from about January to April. It is native to the west of Europe, including the British Isles (not Ireland), where it is locally found in woods, grassy and rocky places, especially on chalk and limestone soils. If its leaves are bruised they emit a foetid odour, as suggested by *foetidus* its specific name. Besides being taken in medicine for many of the ailments listed above, the bitter root of this plant was occasionally resorted to 'as a sure but powerful purgative' to 'rid the body of the persistent worm', a very dubious procedure indeed, having caused many deaths over the centuries because of its improper use.

The fresh roots are still used by homoeopaths, mainly in the form of a tincture, as are the roots of the Lenten Rose (*H. orientalis*) from Greece, which bears flowers in various shades of purple-pink and grey from February to April. Tinctures of the latter plant are generally given in the treatment of indigestion and diarrhoea.

The Green Hellebore, also known as the Bear's Foot (*H. viridis*), a low hairless perennial 20–40cm/7–15in. tall, with deciduous leaves, and bearing half-drooping clusters of greenish cup-shaped flowers from March to May, was formerly used in place of the other species. It is found locally, sometimes in colonies, in the woods and thickets of much of Europe, including the British Isles, although naturalized in several other countries, for example, Poland, Czechoslovakia, and sparsely in parts of the United States.

All the plants mentioned above are poisonous if eaten, and in some cases even a piece of the root applied to the skin will cause irritation.

HERNIARIA
Caryophyllaceae, the Pink family
Rupturewort

Of the 15 species of Herniaria known to grow wild in Europe, only one, the Rupturewort or Burstwort (*H. glabra*), was prescribed to any extent in medieval medicine. This mat-forming perennial plant, also known as Herniary or Breastwort, has tiny fresh green coloured leaves and bears clusters of minute greenish flowers ranging along the stems in summer, and is found in much of Europe, including the British Isles, and northern and western Asia, mainly in fallow or sandy soils. One of the principal uses of this particular species is referred to in Herniaria its generic name, which is derived from the Greek word *hernos*, meaning hernia. Gerard wrote: 'It is reported that being drunke it is singular good for Ruptures and that very many that have been bursten were restored to health by the use of this herbe ...' It would likewise kill worms in children – help stitches in the sides – pains of the stomach and belly – helps all fluxes – vomitings also – those that have the stranguary – and wasteth the stone in the kidneys and expelleth them'.

During the sixteenth and seventeenth centuries the fresh juice or the water distilled from the whole herb was administered 'to help the gonorrhoea'.

It contains an alkaloid known as Paronychine, and herbalists still prescribe it, mainly in infusions, for treating catarrhal affections of the bladder, and for ruptures. Its action is astringent and diuretic.

A similar European species, the Hairy Rupturewort (*H. hirsuta*), was sometimes substituted for the above, and as both its common and specific name suggests, is covered in dense stiff hairs.

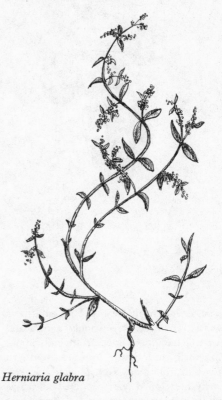

Herniaria glabra

HUMULUS
Cannabaceae, the Hemp family
Hop

The Humulus genus consists of only one or two annual or perennial twining climbers, indigenous to most of Europe, western Asia and Japan.

The most important and by far the most common species is the Hop (*H. lupulus*). This herbaceous perennial, although native to

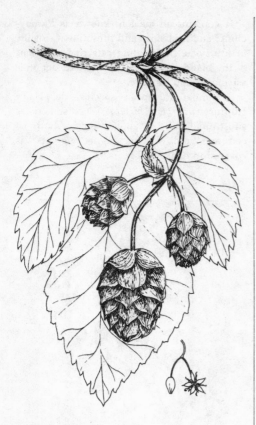

Humulus lupulus

Europe, including the British Isles, and parts of western Asia, is now widely naturalized elsewhere, having escaped from cultivation, as in North and South America, southern Russia, Australia and New Zealand. Several specially developed varieties are nowadays grown as field crops, mainly for the sake of their aromatic glandular fruiting 'cones', which help to preserve and add the bitter flavour to beer. In Sweden a coarse type of cloth is manufactured from the stem fibres and these are occasionally employed in the making of paper.

In its wild state, the Hop is usually found in hedges and damp thickets, where its rough coarsely-toothed opposite pale-green leaves and slender, angular, clockwork climbing stems reach 7m/23ft or more in height. It bears from June to September small greenish yellow flowers in loose axillary panicles, the males and females on different plants, th female sort developing into leafy pendulou cone-like catkins, consisting of a number o overlapping papery pale-green oval bracts covered by an aromatic and bitter yellow dust The latter, known as Lupulin, found its wa into the *Pharmacopoeias* of both Britain an the United States.

The plant has been known for thousand of years. Traditionally, the Jewish captives i Babylon drank barley beer with Hops and s managed to stay clear of 'leprosy'. Pliny als records that the Romans cultivated the specie as a garden plant, and in spring ate the youn shoots as a vegetable dish.

Little is recorded of Hops' use in brewin until 1097, when Hildegard the Abbess o Rupertsburg recorded that Oat beer wa prepared with Hops. The name Hop i derived from the Anglo-Saxon *hoppan* or th Middle English *hoppe*, meaning to climb, an refers to the plant's rambling nature. By th early fourteenth century, the Dutch brewer of the Netherlands were employing the bitte cone-like catkins in their beers, although thi use was forbidden in Britain. Henry VI o England (1422–61) forbade its cultivation an during his reign proceedings were take against any person who dared put thi 'unwholesome weed called an hopp', int beer. A prohibition continued by Henry VIII and not until the reign of Edward VI was thi relaxed. John Evelyn in the 1670s was sti rather uncertain of its virtues: 'This on ingredient, by some suspected not unworthily preserves the drink indeed, but repays th pleasure in tormenting diseases and a shorte life.'

Nevertheless during the seventeenth cen tury, the hop became regarded as an importan medicinal herb. The decocted tops take inwardly, or externally applied as a foment ation, 'cleanses the blood – cures the venerea disease – the scab and itch – abscesses an boils – the morphew – and discolourings an breakings out in the skin'. Decoctions of th flowering tops 'help to expel poisons' whil half a dram of the seed taken in wine 'bring down women's courses – kills the worms o the body – and surely expels the urine. The juice in a syrup 'relieves the yellov jaundice – cures the headache coming of heat – and tempers long and hot agues'. The young shoots may be used as a potherb, and the leaves and flowers yield a brownish dye.

During the late nineteenth century the Hop was prescribed in the United States for its 'tonic, hypnotic, febrifuge, antilithic, and anthelmintic' principles, but was principally used for its sedative or hypnotic action, to 'produce sleep – remove restlessness – and abate pain, but is recorded as sometimes failing to do so'. In Europe and Asia a pillow stuffed with Hops became a favourite remedy for relieving earache, toothache and again for producing sleep. A Tincture of Lupulin was also given in the treatment of 'delirium tremens, nervous irritation, anxiety and exhaustion' which 'does not disorder the stomach, nor cause constipation, as with opium', and is 'useful in after-pains, to prevent chordee, suppress venereal desires, etc.' Externally applied 'in the form of a fomentation alone, or combined with Boneset [*Eupatorium perfoliatum*] or other bitter herbs, it has proved beneficial in pneumonia, pleurisy, gastritis, enteritis and as an application to painful swellings and tumours.' An ointment of Hops and Stramonium leaves 'in lard, is an excellent application in salt rheum, ulcers and painful tumours. It is a powerful antaphrodisiac, composing the genital organs' and 'quieting painful erections in gonorrhoea, etc.'

The flowers (or strobiles) are still prescribed for their tonic, anodyne, diuretic, nervine and aromatic bitter effects, and are generally combined with other remedies mainly in the treatment of debility, indigestion, atonic dyspepsia, nervous complaints, insomnia, intestinal worms and as a general tonic and sedative.

The more popular varieties commercially grown for their use in brewing are known as Grapes, Goldings and White Blues.

A second species, the Japanese or Annual Hop (*H. japonicus*) which is native to Japan, Manchuria and China, was at one time prescribed, although to a much lesser extent, for some of the illnesses listed above. This climber reaches 5m/16ft or more in a season.

HYDROCOTYLE
Umbelliferae, the Parsley family
Common Marsh Pennywort, Indian Pennywort

This small genus consists of a number of creeping perennial plants, native to much of Europe, including the British Isles, parts of Asia, New Zealand, southern Africa and the southern parts of the United States.

The most familiar species, the Common Marsh Pennywort (*H. vulgaris*), a slender prostrate creeping perennial, having long stalked, almost circular shining green leaves and bearing inconspicuous whorls of pinkish-white or greenish flowers from about June to September, was prescribed during the latter part of the medieval period 'as a dissolver of gravel' and 'breaker of stone' throughout Britain and much of Europe, where it is generally found in damp meadows, bogs, marshes and the banks of rivers and streams. This liking for a damp habitat is alluded to in

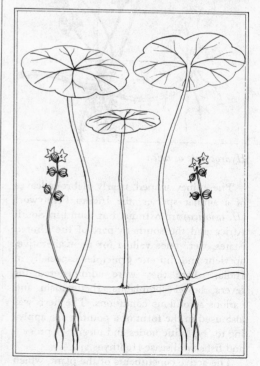

Hydrocotyle vulgaris

Hydrocotyle the generic name, which is derived from the Greek *hydor*, meaning water, and *kotyle*, the Greek for a platter or cup, referring to the shape of the leaves.

The Marsh Pennywort's other common names include Marsh Penny, White Rot and Common White Rot. The last two names came into use because the plant was formerly believed to cause footrot in sheep. It is rarely prescribed nowadays.

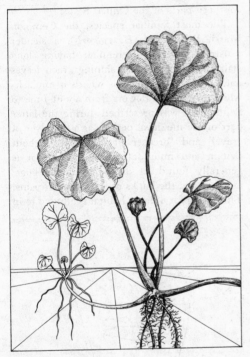

Hydrocotyle asiatica

The kidney shaped, nearly glabrous leaves of a similar species, the Indian Pennywort (*H. asiatica*) from India, but found in South Africa and the southern part of the United States, were once valued for their alterative, aperient and diuretic principles especially in India, where they were administered for fevers, bowel complaints, rheumatism and various scrofulous conditions. The herb was also used in the form of a poultice for applying to 'syphilitic nodes and ulcers – leprosy – and fishskin disease [Ichthyosis]'.

The active constituents of the plant, which appears to be little used nowadays, are tannic

acid, and a bitter, pungent, oily, volatile liquid known as Vellarin. When correctly prescribed in small amounts this acts as a stimulant, although large doses are narcotic, causing headache, stupor, dizziness and occasionally coma.

HYOSCYAMUS
Solanaceae, the Nightshade family
Common Henbane, White Henbane

The Hyoscyamus genus consists of a small group of annual, biennial or perennial herbs, native to the Canary Islands, parts of Europe, Asia and India. Of these, the principal species prescribed in medicine was and still is, the Common Henbane (*H. niger*). This very poisonous, coarse, softly haired, sticky and unpleasant smelling annual or biennial reaches 20–80cm/7–31in. in height, has alternate leaves, and bears greenish-yellow funnel-shaped flowers with purple veins from about May to September. It grows in waste and sandy places, often near the sea, in farmyards and on rubbish dumps in most of Europe, North Africa, western Asia and from Siberia to India.

The use of this herb dates back to the time of the ancient Greeks, the generic name Hyoscyamus having evolved from the Greek *hyoskyamos*, with *hys* meaning hog, and *kyamos*, bean, thus Hog's Bean or Bean of the Hog, so-called according to Dioscorides, because pigs could eat its poisonous seed. The specific name of *niger*, meaning black, could refer either to the plant's poisonous principles, or to the ancient belief that if it was applied to any part of the human body, the part touched would turn black and rot. The Anglo-Saxons knew the herb as Belene, probably referring to its bell-shaped flowers, and this appears to have evolved into the English Henbane by the late medieval period, with the 'bane' part again alluding to its poisonous nature.

As an early and most unreliable anaesthetic, the juice of the plant was included in the Soporific Sponge, which was administered to the sick before painful operations such as

mputations were performed. Dioscorides
rescribed the herb as a procurer of sleep and
s a reliever of pain, as did Celsus, who also
sed it as an external application.

During the Middle Ages small doses of
Ienbane were employed in witchcraft, to
ause insanity, frenzy, convulsions, and to
ive visions. The seed was either roasted or
he leaves burnt and the fumes given off
nhaled. Its use often deranged the taker's
enses, causing maniacal delirium, near blind-
ess and unbearable pain.

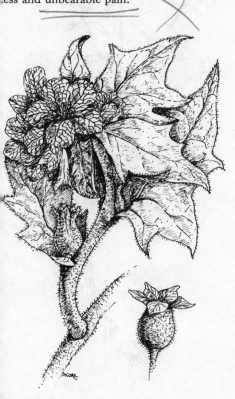

Hyoscyamus niger

In contrast, however, small pieces of root
vere hung around the necks of children 'as a
reventer of the fitte' and about infants 'to
ause an easy breeding of the teeth'. In
upgrown people', the seeds were sometimes
moked 'for relieving the pains of the tooth-
che'.

The White Henbane (*H. albus*), so-called
ecause it has paler coloured flowers, a
imilar but less fetid, hairy annual or biennial,
native to parts of the Mediterranean region
where it is generally found in waste places,
was often indiscriminately mixed and prescribed with the species above.

Gerard observed of both species: 'Henbane
causeth drowsinesse, and mitigateth all kinde
of paine: it is good against hot and sharp
distillations of the eyes and other parts. The
leaves stamped with the ointment Populeon,
made of Poplar buds, asswageth the pain of
the gout. To wash the feet in the decoction
of Henbane causeth sleepe; and also the often
smelling of the floures.'

Culpeper writing of the Common Henbane
said: 'The leaves cool inflammations of the
eyes and any part of the body, and are good
for the swellings of the testicles, or womens'
breasts, or elsewhere, if they are boiled in
wine, and either applied themselves, or the
fomentation warm . . . The oil of the seed is
good for deafness, noise and worms in the
ears, being dropped there; the juice of the
herb or roots act the same.'

In North America the common Henbane
became valued for its 'calmative, hypnotic,
anodyne and antispasmodic principles'. It
had escaped from cultivation in the 1670s and
has since naturalized itself in waste places and
sandy soils from eastern Quebec to Ontario
and Michigan. One physician writing of its
use there in the late nineteenth century says:
'It is much better than opium, as it does not
produce constipation.' Combined with other
preparations 'it is most excellent for gout,
rheumatism, asthma, chronic cough, neuralgia, irritation of the urinary organs, etc. The
leaves make fine external preparations for
glandular swellings or ulcers, etc.'

The fresh or dried leaves, the flowering tops
and the seed of the Henbane, generally
obtained from cultivated biennial plants, and
which contain the alkaloids Atropine, Hyoscine and Hyoscyamine, are still officially listed
in several Pharmacopoeias. All three are able
to withstand boiling and drying, and when
correctly administered medicinally in extracts
and tinctures by doctors, have a calminative,
hypnotic and mildly diuretic effect. These are
chiefly given in narcotic medicines, as a
tranquillizer and sedative in cases of nervous
infections, whooping cough, asthma, etc., and

in tablet form for sea-sickness. Solutions are also applied to the eyes as a mydriatic to dilate the pupils. But unless administered under strict medicinal supervision the Henbane is best left well alone. In countries where the White or Russian Henbane was employed in medicine, as in France, only the seeds were officially listed.

The three alkaloids mentioned above are also extracted from the Egyptian Henbane (*H. muticus*) which is grown there for its narcotic uses, as it is in several other countries, such as India and the East Indies. The Golden Henbane (*H. aureus*) from the islands of Greece has occasionally been employed in the medicine of that region.

HYPERICUM

Hypericaceae (or Guttiferae) the St John's Wort family

St John's Wort, Tutsan

This large genus consists of about 200 species of evergreen or deciduous shrubs, sub-shrubs and herbaceous perennials, and has simple opposite or whorled leaves and usually golden-yellow many stamened flowers. They are native mainly to North America, Europe, Asia Minor, the Soviet Union, India and China.

One of the principal species valued in medicine, the Common or Perforated St John's Wort (*H. perforatum*), is a hairless perennial 20–100cm/7–39in. tall, has spreading branches, with small deep green glabrous oblong-ovate leaves, perforated by many translucent glandular dots (which are referred to in *perforatum* the specific name), and bears from May to August branched clusters of golden yellow flowers with tiny black spots. It is found in open woods, dry meadows and fields, on grassy banks, in thickets and by the wayside, throughout Europe (except Iceland), Asia and North Africa, and is now naturalized in many other countries.

As a medicinal herb this particular St John's Wort has been used in the treatment of wounds at least since the time of Dioscorides. He knew of it as *Hypereikon* the old

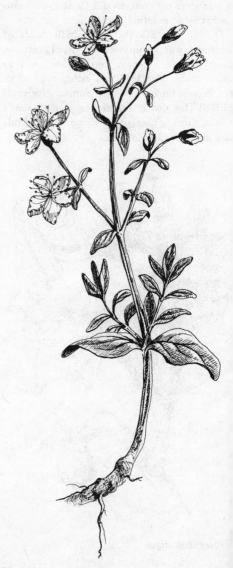

Hypericum perforatum

Greek name, which is perhaps derived from the words *hypo*, meaning under and *ereike*, heath or heather. Other authorities believe the name refers to the ancient Greek belief that the herb was distasteful to evil spirits and that the smell of it would cause them to fly away.

In Europe the plant became closely associted with the early Crusaders, who used it as a styptic on the battlefield. It was noticed that the herb's juice turned red on exposure to air, and this was likened to the blood of St John the Baptist.

As the herb was credited with such protective powers against evil spirits and witches, it became a common custom to hang sprays of it above the doors of houses and churches on the Eve of St John's Day (24 June), when witches were believed to be most active. The possessed or insane were also obliged to inhale the odour of the crushed leaves and flowers, or drink a potion of it, in an effort to rid them of their madness.

During the late nineteenth century, the herb was prescribed both in Europe and North America for its astringent, diuretic and sedative principles. It was described as 'very applicable in chronic urinary affections, diarrhoea, dysentery, jaundice, menorrhagia, hysteria, nervous affections, hemoptysis and other hemorrhages. Externally in fomentation, or used as an ointment, it is serviceable in dispelling hard tumors, saked breasts, bruises, etc.'. The recommended dose at that time: 'Of the powder, from half a drachm to two drachms' and of the 'infusion, one or two ounces'.

Infusions are still given by herbalists for their slightly astringent, diuretic and expectorant principles, mainly in the treatment of urinary complaints, and for coughs and colds, etc. The 'Oil of St John's Wort', which is made by infusing the fresh flowers in olive oil, makes a useful application for wounds, ulcers, sores and slight burns. The active constituent of this and other plants of the genus, is a volatile oil known as Hypericum Red, and this taken in small amounts is said to relieve general body pain.

Other names for the common St John's Wort include Amber, Cammock, Penny John, John's Wort and the Grace of God.

A second species, listed as the Woolly St John's Wort (*H. tomentosum*), was substituted for the above in medieval medicine. A Siberian Hypericum known as St Peter's Wort (*H. ascyron*) was prescribed in Russia in the treatment of burns and scalds and was introduced in England in the early 1770s.

The Tutsan (*H. androsaemum*), a native of the damp woods and shady places of much of western Europe although naturalized elsewhere, formerly had several medicinal uses, and is a small, shrubby half-evergreen perennial ½–1m/1½–3ft high, with large broad oval opposite stalkless leaves, and bearing in June and July, terminal, more or less flat-topped clusters of yellow flowers, followed by fleshy berries, red at first, but turning blackish-purple when ripe.

As with the previous species, the pores (or glands as they are sometimes called) of this plant were likened to wounds in the skin, for which it was prescribed by Paracelsus and other believers of the Doctrine of Signatures. The specific name of *androsaemum* is derived from the Greek *andros*, meaning man, and *aima*, blood.

According to Culpeper 'It purges choleric humours, helps the sciatica and gout, and heals burns; it stays the bleeding of wounds, if the green herb bruised, or the powdered herbe be dried and applied. It is a sovereign remedy for either wound or sore, either out-

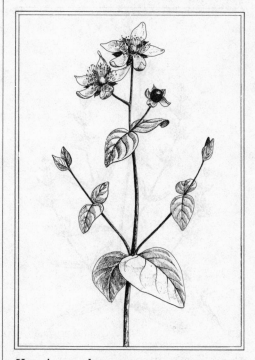

Hypericum androsaemum

wardly, if used in drinks, lotions, balms, or ointments and also in any other sort of green wounds, old ulcers, etc.' Variations of its common name include Tutseyn, Tipsen and Tutzen. The leaves were sometimes dried for their scent; they were thought to bring good luck, and were used as bookmarks in prayer books and bibles.

HYSSOPUS

Labiatae, the Mint family

Hyssop

The Hyssop (*H. officinalis*) is an almost ever-green, aromatic, much branched sub-shrub 20–60cm/7–23in. tall, having angular stalks and oblong lance-shaped leaves, and bearing whorls of small purplish-blue flowers for much of the summer. It is native to parts of the Mediterranean region and temperate Asia, and grows mostly on dry banks and among rocks and ruins, although now naturalized, generally as a result of its culti vation as an ornamental, in many othe countries, such as Canada and the Unite States.

The generic name of Hyssopus is derive from the Hebrew *ezoph*, which was known t have been an aromatic herb anciently use for cleaning sacred places, although man scholars now believe that the Hyssop liste here is not the one referred to in the Bible.

Several of the ancient physicians mad good use of the plant in medicine, includin Hippocrates, who prescribed it for pleuris and bronchitis. Galen burnt it with brim stone and certain other substances, th patient having to inhale the fumes given off t relieve quinsy and inflammations of th throat, while the Salerno School recom mended the boiled herb with honey to hel in pulmonic complaints of the lungs and t evacuate the mucus.

Although not indigenous to Britain, it wa certainly known to the Cistercians by th middle of the thirteenth century. The favoured it as a bee plant, the honey from having a delicious taste and smell. Th religious also extracted the oil and used it t add a spicy taste to their soups and sauces.

Gardener in the 1440s described its culti vation in his *Feate of Gardening*. Turne wrote that: 'The brethe or vapor of Hiso driveth away the winde that is in the ears, they be holden over it.'

By this period the shrub had become a essential herb for the gardens of large houses. The clippings were employed fo strewing floors and closets, while infusions o the leaves made a useful wash to kill off bod and hair lice and to take away 'the nits an itchings of the beard'. Gerard recommended 'A decoction of Hyssope made with figge water, honey, and rue and drunken, helpet the old cough.' Parkinson described it as country peoples' medicine 'for a cut or green wound, being bruised with sugar an applied'. It was also prescribed with honey t 'kill worms in the belly', with oxymel 't purge gross humours by stool', with Fig 'to loosen the belly' and with nitre added 't help the dropsy and spleen'. As a wash ' taketh away the black and blew marks, tha

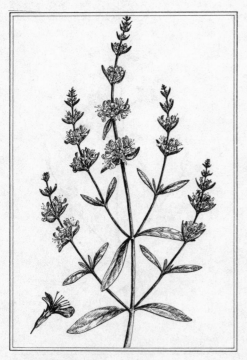

Hyssopus officinalis

ome by bruises, strokes and falls' and with
vinegar added, gargled 'it helps to cure the
toothache'. Culpeper said: 'The hot vapours
of the decoction taken by a funnel in at the
ears, eases the inflammations and singing
noise in them.'

In both Canada and the United States
during the nineteenth century the leaves were
Generally used in quinsy and other sore
throats – as a gargle with sage' and as a
beneficial expectorant 'in asthma, coughs,
etc.' Infusions of the leaves were also applied
to relieve the pains of muscular rheumatism'
while 'the leaves applied to bruises speedily
relieves the pain' and 'removes the dis-
colouration'.

The leaves of the Hyssop are still pres-
ribed, mainly infused, for their carminative,
stimulant and pectoral principles, in coughs
and colds in babies, chronic catarrh and other
chest complaints and is sometimes combined
with Horehound. The fresh green tops served
in the form of a tea, taken three or four times
a day, are said to be good for relieving rheumatism and similar aches.

The aromatic oil extracted from the leaves,
stems and flowers is also employed in the
manufacture of Chartreuse and other liqueurs, and is added to perfumes such as Eau
de Cologne.

ILEX

Aquifoliaceae, the Holly family

Holly, Maté, Yaupon,
Black American Alder

About 300 species of Ilex are known, consisting mostly of small trees and shrubs, with
deciduous or evergreen, often spiny leaves,
and bearing small greenish-white flowers,
followed by yellow, red or black berry-like
fruits, which often remain on the branches
for the winter. They are native to the tropical
and temperate regions of both hemispheres.

The use of one of the better known species,
the Holly (*I. aquifolium*), dates back to
ancient times. A small tree or dense shrub
–15m/10–50ft high, it has smooth grey
bark and dark shiny evergreen, spiny, oval-

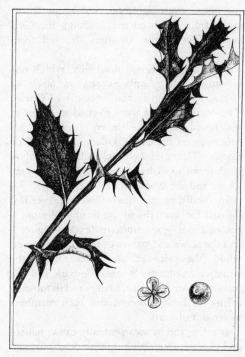

Ilex aquifolium

elliptic, leathery leaves, and bears axillary
clusters of small white flowers from about
April to May, followed by scarlet berries.
Native to the woods, thickets and hedges of
most of Europe, it is now widely cultivated,
together with its numerous forms and
ornamental varieties, in many other regions,
including North America where it is found
on the Pacific coast from British Columbia
south to California.

The origin of this common Holly can be
traced back to the time of the Druids, for this
was one of the evergreen shrubs they used to
decorate their huts to give shelter to the spirit
or deity of the woods during the winter
months. Pliny referred to the Holly as
aquifolium, now its specific name, a Latin
word derived from *acus*, a needle, and *folium*,
a leaf, hence Needleleaf or Needleaf, and
goes on to say that if it was planted near a
house it would give protection from witchcraft and lightning, besides repelling poison.
Parkinson recorded that the branches with
berries on, were used at 'Christ Tide' to 'deck
houses withall' and 'that they should defend

the house from lightning, and keepe themselves from the witchcraft', adding this 'is a superstition of the Gentiles, learned from Pliny'.

According to legend the Holly, which was known to the Anglo-Saxons as *holen* or *holegn*, sprang up in the footsteps of Christ. The scarlet berries were likened to drops of his blood, and the thorny leaves to his sufferings on the Cross. Other names include Christ's Thorn, Holy Tree, Holm and Hulver Bush (both used by Culpeper), Hulm, Holme Chase and the Needle-Leaved Holly.

In medicine, the leaves were prescribed infused for 'catarrhs of the head – pleurisy – the smallpox – intermittent fevers – agues – and the aches and paines of the joints all over' while 'the juice of the leaves helps the jaundice'. Culpeper wrote 'the bark and the leaves also are excellent, being used in fomentations for broken bones, and such members as are out of joint.'

If eaten, the berries generally cause nausea and excessive vomiting, followed by purging, but were formerly regarded as 'beneficial in dropsies', and when powdered as an astringent 'to stay bleedings'.

The leaves, which contain an alkaloid known as Ilicin, are still prescribed decocted or infused for their diaphoretic, febrifugal and tonic principles, mainly for relieving fevers and rheumatism. The berries are still sometimes administered as a cathartic in dropsy.

The very dense, strong wood of the species is frequently substituted for Boxwood (*Buxus sempervirens*) in inlaywork, the making of scales, rules, printing blocks, carving, engraving and in turnery. The handles of coffee pots, tea pots and walking sticks are also made from this wood, while the sticky substance extracted from the bark is made into birdlime.

The leaves of a South American Ilex, the Maté or Yerba (*I. paraguayensis*), a large shrub or small tree up to about 7m/23ft tall, with oval or lanceolate, broadly toothed evergreen leaves, and bearing white flowers followed by red berries, were and still are widely used in that region to make a bitter but sustaining drink. The leaves and young shoots of the plant were collected by the Indians, slowly dried over a fire until brittle, then powdered and prepared in much the same way as tea. The resulting liquid was generally sucked through a tube or straw inserted into a small hole at the top of a calabash or gourd. This container was known to the Incas as a Maté, hence one of the plant's more common names. Others include Yerba Maté, Jesuit's Tea, Jesuit's Brazil Tea, Houx Maté, Brazil Tea and Paraguay Tea.

The consumption of Maté as a beverage in South America now runs into several million pounds weight annually, and like tea, it is drunk at any time of the day. Its stimulant and refreshing effects have since been found to be largely due to the presence of caffeine.

The leaves are medicinally used for their diuretic and tonic principles, and were at one time recommended for rheumatism and gout. Large doses are said to be antiscorbutic, but tend to cause purging. The leaves are still prescribed in the form of a liquid extract.

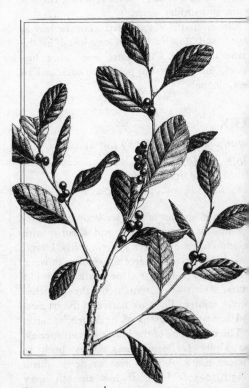

Ilex paraguayensis

The leaves of at least two other South American species, *Ilex gongonha* and *I. theezans* were infused and taken like tea or prescribed in medicine for their diaphoretic and diuretic effects.

A similar beverage to that of the Maté was obtained from the Yaupon (*I. vomitoria*) a native of the southern part of the United States, where it grows by the banks of streams and in swamps as a small tree, or more often than not as a thicket forming shrub. It has small evergreen, elliptic leaves, and bears small white flowers in short axillary clusters, followed by red berries. From the dried, roasted leaves of this plant, the North American Indians made their famous black drink. This was in such demand at one time that the leaves formed an important article of trade among the different Indian tribes. Very strong doses were also administered in medicine for their emetic effects. The leaves are still substituted for tea in parts of the United States, especially along the south Atlantic coast. In Texas, where the shrub is common, it is generally known as Yaupon; other names include Cassena and Indian Black Drink.

The dried powdered leaves of the Dahoon Holly (*I. cassine*), a shrub native to the Atlantic and Gulf coasts of America, from Virginia to Louisiana, were also infused as a tea, and this was especially liked by the Creek Indians and, like the previous species, was administered in strong doses as an emetic.

Other Hollies used in North America as substitutes for Paraguay Tea include the Appalachian Tea or Evergreen Winterberry (*I. glabra*) which grows from Nova Scotia to Florida generally near the coast, and the Black American Alder (*I. verticillata*, syn. *Prinos verticillatus*).

The latter, a deciduous shrub, is found from Nova Scotia to Wisconsin, then south to Florida and Missouri and reaches from 1–3m/6–9ft in height. It has thin oval-lanceolate leaves bearing white flowers from May to July, followed by bright scarlet pea-sized berries in the autumn. The brownish-grey bark, collected before the first autumn frosts, was used by the North American Indians for its very astringent effects, and was

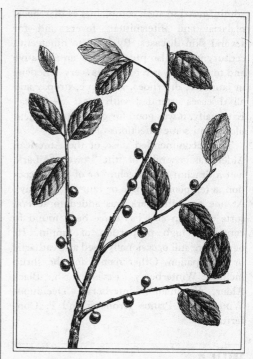

Ilex vomitoria

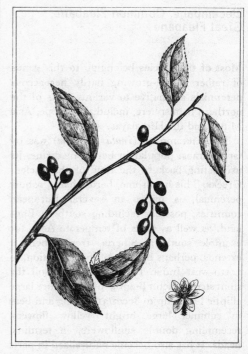

Ilex verticillata

administered in such complaints as diarrhoea, malarial and intermittent fevers and for several skin diseases. By the late nineteenth century it was also prescribed as an alterative and tonic, and was regarded as 'very beneficial in jaundice, diarrhoea, gangrene, dropsy and all diseases attended with great weakness'. Externally, it was good for gangrene, indolent ulcers and some infections of the skin.

The recommended dose of the American Alder was generally of the 'Powdered bark, half a drachm to a drachm' or of the 'decoction, a teaspoonful three or four times a day'. At one time the bark was added to several sorts of syrup and has since been found to contain a high proportion of tannin. Its berries are still occasionally used as a cathartic in constipation. Other names for the shrub include Winterberry, Fever Bush, Black Alder, Virginian Winterberry, Deciduous Winterberry, Prinos Gronovii and P. Confertus.

INULA

Compositae, the Daisy family
Elecampane, Common Fleabane,
Great Fleabane

Most of the species belonging to this genus of rather coarse-growing hardy herbaceous perennials are native to various parts of the northern hemisphere, including Europe, Asia Minor and the Himalayas.

The Elecampane (*Inula helenium*) was by far the most popular in herbal medicine, its use dating back to the time of the ancient Greeks. This handsome, hardy, hairy, robust perennial, is native to several European countries, possibly including southern England, as well as parts of temperate Asia, for example southern Siberia, from where it extends, perhaps because of its cultivation, to north-west India. In a good moist soil the stout stems reach 1½–2m/5–6½ft, produce large elliptic leaves up to 80cm/31in. long and bear in summer large bright yellow flowers, resembling double sunflowers, in terminal heads. It has also become naturalized in parts of North America, having escaped from

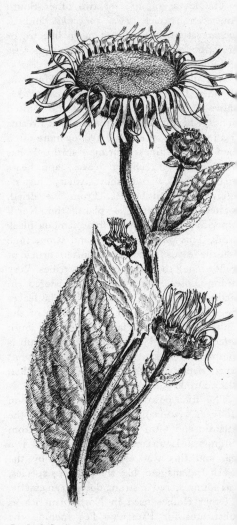

Inula helenium

cultivation. As in Europe, it is found main in damp meadows, pastures, copses an woods.

The generic name of this plant, Inula, i believed to be derived from the Gree *helenion*, the Latin version *helenium* formin its specific name. Several ancient legends exis as to the origin of this word, Gerard writin that it 'took the name Helenium of Helen wife of Menelaus, who had her hands full o it when Paris stole her away ...' Anothe version says 'it sprang from her tears'.

Both Galen and Dioscorides extolled it

medicinal virtues and Pliny prescribed the root 'being chewed fasting' to fasten the teeth, while Galen said it was good for sciatica, or as he called it 'passions of the hucklebone'. Other writers of this period prescribed the root for women's diseases, dropsy and phthisis, a wasting disease. The Romans ate the bitter brownish-grey fleshy root as a vegetable, or carefully preserved them for use as a condiment, or simply took them regularly for their soothing digestive effects.

The Anglo-Saxon chroniclers wrote of this plant as Hors-helne and made good use of it as a general tonic, both for themselves and their horses. It was widely cultivated in Norman England, as it was throughout the rest of Europe and parts of Asia, in kitchen and monastic gardens, and was given for all manner of ills and complaints. Decoctions of it were given 'to cure the scab of sheep', hence Scabwort, another common name, with Horse-Heal referring to its virtues in the treatment of cutaneous diseases of horses and cattle. The religious orders also used the root to help relieve a number of skin diseases, including 'leprosy, scab, the itch, putrid sores and cankers'.

Gerard prescribed it 'for shortnesse of breathe – and old cough', and for those that cannot breathe unless they hold their neckes upright'. He added: 'It is good for them that are bursten and troubled with cramps and convulsions.' Culpeper considered the fresh roots preserved with sugar, as 'one of the most beneficial roots nature affords for the help of the consumptive'.

The powdered root or extracts are still prescribed for coughs, often in combination with other herbs, and for similar pulmonary complaints. A pleasant tasting candy can be made from the roots, which is said to be good for asthma. The action of the root is said to be antiseptic, alterative, diaphoretic, diuretic, expectorant, stimulant and tonic.

In the United States, the root was administered both externally and internally in the treatment of skin diseases and as an embrocation for 'facial neuralgia – sciatica – and for other pains of the nerves'. One nineteenth-century writer said: 'It is much used in chronic pulmonary effections, weakness of the digestive organs, hepatic torpor, dyspepsia, etc.' The recommended internal dose at that time was: 'Of the powder, from one scruple to one drachm; of the infusion, one to two fluid ounces.' Joseph Taylor in *Nature the Best Physician* (1818), recommended the plant for coughs. The seed was also included in John Winthrop Junior's seed list.

The species' other names include Elf-Wort, Elf-Dock, Velvet-Dock and Wild Sunflower. The Welsh Physicians of the thirteenth century referred to it as Marchalan.

The dried, bitter, hoary leaves, or the root of the Common or Middle Fleabane (*I. dysenterica*, syn. *Pulicaria dysenterica*) were

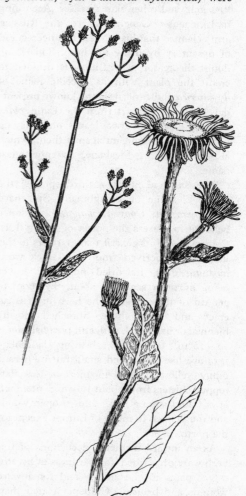

Inula dysenterica (right) and *I. conyza* (left)

formerly prescribed decocted or infused for their astringent principles. This is an erect and leafy, rough or shaggy looking perennial 20–60cm/7–23in. tall, the lance-shaped leaves clasp the stem with conspicuous basal lobes and bears from July to September long rayed, bright yellow daisy-like flowers, borne in loose more-or-less flat-topped clusters. It is found, often massed, in ditches, marshes, in wet meadows, by damp roadsides and in salt rich soils throughout most of Europe and temperate Asia, except for the north.

As a medicinal herb this species appears to have been little used in Britain, although once held in high regard by continental physicians, who prescribed it for relieving 'the itch' and other skin diseases. According to Linnaeus a General Keit of the Russian army claimed that his soldiers had been cured of dysentery by using the herb. This is no doubt the reason why Linnaeus decided to credit the plant with its specific name of *dysenterica*. Pulicaria, its better known present-day name, is derived from the Latin *pulex* meaning flea, the dried leaves once having been used as a fumigant against them, which also accounts for Fleabane, its commonest name.

The smell alone of a third species, the Great Fleabane or Ploughman's Spikenard (*I. conyza*, syn. *Conyza squarrosa*), was once believed to possess the power of killing fleas. Conyza, one of its generic names, refers to this use, and is derived from the Greek word meaning dust, its dried powdered leaves being burnt or scattered about the room to get rid of these pests. The herb itself is an erect and leafy, little branched downy biennial or perennial, with stiff purplish stems 20–120cm/7–47in. tall, bearing lanceolate foxglove-like leaves and small but numerous dingy yellow flowers in more-or-less flat-topped clusters from about July to September. It is found among rocks and in open woods and rough grass in much of Europe except for the north.

As an inward medicine decoctions of this herb were prescribed 'for hardness of breathing – pains in the side – and for inward wounds and bruises.' Culpeper stated that: 'The leaves when bruised, emit a quick and

aromatic smell. They are bitterish to the taste, with some sharpness ... A weak tea made of this herb is good to promote the menses, and much preferable to any mineral.'

Today, the Elecampane gives its generic name to a chemical substance known as Inulin, a white polysaccharide found in its roots, which is prescribed in the treatment of coughs.

IRIS
Iridaceae, the Iris family
Stinking Iris, Yellow Flag, German Iris, Florentine Iris, Blue Flag

The Iris genus as a whole consists of about 180 flowering species, native mostly to the temperate regions of Europe, Asia, Japan and America, which grow from bulbs, rhizomes and thickened rootstocks.

As cultivated herbs the use of the genus dates back to ancient times. One species, possibly *Iris florentina*, was represented in the Temple of Thutmosis III (1501–1447 B.C.) The Egyptians regarded the Irises as symbols of eloquence, carving them on the brow of the Sphinx and on the sceptres of their kings. Due to the beauty and colouring of the flowers the genus was named in honour of Iris, who in Greek mythology was the personification of the rainbow, and in Homer's *Iliad* the gods' messenger.

One of the species prescribed in ancient medicine and known to Theophrastus in 300 B.C., was the Stinking Iris or Gladwin (*I. foetidissima*) a native of the woods, shady banks and similar places of much of western Europe, including parts of the British Isles. With narrow, dark evergreen sword shaped leaves, it bears from May to July dull purplish occasionally yellowish, flowers on stems 50–80cm/19–31in. tall, followed by seed capsules which when ripe, split open to reveal their beautiful orange-red seeds. The common name of this hardy perennial refers to the smell its leaves emit if bruised or crushed, as does *foetidissima* its specific name. Culpeper writing of its odour, said the root, the part prescribed in medicine is 'very sharp and ho n the taste, and as evil scent as the leaves'. Hanbury on the other hand appears to have found the smell rather pleasant and described t as like a 'piece of roast beef'. By this period t had become commonly known as the Roast Beef Plant. Its names of Gladdon, Gladwyn and Gladwin evolved from the Anglo-Saxon *laedene* to *gladene* or *gladine* by Chaucer's time. Turner, writing in the sixteenth century, knew of it as the Xyris or Spourgewort (Spurgewort).

Medicinally the root had several uses. Decoctions would 'purge corrupt phlegm and choler'; the sliced roots and leaves added to ale 'serve well for weak stomachs'; and the juice 'snuffed up the nose causes sneezing and draws corruption from the head'. The powdered root added to and drunk in wine helps those that are troubled by cramps or convulsions – gout and sciatica – eases the griping pains of body and belly – helps the stranguary – and stays fluxes, by cleansing and purging them'. Culpeper advised that: 'The root boiled in wine procures womens' courses; and, used as a pessary works the

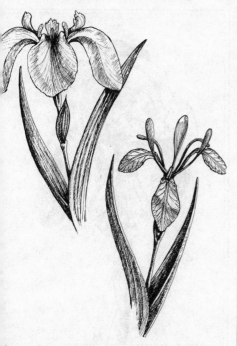

is pseudacorus (left) and *I. foetidissima* (right)

same effect but causes abortion to women with child.' He also wrote: 'The root used with a little verdigris and honey, and the great centuary root [*Centaurium*] is very effectual in all wounds, especially in the head, as also to draw forth any splinters or thorns, or any other thing, sticking into the flesh, without causing pain.'

The thick creeping fibrous rhizomes of this plant are still occasionally prescribed infused, or in powder from five to thirty grains, for their antispasmodic, anodyne and cathartic principles, mainly for relieving pain, cramps and convulsions, and for hysterical and other nervous conditions. It should however be used with caution, as it can act as a powerful purgative.

A more familiar species, the Yellow Flag (*I. pseudacorus*), is found in marshes, swamps, ditches and by the banks of lakes and ponds, throughout the whole of Europe (except Iceland), including the British Isles, western Asia, Siberia and North Africa. Its stiff, sword-shaped leaves reach 40–150cm/15–59in. growing from a fleshy rhizome, and from May to July, lateral terminal clusters of two or three yellow flowers with green spathes, are borne on stalks a little longer than the leaves.

The specific name of this Iris, *pseudacorus*, is derived from the Greek *pseudo*, meaning false, and *acorus*, because it resembles when not in flower *Acorus calamus*, the Sweet Flag or Sedge, a pleasantly scented plant once widely used for strewing floors, hence another of its names, False Acorus. In the past the Yellow Flag has been listed by many alternative names, from the Latin *Radix pseudacori* (*Radix* – root) to the Anglo-Saxon *Segg*, a small sword, *Cegg* and *Skegg*. Other names include Jacob's Sword, Flaggon, Meklin, Myrtle Flower, Myrtle Grass, Myrtle Root, Yellow Iris, Fliggers, Daggers, Gladdyn, Levers, Shalder, Dragon Flower and Fleur de Luce. The last name refers to the fact that the plant, as is generally accepted, was the origin of the Fleur de Lys, or Luce, of the French kings.

During the medieval period, the juice of the roots was prescribed throughout Europe much as for the previous species, as 'a reliable cure for the obstinate cough – convulsions and cramps' and on snuffing up the nose 'to cause violent sneezing'. Gerard wrote: 'The root of the common Floure de-luce cleane washed, and stamped with a few drops of Rose-water, and laid plaisterwise upon the face of man or woman, doth in two daies at the most take away the blacknesse or blewnesse of any stroke or bruse.'

Culpeper in the 1650s wrote that: 'The roots, which only are used, are hot and dry, opening and attenuating, and good for the obstructions of the liver and spleen.' They 'provoke urine and the menses, help the colic, resist putrefaction, are useful against pestelential contagions and corrupt noxious air . . .'

The very acrid tasting rhizomes of this plant, like those of the Stinking Iris can, if eaten, cause gastro-enteritis. It is only occasionally used internally nowadays, but is still administered as a lotion for its cooling and astringent principles, mainly in the treatment of leucorrhoea and dysmenorrhoea. Its ripe seed if roasted and ground makes a good coffee substitute. At one time a yellow dye was obtained from the flowers, while the root with sulphate of iron provided a Sabbath Black. The latter was also used as an ink in Scotland.

The German or Common Iris (*I. germanica*) had several medicinal uses. It is a handsome robust perennial, with bluish-green sword shaped leaves, and bears from April to June clusters of two or three large, scented, deep blue or bluish-violet flowers on stems up to 1m/3ft high. Native to southern Europe, it is now, however, often found naturalized elsewhere.

The sliced roots of this plant, like those of the Yellow Flag, were applied to the skin for their cosmetic effects, especially for the removal of freckles, while the crushed root 'taken in any convenient wine' became highly esteemed in the relief of dropsy. Culpeper wrote: 'boiled in water and drunk, it provokes urine, helps the colic, brings down womens' courses; and made up into a pessary with honey, and put up into the body, draws forth the dead child.'

Its other common names include Blue Flag, Garden Flag, Flag Iris, Common German

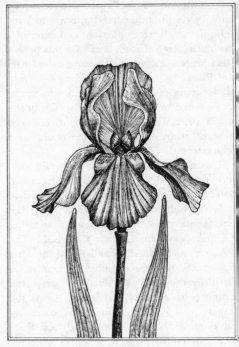

Iris germanica

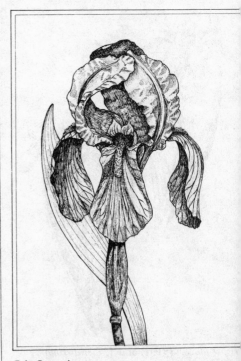

Iris florentina

Flag, Blue Flower de Luce or Blue Fleur de Lys.

A similar species, the Pale Iris (*I. pallida*), a native of the eastern Mediterranean region with delicate, pale blue sweetly scented flowers, was often used as a substitute for the German Iris. It is sometimes found naturalized, mostly in other parts of Europe.

The Snake's Head Iris or Widow Iris (*I. tuberosa*, syn. *Hermodactylus tuberosus*), also from the Mediterranean region, was prescribed as a cathartic in medicine and grows about 30cm/11in. tall, bearing in early spring purplish-brown flowers marked with greenish-yellow. It is occasionally found naturalized, for example, in southern England.

The Florentine Iris or Orris (*I. florentina*), robust perennial up to 60cm/23in. tall, bears from March to May large sweetly scented white flowers, tinged with pale blue. The powdered rhizomes of the plant were, and still are, added to many cosmetics. Although native to such countries as Spain, Italy, Greece and Yugoslavia, it is widely cultivated elsewhere and is sometimes found semi-naturalized.

The rhizomes of this plant when dug out of the ground, have very little smell, but as they gradually dry they develop their characteristic violet odour. When ready these were applied in toilet waters or plaisters' to 'clear bruises and minor skin diseases' and in the house 'were put upon the linnens as a perfume' and sometimes mixed with Anise (*Pimpinella anisum*), as mentioned in 1480 in the Wardrobe accounts of Edward IV of England.

As the common name of Florentine Iris, and the specific *florentina* suggest, this plant was, and still is, widely cultivated in Italy, although some of today's commercial crops are produced in other parts of Europe, and in Morocco, Mexico, and even India. The main present-day use of the dried root is as a fixative in perfumes and with its distinctive violet fragrance nearly all 'violet' perfumes are based on Orris Root.

Medicinally, the juice was prescribed often under the name of White Flower de Luce or Flower de Luce of Florence, as a powerful cathartic 'in the dropsy' and in a dry state for 'disorders of the lungs caused by sharp humours'. Millar wrote that 'it helps coughs, hoarseness and soreness at stomach – It is likewise commended against the gripes in children.' Well dried pieces of Verona Orris were occasionally given to teething babies to chew on, or were chewed 'to disperse bad breath'.

The fresh and acrid tasting roots, although classed as cathartic and diuretic, are rarely prescribed in internal medicines now as they can cause violent vomiting, nausea, colic and purging. The present day crops of Orris Root (*Rhizoma iridis*) are obtained from *Iris germanica*, *I. pallida* and *I. florentina*.

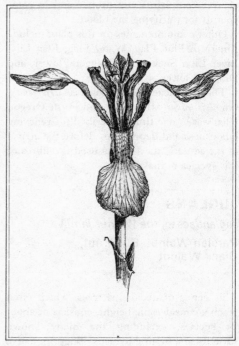

Iris versicolor

The fleshy, fibrous rhizomes of the Blue Flag (*I. versicolor*), a perennial native to the swamps and moist places of much of Canada and the United States, having sword shaped leaves 60–90cm/23–35in. high and bearing from May to July, large bluish-purple flowers, were formerly dried and used by the North American Indians as a cathartic and emetic.

During the latter half of the nineteenth century, this species became regarded as one of America's 'most valuable medicinal plants, capable of extensive use' and was widely prescribed as 'an alterative, cathartic, sialogogue, vermifuge and diuretic', and in scrofula and syphilis, acting 'as a powerful and efficient agent', and as useful 'in chronic hepatic, renal and splenitic affections'.

The active principle of the plant, which was officially prescribed in the medicine of the United States, was an oleo-resin known as Iridin, a nauseous and bitter substance with diuretic and aperient properties that act directly on the liver.

Liquid or solid extracts of the powdered root, or Iridin, is still given in the treatment of liver complaints and dropsy and in compounds for purifying the blood.

Other common names for this plant include American Blue Flag, Water Flag, Flag Lily, Liver Lily, Snake Lily, Dagger Flower, and Dragon Flower.

The American plant known as *Iris lenax*, syn. *Iris minor*, which is found in the Oregon hills, was at one time prescribed for relieving biliousness and depression. Before the arrival of the settlers, the Indians used the fibres of this species to make rope.

JUGLANS

Juglandaceae, the Walnut family
Persian Walnut, Butternut,
Black Walnut

This genus of deciduous trees, which often reach a considerable height, consists of about 15 species, excluding the many known varieties and natural hybrids. They are native mainly from south-east Europe to the Himalayas, through China and Manchuria to Japan and in both North and South America, besides being cultivated in many other countries, for example the West Indies, India and the British Isles.

The majority of the family are fairly large, generally rough-barked, nut-bearing trees, valued not only for these edible fruits, but also for their hard, dark, finely grained wood, while others are planted in gardens and parks simply as specimen trees.

The commonest Walnut of all is the Persian or English Walnut (*J. regia*), a large and handsome tree with a smooth, cool grey bark when young, which later becomes fissured and furrowed. It has large pinnate leaves divided into leaflets, which exude an aromatic fragrance if crushed; unisexual flowers are borne in early spring, just before or as the leaf-buds burst; the males form conspicuous pendulous catkins 5–15cm 2–6in. long, while the females are insignificant and succeeded by wrinkled nuts enclosed in a husk. In all probability this particular species is native to parts of south-east Europe, from Greece to Asia Minor, Iran, the Lebanon and the Caucasus through to the Himalayas, but is often found naturalized and widely cultivated elsewhere.

According to legend the gods lived on walnuts; hence *Jovis glans* – the Nuts of Jupiter or Jupiter's Nuts – which evolved to Juglans, the present-day generic name. The almost universal name of Walnut is believed to have evolved from Walsh-Nut, a name derived from the German *Wallnuss, Walshe nuss* or *Welsche Nuss, Welsche* meaning foreign. In Holland it is known as *Wallnoor*

It is uncertain when the tree was introduced into Britain; some authorities believing it was the middle of the sixteenth century. It was however, probably earlier, for Gerard writing at the close of that century described it as common in orchards and fields near the highways. It was certainly regarded as a very important tree in parts of Europe during the seventeenth century, for Evelyn observed that it abounded in Burgundy, saying: 'In several places betwixt Hanou and Frankfort in Germany no young farmer is permitted to marry a wife till he bring proof that he hath planted and is a father of such a number of trees.'

As a medicinal herb the Walnut was prescribed in several different forms. The dried and powdered bark, taken internally was regarded 'as a useful purgative' and at the same time was externally applied 'for varicose veins and their ulcers – herpes – eczema – carbuncles – the smallpox – scrofulous infections' and even 'leprosy and gangrenes'. The fresh green leaves in white

Juglans nigra (left), *Juglans regia* (centre),
Juglans cinerea (right)

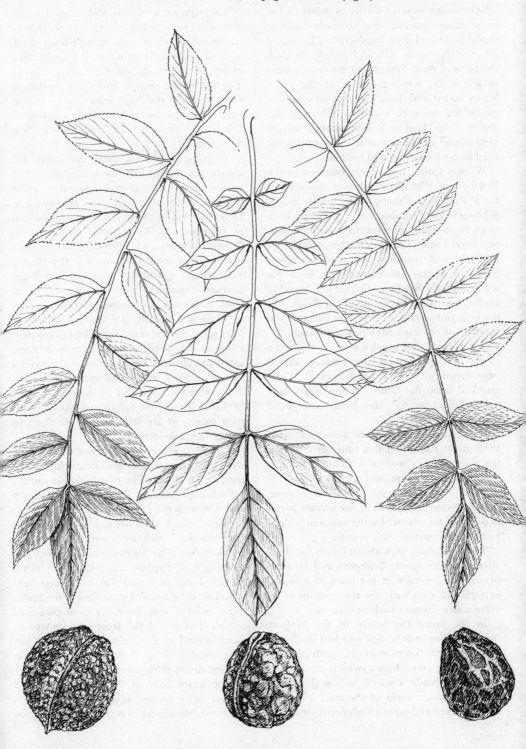

wine 'moves the belly downwards' and 'removeth the broad and other worms thereof'. The older leaves were harder to digest and in some cases 'grieved' the stomach 'causing choler – and violent headache'. The leaves taken with onions, salt and honey, 'helpeth the bites of mad dogges – or poisonous bites of any kind', while the juice of the green leaves boiled with honey 'makes an excellent gargle for the sore mouth – ulcers of the throat – the heat and inflammation of the same – and of the stomach'. The nuts were used in confectionery and baking.

William Coles, who firmly believed in the Doctrine of Signatures, likened the seed of the Walnut to the shape of the human brain. Writing in 1657 he observed: 'The outer husk or green covering represents the Pericranium, or outward skin of the skull, whereon the hair groweth, and therefore salt made of those husks or barks, are exceedingly good for wounds in the head . . .' The inner 'wooddy shell . . . hath the Signature of the Skull, and the little yellow skin, or Peel, that covereth the Kernell, of the hard Meninga and Pia-mater, which are the thin scarfes that envelope the brain.' He prescribed the bruised kernal 'moystoned with the quintessence of Wine, and laid upon the Crown of the Head' as a way of comforting 'the brain and head mightily.'

The root and bark were also prescribed throughout Europe at this time for 'fainting fits – hysteria in women – flatulent colic – rheumatism – stone and gravel – gout – jaundice – as a provider of milk in nursing mothers – for complaints of the private parts' and even for those having evidently 'exhausted themselves' with women.

The bark and leaves are still used for their alterative, astringent, detergent and laxative principles, generally in the form of a liquid extract and externally in the treatment of certain skin diseases such as eczema.

In the home the leaves of the Walnut 'repelleth flies and the flea' and laid in closets and cupboards 'keeps away the moth'. Boiled in water the green husks (which are rich in vitamin C) made a useful yellow dye. The light but tough wood of the tree, which is easily worked and takes a high polish, was and still is employed in the making of furniture and in inlaywork.

The ripe nuts of this and other species, although consumed as a food, also provide an edible oil, which is used for polishing wood, in cooking, or as lamp oil, in the preparation of artists' paints, and in the making of soap. The green and unripe fruits are pickled in vinegar, while the fresh leaves or green nut rind form the basic ingredient of Walnut Cordial or wine, both making excellent aperitifs.

A second Walnut, the Butternut (*J. cinerea*), a native of North America, had several medicinal uses and is found, often in cold and rocky soils, from New Brunswick to Delaware and in the mountain regions south to Georgia and Mississippi, then west to Dakota, Kansas and Arkansas. This species reaches from about 15–20m/49–65ft high, has a few wide spreading branches, and bears alternate compound leaves 40–60cm/15–23in. long, with each leaf composed of from eleven to seventeen leaflets. Its catkins appear in May when the leaves are about half developed, followed by hard, deeply furrowed nuts, usually in clusters of two to five, each covered by a thin husk with numerous sticky hairs. These when still soft and green are made into 'pickled oil nuts' for eating as a winter relish with meats, or are left to ripen on the tree before being collected.

The parts generally prescribed in medicine were the bitter, slightly acid inner bark of the root, or the leaves. The root bark was usually collected in May or June, powdered down and administered 'as a gentle and agreeable cathartic' which 'does not induce constipation after its use' and is recorded as having considerable value 'in habitual constipation – dysentery – hypatic congestions – other intestinal diseases' and 'for old ulcers and syphilitic conditions'. Decoctions of the leaves 'relieves fever' and 'the murrain or plague of cattle'. The oil of the fruit was sometimes administered as a vermifuge to 'remove the tapeworm' and as a counter-irritant, was applied direct to the skin.

The inner bark of the root of this and several other species, is still prescribed as a cathartic, tonic and vermifuge, generally in liquid or solid extracts or in syrups and pills. The sweet sap of the tree is sometimes added to that of the Sugar Maple or Bird's Eye Maple (*Acer saccharinum*) in the making of sugars and syrups.

The inner bark was often employed by the early immigrants to dye wool a dark brown or tan. The husks of the fruits of both this and the Black Walnut were also used for this, particularly by some of the regiments during the American Civil War to dye their army uniforms. Other names for the Butternut include the White Walnut and Oil Nut.

The Black Walnut (*J. nigra*), another North American species, had several uses besides being valued for its timber. It is usually found alongside hedges and roads, or in the borders of woods from Massachusetts to Minnesota, south to Florida and Texas. It often reaches 35m/113ft or more in height, develops large wide spreading branches, a dark brown, ridged and furrowed bark, and bears large, dark green compound leaves. Its catkins resemble those of the Butternut, although the shells of the nuts are generally so thick and hard they are difficult to crack open. The nuts were eaten by the Indians, while their aromatic husks were used in dyeing and tanning. The kernels are nowadays added to ice-cream and confectionery, mostly in the United States. During the nineteenth century the Black Walnut was precribed more or less as for the previous species, while the 'juice of the rind' cures 'herpes, eczema, porrigo, etc., and a decoction of it has been used to remove worms'.

Other species used by the North American Indians, include the Texas Walnut (*J. rupestris*) which has small, thickly shelled nuts much liked by the Mexicans and Indians of that region; the California Walnut (*J. califronica*) with small, sweet tasting, thinly shelled nuts, and *J. kindsii*. The latter is mainly found growing in the vicinity of old Indian camp sites in central California. Certain other species have from time to time been prescribed in medicine, including the Japanese Walnut (*J. sieboldiana*).

KRAMERIA
Polygalaceae, the Milkwort family
Rhatany

Most of the species belonging to this genus, named after J. G. H. and W. H. Kramer, the German botanists, are bushy many-stemmed shrubs, native to various parts of South America.

The most familiar medicinal kind, the Rhatany (*K. triandra*), a native of the dry sandy and gravelly hills of Peru and parts of Bolivia, is a fairly low-growing shrub, with hoary alternate leaves, and a long more-or-

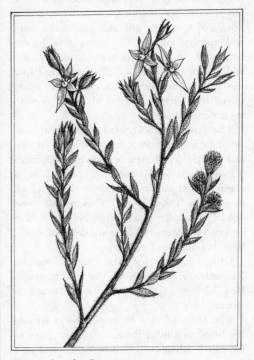

Krameria triandra

less horizontal root. It has a round procumbent stem with branches up to 1m/3ft long and bears for much of the year large red flowers on short stalks, followed by dry hairy fruits or drupes.

The roots of this plant provide the medicinal part and were first made official by Ruiz in 1780, although the natives of Peru and

Bolivia had used them for many years for their astringent principles in the treatment of 'various diseases, afflictions, maladies and complaints'. They were dug up after the rains, and more often than not exported in bulk to Portugal, where they were used to adulterate red wines. Strong tinctures in brandy are still used there to add roughness to various ports.

Extracts of the powdered root were prescribed for its 'powerful astringent and slightly tonic effects.' Taken internally it was 'found useful in chronic diarrhoea and dysentery – mucous discharges and menstrual disorders – menorrhagia – haematuria – incontinence of urine – and passive haemorrhages'. Infusions were also used as a wash for 'the mucous membranes of the eyes and nose' and to relieve 'the bleeding of the teeth and spongy gums'. The same was locally employed 'in prolapsus ani – leucorrhoea – and fissure of the anus'. The powdered root was at one time used as a dentifrice, when mixed with Orris Root and charcoal, or with myrrh and chalk.

The principal constituent of the root, once listed in both the Pharmacopoeias of Britain and the United States, is known as Rhatania Tannic Acid or Krameria Tannic Acid, a compound crystalline substance closely allied to Catechu Tannic Acid. This is still prescribed, generally as an intestinal astringent, in syrups, lozenges, concentrated solutions, tinctures and solid extracts.

Other names for this shrub include Rhatanhia, Krameria Root, Peruvian Rhatany, Red Rhatany, Pumacuchu and Ratanhiawurzel.

The roots of two other Krameria species are listed as official in medicine, the Para or Brazilian Rhatany (*K. argentea*) and the Savanilla Rhatany (*K. ixene*). The Texan Rhatany (*K. lanceolata*) is very rich in tannin and was at one time used as an astringent by the North American Indians.

LEONURUS
Labiatae, the Mint family
Motherwort

This small genus of biennial or perennial herbs is native principally to parts of Europe, where they are found in waste places, in hedges and by the wayside. Of these only one, the Motherwort (*L. cardiaca*), appears to have been prescribed in medicine. Stout, erect and slightly downy, this dark green,

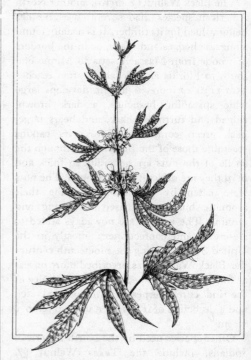

Leonurus cardiaca

leafy, unbranched perennial 50–120cm/19–47in. tall, bears from June to September aromatic whorls of spotted two-lipped pinkish, white or pale purplish flowers in leafy spikes.

The specific name of this plant, *cardiaca*, a Latin word, points to one of its more ancient medicinal uses and is derived from the Greek *kardia*, the heart, for which the whole of the bitter-tasting herb was prescribed throughout Europe and parts of the Mediterranean region, for, as Gerard said: 'Divers commend it against infirmities of the heart.' Other apothecaries agreed and prescribed it to 'help women in sore travail – for inward tremors – as a tonic in female diseases' and 'for the suffocating or rising of the mother'. The same 'provoketh womens' courses – cleanseth the chest of cold phlegm – warms and dries up cold humours that settle in the body – helps cramps and convulsions – and kills the worms of the belly'.

This particular species was introduced as a medicinal herb to North America from Europe, where it soon escaped from cultivation and naturalized itself in the wild, mainly in the eastern parts of the United States, where it is now found in fields and pastures. It was prescribed there much as it was in Europe for its 'emmenagogue, nervine and laxative principles'. During the nineteenth century it was regarded in both Britain and the United States as a valuable and versatile remedy.

It is still prescribed infused, or in powders and as liquid and solid extracts, in the treatment of some of the womens' complaints listed above, and in tonics for weakness and hysteria, irritability and various uterine complaints.

The botanical name of this genus, Leonurus, a Greek word, refers to a lion's tail which the different species supposedly resemble, hence Lion's Tail and Lion's Ear, two more common names.

LEVISTICUM
Umbelliferae, the Parsley family
Garden Lovage

Although found wild in the hedges and meadows of the mountainous districts in most of Europe and western Asia, the Garden Lovage (*L. officinale*, syn. *Ligusticum levisticum*) probably originated from such Mediterranean areas as the mountains of southern France, northern Greece, Liguria in Italy and the Balkans. Its erect and robust stems reach 1–2m/3–6ft high, have large bipinate leaves, and bear umbels of greenish-yellow flowers from July to August.

The leaf-stalks and the bases of the stem

were blanched and added to salads as a vegetable, while the young stems were candied like angelica, or were added to give a celery-like flavour to soups and stews.

As a medicinal herb the whole of this odorous plant, with its warm, aromatic taste, was put to good use. Culpeper wrote that: 'It opens, cures and digests humours, and provokes womens' courses and urine. Half a dram at a time of the dried root in powder taken in wine, warms a cold stomach, helps digestion and consumes all raw and superflous moisture therein; eases all inward gripings and pains, dissolves wind, and

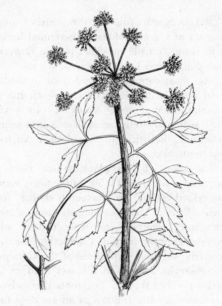

Levisticum officinale

resists poison and infection.'

Gerard advised that: 'The distilled water of Lovage cleareth the sight and putteth away all spots, lentils, freckles and rednesse of the face, if they be often washed therewith.' Lovage cordial was also prescribed for children suffering from colic, obstruction, feverish attacks, various stomach disorders and to promote perspiration. The fresh leaves eaten in salads, or dried and later infused as a tea, were said to promote the menstrual flow.

The thick and fleshy carrot-like root of the Lovage has a sweet but slightly bitter taste, and is still administered for its diuretic and carminative principles, mainly in the treatment of febrile and stomach disorders, and in dysmenorrhoea.

Other names for the plant include English Lovage, Old English Lovage, Italian Lovage and Cornish Lovage. (For the Sea or Scotch Lovage, see *Ligusticum*).

LIATRIS

Compositae, the Daisy family
Blazing Star, Button Snakeroot, Deer's Tongue

Native to North America, the Liatris family consists of a group of hardy perennial herbs with showy purple or violet-purple flowers, arranged in long loose spikes.

The most common species used in medicine, the Blazing Star (*L. squarrosa*), has a tuberous root, stout stems 1–1½m/3–5ft high with many long narrow leaves, and bears flowers of a beautiful purple colour in August and September.

The roots of this plant, which have a turpentine odour and a hot bitter taste, were prescribed during the nineteenth century for their diuretic, emmenagogue, tonic and stimulant principles and were usually administered in the form of a decoction 'for the gonorrhoea – gleet – affections of the kidneys' as 'of service in uterine diseases' and as 'a gargle for sore throat'. The roots themselves were used by the Indians as an antidote for rattlesnake bite, this giving rise to Rattlesnake's Master, one of its more common names. Other names include Gay Feather, Devil's Bit and Colic Root.

A second and similar species also known as Gay Feather or Blazing Star (*L. spicata*), again referring to its handsome flowers, was administered in the herbal medicine of North America, where it is mostly found in moist fields from Minnesota and southern Ontario southwards, growing up to 1m/3ft high.

Its somewhat tuberculate rhizomes have a warm, bitter taste and, medicinally, were regarded as stimulant and diuretic. They were 'locally applied in the treatment of sore throat – gonorrhoea – snakebite – and as

beneficial in Bright's Disease [a kidney infection] and other diseases of those parts.'

The decocted or infused roots of the herb, which is also known as Button Snakeroot, Backache Root, Devil's Bit or Colic Root, are still prescribed and are generally taken internally, three or four times a day as a diuretic.

The tuberous roots of a third Liatris (*L. scariosa*), again known as Gay Feather, were

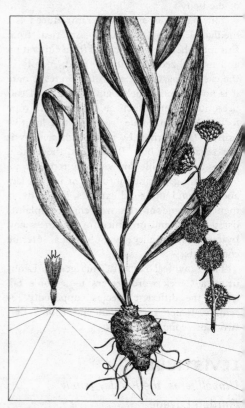

Liatris squarrosa

formerly prescribed for snakebites much as the other species. The leaves of a fourth species, the Deer's Tongue (*L. odoratissima*, syn. *Trilisia odoratissima* or *T. odorata*), were administered for their demulcent, diaphoretic, diuretic, stimulant and tonic effects. The fleshy oblong basal leaves, along with those of several other kinds, were and still are, used to flavour tobacco, having when dried a sweet smell of new mown hay, due to the presence of Coumarin. This plant is often listed as Vanilla Leaf or Wild Vanilla.

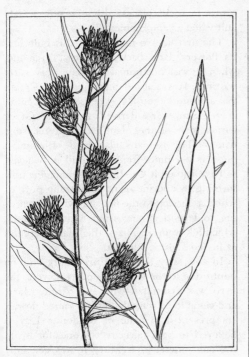

Liatris scariosa

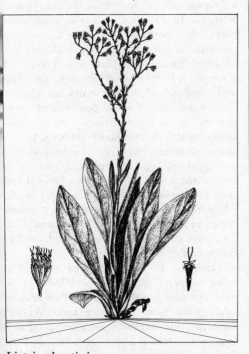

Liatris odoratissima

LIGUSTICUM
Umbelliferae, the Parsley family
Sea Lovage

Only one or two of the Ligusticum genus appear to have been prescribed in the medicine of medieval Europe, one of the more familiar species being the Sea Lovage (*L. scoticum*). This stocky, bright green, glossy,

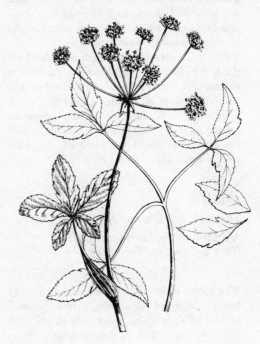

Ligusticum scoticum

leathery-leaved, leafy perennial 15–80cm/ 6–31in. tall, with a stout, strongly scented rootstock, and stiff, ribbed, little branched stems, usually purplish coloured near the base, bears umbels of greenish-white or pink flushed flowers in July. A native of Scotland and northern Europe, it grows mostly on cliffs by the sea, by rocky shorelines and river mouths.

In the past the rather unpleasant tasting leaves of this species, under the name of Shunis, were eaten as a vegetable in parts of Scotland, including the Hebrides and the Isle of Skye. It is still occasionally used there to add a strong celery-like flavour to soups and stews.

As a medicine only the aromatic roots of the Sea Lovage, also known as the Northern Lovage and Scotch Parsley, were prescribed and then mainly for 'easing the griping pains of the stomach – expelling flatulence – and for hysterical and uterine complaints in women'. The boiled leafstalks eaten as a vegetable were regarded as 'most beneficial' for relieving the scurvy in sailors. The seeds also had their uses and were given for their stimulant and carminative principles, and are still employed by herbalists to improve the flavour of some of their medicines.

Other species once used medicinally include the Colorado Root (*L. filicinum*), a native of the north-western parts of the United States, administered for its stimulant and expectorant principles, and the root of the perennial known as Kao-Pau (*L. sinense*) which is still prescribed in China for some of the complaints listed above (see *Levisticum*).

LILIUM

Liliaceae, the Lily family

Madonna Lily, Martagon Lily, Turk's Cap Lily, Tiger Lily

The Lilies make up a large genus of mostly hardy, beautiful flowering plants, characterized by scaly bulbs, erect leafy stems, with bell-like, cup or funnel shaped flowers. They are native to the temperate regions of both hemispheres, although the greatest number come from Asia Minor. About 85 species are known, their habitats varying from very poor soil in full sun, to shady positions in rich forest leaf-mould, while a few prefer swamps or alpine country. The length of their flower stems also varies, from a few inches to over 3m/9ft, for example the Giant Himalayan Lily (*L. giganteum*).

The aristocrat of the genus is generally regarded as the Madonna Lily (*L. candidum*) from the Mediterranean region. Its erect leafy stems reach 1½m/5ft and bear from May to July very large, sweetly scented brilliant white funnel shaped flowers. It generally grows in rocky places, although now widely cultivated as an ornamental.

The first known mention of this bulb and its flowers dates back to at least 2350 B.C. when it was mentioned in some very early writings. It was also depicted on some Cretan vases around 1500 B.C. The generic, Lilium, is a Latin word derived from the Greek *leirion*, one of the plant's earliest recorded names. The Romans also made Lirium, a popular perfume, from it. Virgil is believed to have named it Candidium – *candidum* now forming its specific name – meaning pure or white, referring to the flowers, which according to legend sprang from a drop of milk which fell from the lips of the infant Hercules as he fed at Juno's breast.

In the early days of Christianity and no doubt due to the whiteness of its flowers, the herb was associated with the Virgin Mary, and came to be regarded as her sacred flower. Its present-day name of Madonna Lily is believed to be a fairly recent one, for up to the late nineteenth century it was generally known as the White or White Garden Lily.

As a medicinal herb the use of the Madonna Lily goes back to the time of the Greeks and Romans. In Pliny's day it was a common plant, the Romans employing it for the complexion and feet complaints. During the medieval period, the plant was prescribed throughout Europe for its 'emolient, suppling and anodyne' effects for many complaints. The roots and flowers first boiled were applied 'to dissolve and ripen hard tumours, inflammations and swellings – to break boils – imposthumations' and 'to cleanse foul and rotten ulcers'. As an 'excellent remedy in pestilential fevers' the roots were bruised and boiled in wine and the decoction drunk, while the roasted roots with hog's grease 'ripen and break plague and fever sores'. The latter was also applied to 'scald heads' and to 'unite cuts or contracted sinews'.

According to Culpeper: 'the juice of it being tempered with barley meal baked, is an excellent cure for the dropsy.' This remedy could have been borrowed from William Godorus, the Sergeant Surgeon to Queen Elizabeth I, who is known to have baked the juice into cakes for treating this particular

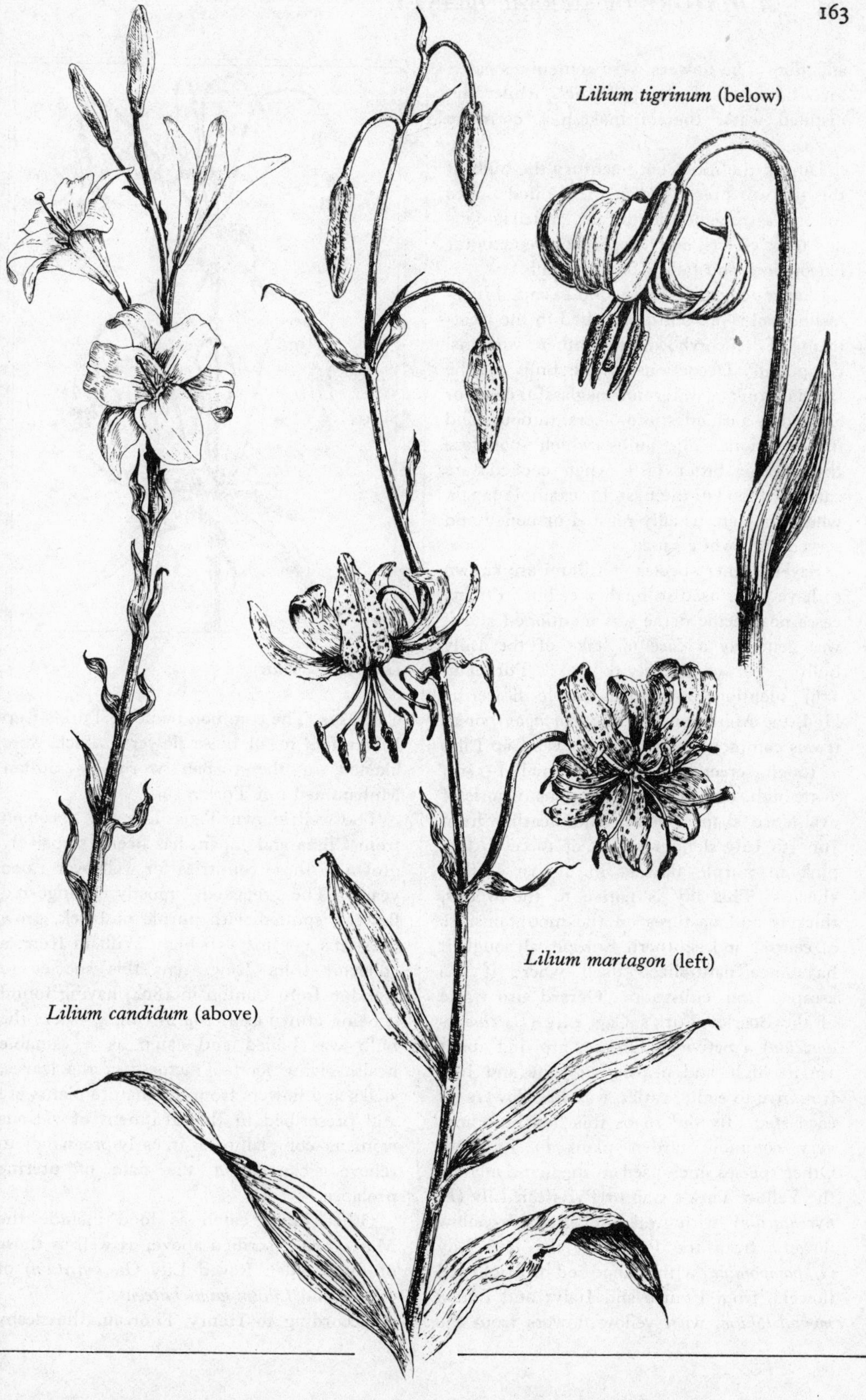

Lilium tigrinum (below)

Lilium martagon (left)

Lilium candidum (above)

affliction. The flowers were sometimes eaten for 'the fittes of the epileptic', while 'the distilled water thereof maketh a cosmetic wash'.

During the nineteenth century the bulb of this lily was prescribed in the United States for its 'astringent, demulcent, mucilaginous and tonic effects' and 'as a certain remedy for leucorrhoea and falling of the womb.'

The mucilaginous and unpleasant, bitter-tasting bulbs are still prescribed in the treatment of leucorrhoea and other womens' complaints. Decoctions of the bulb can be taken in milk or water in wineglassful doses or applied as a cataplasm to ulcers, tumours and inflammations. The bulbs, which soon lose their rather bitter taste when cooked, are eaten as a food in the East, for example Japan, where they are usually roasted or boiled and served with white sauce.

Several other species of Lilium are known to have been used in medicine, but in many cases no specific name was mentioned and it was generally a case of 'take of the Lilly bulb . . .' or 'of the Lily root . . .'. Turner in 1568 mentions a reddish-purple flowering kind, the Martagon Lily (*L. martagon*), or as it was commonly called the Turk's Cap Lily, a rough, erect, hairless perennial 1–1½m/ 3–5ft high, with red-spotted stems, whorls of oval-lance shaped leaves and bearing from June to July slender spikes of three to ten, pink to purple flowers in almost leafless clusters. This lily is native to the woods, thickets and pastures on the mountainsides of central and southern Europe, although it has since naturalized itself where it has escaped from cultivation. Gerard also wrote of the Scarlet Turk's Cap Lily (*L. chalcedonicum*) a native of Greece, growing about 1m/3ft high, and bearing in June and July from five to eight scarlet, wax-like flowers on each stem. By the 1630s this had become a very common garden plant in England. Other species once used in medicine include the Yellow Turk's Cap or Pyrenean Lily (*L. pyrenaicum*) with wax-like greenish-yellow flowers, from the Pyrenees; the Red Lily (*L. pomponium*) with orange-red or bright red flowers, from France and Italy; and *Lilium monadelphum*, with yellow flowers from the

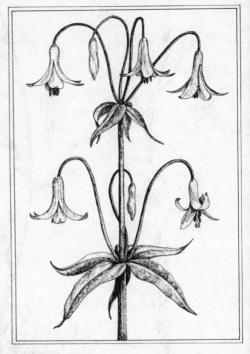

Lilium canadense

Caucasus. The common name of Turk's Cap Lily refers to all these flowers, which were likened to the turban worn by Sultan Muhammed I of Turkey.

The well known Tiger Lily (*L. tigrinum*) from China and Japan, has been extensively grown in those countries for well over 1,000 years. The reflexed, mostly orange-red flowers, spotted with purple or black, grow on stems 1–1½m/3–5ft high. William Kerr, a collector from Kew, sent this species to London from Canton in 1804, having found it being grown as a crop in China, where the bulb was boiled and eaten as a valuable health-giving food. Tinctures of the leaves, stalks and flowers from the mature plants are still prescribed in the treatment of various womens' complaints, as in early pregnancy to relieve sickness, or the pain of uterine prolapse.

Other bulbs eaten as food include the Martagons described above, as well as those of the Golden Rayed Lily (*L. auratum*) of Japan, and *Lilium kamschatcense*. According to Henry Thoreau, the fleshy bulbs of the Swamp or American Turk's Cap Lily (*L. superbum*) were eaten by the North American Indians, who sometimes used them to thicken soups and gruels. This beautiful Lily produces orange-red flowers flushed with crimson in July and August, and is generally found on the banks of streams and similar places, from New Brunswick to Minnesota, south to North Carolina and Missouri. The bulbs of a second North American species, the Wild Yellow or Canada Lily (*L. canadense*), were also cooked and eaten by the Indians, and like the previous plant, were bruised and applied to inflammations, tumours and swellings. This beautiful Lily is found in woodlands, meadows and low ground, from Nova Scotia to Minnesota, south to Georgia and Missouri, and flowers in July. There are two distinct forms of this plant, one with golden yellow flowers, the other with orange-red.

LINARIA

Scrophulariaceae, the Figwort family

Common Toadflax, Ivy Leaved Toadflax, Male Fluellin, Sharp Leaved Fluellin

At least 130 species of Linaria are known. This genus of hardy annual, but mostly perennial herbs and a few sub-shrubs with whorled or opposite leaves is widely native in the northern hemisphere and South America.

The generic name of this group, Linaria, is derived from the Latin *linon* or *linum*, meaning Flax and refers to *Linum usitatissimum*, because the leaves of some of the species resemble that plant. This is especially marked in the Common Toadflax (*L. vulgaris*), an erect and handsome glaucous perennial 30–80cm/11–31in. tall, with linear leaves and several erect leafy stems, which bear from June to the end of the summer bright spikes of rich yellow orange-tipped flowers. It is found throughout Europe on banks, in hedges, waste places and by the wayside, generally in sandy, gravelly or chalky soils. On its introduction into North America,

possibly in shipments of grain or coal, it soon spread to become a troublesome weed along roadsides and railways.

Its commonest name, Toadflax, is believed to refer to its flowers, as these are fashioned like a 'a toad or frog's mouth . . . from whence it has taken like the Antirrhinum, the name of the Snapdragon'. Gerard called the Linaria 'a kind of Antyrrhinum,' having small, slender, blackish stalks 'from which do grow many long narrow leaves like flax. The flowers be yellow with a spurre hanging at the same like unto a Larkesspurre, having a mouth like unto a frog's mouth, even such as it is to be seene in the common Snapdragon.' Coles believed the plant was called Toadflax because toads sometimes sheltered 'themselves among the branches of it'. Other names include Pattens and Clogs, Eggs and Bacon, Churnstaff, Brideweed, Dragon Bushes, Yellow Rod, Devil's Ribbon, Devil's Head, Pedlar's Basket, Toad, Eggs and Collops, Rabbits, Doggies, Buttered Haycocks, Yellow Toadflax and Ramsted.

As a medicinal herb, Dodoens tells us that the Toadflax was used during the sixteenth

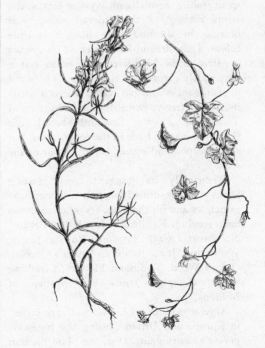

Linaria vulgaris (left) and *L. cymbalaria* (right)

century to relieve the hot swellings of buboes, while Tragus said it removed the obstructions of liver and spleen, and carried away the water of dropsies. The juice alone 'healeth foul ulcers, whether they are cancerous or not – if the parts be washed or injected therewith', and when mixed with 'the powder of lupines' it cleanses the skin of 'spots – pimples – scurf – wheals – morphew – leprosy – and other deformities'. The water distilled from the herb 'is a certain remedy for the heat, redness and inflammation of the eyes, being simply dropped into them', and the 'whole herb chopped and boiled in the grease of old hog until green, maketh an excellent application for the piles, ugly sores and eruptions of the skin'.

The whole of the herb, gathered just as it comes into flower, is still prescribed for its astringent, detergent and hepatic principles, mainly for jaundice, liver troubles and various skin diseases. Its active constituents are two glycosides known as Linarin and Pectolinarian.

The Ivy Leaved or Wall Toadflax (*L. cymbalaria*, syn. *Cymbalaria muralis*) is a small trailing annual with ivy-like leaves, the stems rooting as they spread along, and bearing in summer pale lilac to purple coloured snapdragon-like flowers. This species is native to the Mediterranean region, but is now widely naturalized elsewhere. It is found in damp rocks and old walls, where it seeds itself very freely, hence its name Mother of Thousands. It was first introduced into Britain as a salad herb in the early 1600s, but soon escaped and spread rapidly itself in the wild.

Medicinally its pungent, acrid tasting leaves were prescribed for their anti-scorbutic principles and for diabetes. Its other common names include Kenilworth Ivy, Italian Bastard Navelwort (1633), Ivywort, Roving Jenny, Wandering Jew, Rabbits, Pedlar's Basket, Oxford Weed, Thousand Flowers, Climbing Sailor, Creeping Jenny and Mother of Millions.

At least two other Linarias were prescribed in Europe and Britain during the medieval period as astringents. One, the Male Fluellin or Round Leaved Fluellen (*L. spuria*, syn.

Kickxia spuria), is a low, often prostrate softly haired annual, with roundish or oval alternate leaves, which bears from June to September solitary yellow flowers with maroon upper lips on slender downy stalks at the base of the leaves. It is found in dry places and cultivated ground. The other, the Sharp Leaved Fluellin (*L. elatine*, syn. *Kickxia elatine*), is a similar but more slender plant, with triangular upper leaves and small pale yellow flowers with deep violet-purple upper lips and throats. Both plants can be found in most of Europe, often growing together, although in the north they are introductions.

The Sharp Leaved Fluellin, known also as Fluellin or the Sharp-Pointed Fluellon or Toad Flax, was prescribed during the sixteenth and seventeenth centuries as 'a vulnery plant – and accounted good for fluxes and haemorrhages of all sorts' and was administered 'to hot watery and inflamed eyes – as also fluxes of blood or humours – as the lax, bloody, flux, womens' courses' and to 'stay all manner of bleeding at nose, mouth, or any

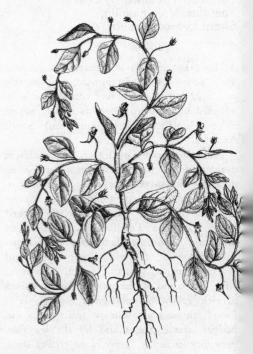

Linaria spuria

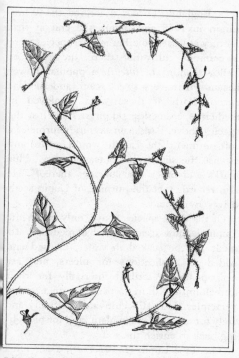

Linaria elatine

other place, or that comes by any other bruise or hurt – or the bursting of veins'.

It is still occasionally prescribed infused for its astringent principles, and is taken or applied for the relief of nose bleeds, internal bleeding and for excessive menstruation.

LUPINUS

Leguminosae, the Pea family

White Lupin, Tree Lupin,
Blue Bean

About 300 species make up this genus of annual, herbaceous or shrubby perennial plants, which have divided leaves and bear long spikes of handsome flowers ranging in colour from white to pink, red to yellow and blue. The majority are native to the western parts of North America, at least 65 to California alone, with others to South America, Europe and western Asia.

The species most frequently prescribed in ancient medicine was the White Lupin (L. *albus*), an erect growing annual 15–100cm/ 6–39in. high, with deeply cut palmate leaves, and bearing lax terminal spikes of white flowers tippéd with blue in May or June, followed by pods 7–10cm/2–4in. long, each containing 3 to 6 white, flattened seeds. Although probably native to the south-eastern parts of Europe and western Asia, this species has since been introduced to several other countries and become naturalized. A sub-species listed as *graecus,* with bright blue flowers, is also found in the Balkans and the Aegean region.

The use of this plant dates back to the time of the ancient Egyptians who are known to have grown it, as did the Romans, who valued it not only as an article of food, but as a general fertilizer on the land and as a cattle food. Their womenfolk used the powdered seed as a skin cosmetic. In the third century B.C. Protogenus, the famous painter of Rhodes, lived on nothing but Lupins and water for seven years while painting a hunting scene, simply to keep his mind active and for inspiration.

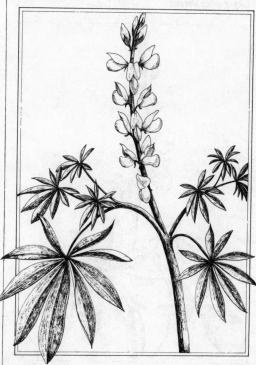

Lupinus albus

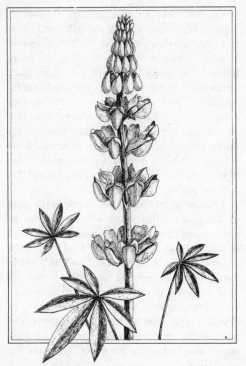

Lupinus arboreus

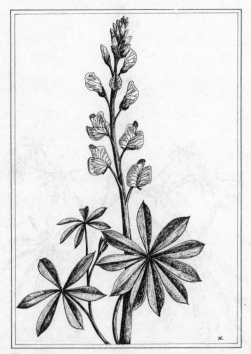

Lupinus perennis

In England, Turner described the White Lupin in 1568 and before the end of that century at least two other annual species were in common cultivation there, the Sweet or Yellow Lupin (*L. luteus*), a popular flower because of its very sweet scent, and *Lupinus varius*. Both of these were employed in medicines, cosmetics and physics much as the species above. Parkinson says in 'a forme of a soft ointment' the Lupin 'would scoure and cleanse the skin from spots, morphew, blue marks and other discolourings thereof'. He also records that the burning of Lupin seeds drives away gnats.

Of the three species above, only the White Lupin is now used in herbal medicine. Its seeds can be soaked in water, bruised and added to applications for ulcers, and are occasionally prescribed internally for their anthelmintic, diuretic and emmenagogue principles. It is still cultivated in Sicily and Italy for use as a forage plant, and for ploughing back to enrich the soil.

The Tree Lupin (*L. arboreus*), a perennial North American species, was not discovered until 1792, when it was found growing in California and subsequently in Oregon. When introduced to Britain and other parts of Europe it quickly became naturalized.

The perennial kinds of Lupin do not appear to have been much prescribed in medicine, although their seed was often added to skin cosmetics, especially during the seventeenth and eighteenth centuries. The seeds of the Wild Lupin, Wild Bean or Blue Bean (*L. perennis*) as it is known, a North American species ranging from Maine to Minnesota then south to Florida and Louisiana, were formerly used in medicine there by the Indians and are still occasionally cooked and eaten like peas. Eating the seeds in any amount, however, can cause poisoning, and in quantity will slow the pace of the heart and cause respiratory troubles. Some of the species contain alkaloids which are not destroyed by drying or storage.

The generic name of Lupinus is derived from the Latin *lupus*, a wolf. The meaning of this is obscure, but it could refer to the early belief that the deep rooting nature of these plants had an impoverishing effect on the soil

Overleaf *Lysimachia vulgaris* (left) and
Lysimachia nummularia (below)

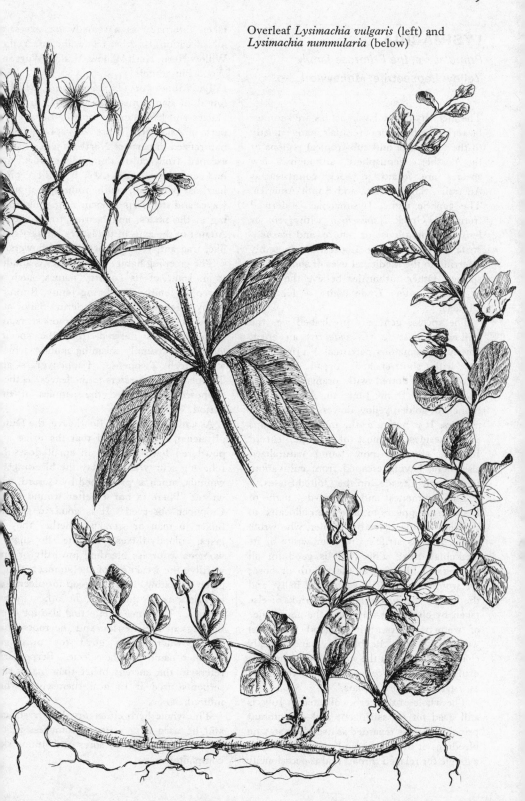

LYSIMACHIA

Primulaceae, the Primrose family
Yellow Loosestrife, Moneywort

The majority of the Lysimachias are summer flowering herbaceous perennials, native mostly to the temperate and sub-tropical regions of the northern hemisphere, although a few species are found in such countries as Australia, South Africa and South America. The generic name, Lysimachia, is derived from the Greek *lysimachion* with *lyein* or *lysis* – meaning loose or relieve, and *mache* – strife or battle, thus Loosestrife, possibly referring to the medicinal uses of some of the species. Other authorities believe the genus is named after Lysimachus, a King of Thracia.

The species generally prescribed was the Yellow Loosestrife (*L. vulgaris*) an erect, downy, rhizomatous perennial ½–1½m/1½–5ft tall with short-stalked, broad lanceolate leaves, often dotted with orange or black, and bearing from June to August, lax, branched, golden yellow flowers in pyramidal clusters. It is native to the marshes, swamps and lakesides of most of Europe, except Iceland, although now found naturalized elsewhere, having escaped from cultivation, for example Canada and the United States.

The commonest and present-day name of Loosestrife appears to have been allocated to the plant in the 1550s by Turner, who wrote of it as 'Lous strife'. Culpeper wrote of its medicinal uses: 'This herb is good for all manners of bleeding at the mouth or nose; for wounds, and all fluxes of the belly, and the bloody flux, given either to drink, or else taken by clyster; it stays also the abundance of womens courses; it is good for green wounds, to stay the bleeding, and quickly closes up the lips of the wound, if the herb be bruised and the juice only applied. It is good as a gargle for sore throats.'

The whole of the herb, collected in July, is still used for its astringent and expectorant principles and is regarded as useful for staying bleedings at the mouth and nose, wounds, as a gargle for relaxed throats and is occasionally taken internally as a remedy for excessive menstruation. Its other names include Yellow Willow Herb, Herb Willow, Willow Wort and Wood Pimpernel.

The Moneywort (*L. nummularia*), which is found in damp meadows, woods, in shady hedges and by water, in most of Europe and parts of Asia, like the previous species is also naturalized in parts of North America having escaped from cultivation. Moneywort, too, had several medicinal uses. It is a creeping hairless perennial, with rounded opposite leaves and stems up to 60cm/23in. long, rooting at the nodes, and bearing from May to August in the axils of the leaves, solitary bell-like, fragrant, yellow short-stalked flowers.

The creeping habit of the species is alluded to in some of its country names, such as Creeping Jenny, Wandering Jenny, Running Jenny, Creeping Joan, Wandering Sailor and Meadow Runagates. Its commonest name, Moneywort, is derived from the specific *nummularia*, simply meaning money, which with Herb Twopense, Tuppenygrass and Twopenny Grass refers to the leaves, as these supposedly resembled the pennies of that period.

As a medicinal plant, Boerhaave, the Dutch physician, recommended that the dried and powdered herb be used in small doses for relieving scurvy and to stay the bleedings of wounds, much as prescribed by Gerard, who wrote: 'There is not a better wound-herb. Culpeper observed: 'It is good to stay all fluxes in man or woman, whether they be laxes, bloody-fluxes, or the flowing of womens' courses; bleeding inwardly or outwardly; the weakness of the stomach that is given to casting. It is also good for ulcers and excoriations of the lungs, or other inward parts . . . The juice is effectual also for over flowings of the menses, and the roots dried and powdered, are good for purgings. Another name for the species, Serpentaria, refers to the ancient belief that snakes and serpents used it to heal themselves when injured.

The whole herb either dried or fresh, can still be used as a wash or compress in the treatment of wounds, sores and minor skin complaints.

MALVA
Malvaceae, the Mallow family
Common Mallow, Dwarf Mallow,
Musk Mallow, Verticillate Mallow

Most of the Malvas are nowadays classed as weeds, and are annual, biennial or perennial plants, native mostly to various parts of Europe, the Mediterranean region and Asia Minor, although several of the species are also found in other parts of the world, having no doubt been introduced in shipments of grain, or as a result of cultivation.

One such plant, the Common Mallow (*M. sylvestris*), a native of Europe, including the British Isles, and parts of Asia, is now naturalized in many countries, such as Canada and the United States. It grows in fields, by the wayside, in waste and similar places, and is a coarse, hairy, very variable, sometimes sprawling biennial or perennial 40–120cm/15–47in. tall, with lobed, crinkly, ivy-like leaves, bearing purplish pink flowers from about May to August.

This particular species was the one generally used by the ancient Greeks in their medicine, and was known to the Anglo-Saxons as *malwe* or *mealwe*, which evolved by the thirteenth century to *malowe* or *malue*, and in time to Mallow, its most familiar present-day name. These, together with the generic Malva, are closely connected with the Greek *malakos*, soft, referring to the plant's emollient effects in medicine. As with the Marsh Mallow (Althaea) the whole of the Common Mallow was put to good use by the Romans, who ate the seed and boiled the leaves like cabbage, serving it at the table as a wholesome vegetable. Pythagorus tells us eating the plant reduced the passions and was a good way of cleansing the stomach and mind. Little else is recorded of its medicinal uses at this period, except that it was held in high repute and widely cultivated in southern Europe, as it was until recent times.

During the medieval period the whole of the herb was used, the root having 'the most benevolent virtues'. Boiled in water, strong decoctions of it 'provoketh lusty urine –

relieves effections of the kidneys – the stranguary – eases bad humours of the bowels – and rids the body of stone'. Culpeper wrote: 'Sweetened with syrup of violets, it cures the dysury or pain of making water with heat, for which a conserve of Mallow flowers is good, or a syrup of the juice, or a decoction of turnips, or willow, or lime tree ashes or the syrup of ground ivy.' The green or dried leaves were also decocted with other herbs

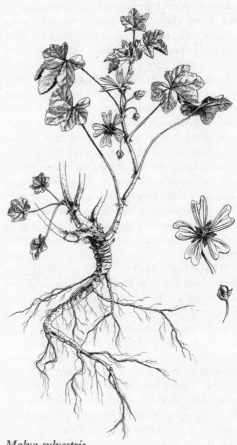

Malva sylvestris

'for the application of clysters' especially during the fifteenth and sixteenth centuries.

In the United States in the nineteenth century, the Common Mallow was regarded as possessing the properties common to other mucilaginous herbs and was prescribed infused as 'an excellent demulcent in coughs, irritation of the air passages, flux, affections of the kidney and bladder . . .'

The leaves and flowers are still prescribed for their demulcent, mucilaginous and pectoral effects, principally in infusions for treating coughs and colds, and as a soothing mucilage for the alimentary canal. The herb's other names include Blue Mallow and Mauls.

The Dwarf or Round Leaved Mallow (*M. neglecta*, syn. *M. rotundifolia*) possessed similar medicinal properties to the above species and was administered during the medieval period throughout Europe for much the same things, including stomach complaints, ulcers and skin infections. This normally prostrate annual has stems 20–50cm/7–19in. long with lobed, rounded, crinkled leaves and bears smallish pale-pink or rose-purple coloured flowers from about June to the autumn. It is native to Europe and Asia Minor, although almost cosmopolitan now, having been introduced to many other countries including Canada and the United States. It grows on grassland, waste places and in farmyards, especially near manure heaps, as it thrives on rich nitrogenous soil. The fresh young leaves of the herb, which is also known as Low Mallow, can be eaten in salads and are rich in vitamin C and pro-vitamin A.

The Musk Mallow (*M. moschata*) was frequently given as a substitute for both the above species. It is a graceful perennial native to most of Europe and Asia Minor, although widely naturalized elsewhere. It grows in grassy and bushy places to about 1m/3ft high, has deeply divided leaves and bears rose-pink or whitish flowers in summer.

The Verticillate Mallow (*M. verticillata*) from Asia, an erect, whitish or pink flowering biennial up to 80cm/31in. tall, was formerly cultivated in southern Europe as a salad herb, and for its medicinal uses which were much the same as for the above species. This species is now found wild throughout Europe and in North America, from Nova Scotia to South Dakota, then south to Pennsylvania, having escaped from cultivation. Under the name of the Whorled or Curved Mallow it was once regarded as an excellent pot-herb.

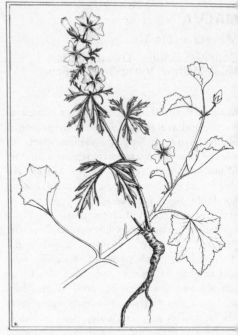

Malva moschata (front), *M. neglecta* (back)

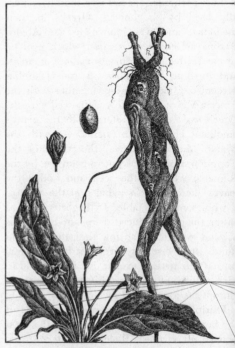

Mandragora officinarum

MANDRAGORA
Solanaceae, the Nightshade family
Mandrake

Only 2 or 3 species belong to this genus of perennial herbaceous plants that are native to the Mediterranean region where they are usually found in stony places and by deserted cultivation.

Of these, the use of the Mandrake (*M. officinarum*, syn. *Atropa mandragora*), a native of southern Europe and the Levant, dates back to the classical period. The large stout taproot is the medicinal portion. Above ground the plant consists of a large flattened basal rosette of leaves; erect, short-stalked, violet bell-shaped flowers rise from the centre, followed by smooth round fruits or berries turning orange or yellow when ripe.

In Pliny's time physicians gave small portions of Mandrake root to patients to chew as a simple painkiller and primitive anaesthetic before operations such as limb amputations. They also administered the plant to give rest and sleep to those suffering from continual pain, for melancholia, mania and convulsions, generally using the juice from the bark of the root, administering it in wine or water. As a very primitive medicine it probably worked, for it contains Hyoscyamine, Mandragorin and several other alkaloids.

Because the roots of the Mandrake sometimes fork, they were once likened to the human form, and among the superstitious beliefs surrounding the plant was that it could only be found by 'virtuous men' for only they were able to detect the light the plant emitted at night. Josephus, in his *Wars of the Jews*, warned that even to touch the plant meant death, except under certain circumstances. But the plant would expel demons from sick people, as the demons could not stand its smell or presence. Bartholomew also refers to its use as an anaesthetic, writing 'the rind thereof medled with wyne' was 'gene to them to drink that shall be cut in their body'.

The leaves of the herb were infused and applied in various forms to ulcers of all sorts, ugly scars and inflammations, and at one time were inserted into the rectum as suppositories. The berries are now regarded as a delicacy in the Mediterranean region, but during the fifteenth and sixteenth centuries, were believed to possess the power of being able to strike a man dumb, and for this and other superstitious purposes were collected by the Arabs and traded to the gullible, under such names as Devil's Testicles, Devil's Apple, Satan's Apple, Apple of the Genie and Apple of the Fool.

The first doubts about the herb's legendary powers first appeared in the *Grete Herbal* of 1526, although it was left to Gerard finally to destroy the myth: 'There hath beene many ridiculous tales brought up of this plant, whether of old wives or some runnagate Surgeons or Physickemongers I know not . . . but sure some one or more that sought to make themselves famous and skilful above others, were the first broches of that errour I speak of . . . All which dreames and old wives tales you shall from henceforth cast out of your bookes and memory; knowing this, that they are all and everie part of them false and most untrue.'

Even so, some fantastic stories were still concocted to keep the common man from harvesting the Mandrake, and roots resembling the human form fetched enormous prices on the markets, especially as they were believed to aid conception and to possess great magical powers.

Culpeper, however, was very down-to-earth about the herb: 'The fruit has been accounted poisonous, but without cause. The leaves are cooling, and are used for ointments, and other external applications. The fresh root operates very powerfully as an emetic and purgative, so that few constitutions can bear it . . . The bark of the root dried, acts as a rough emetic. The root formerly was supposed to have human form, but it really resembles a carrot or parsnip.'

The whole of the fresh herb is still occasionally employed in homoeopathic medicine, in the form of a tincture. Otherwise it is little used.

Mandragora autumnalis, also from the Mediterranean region, was sometimes substituted medicinally for the above.

MARRUBIUM
Labiatae, the Mint family
White Horehound

These many-branched hardy herbaceous perennials are found in nearly all the temperate countries of the world.

The Common or White Horehound (*M. vulgare*) once possessed a considerable reputation in domestic medicine throughout the whole of Europe and the Mediterranean

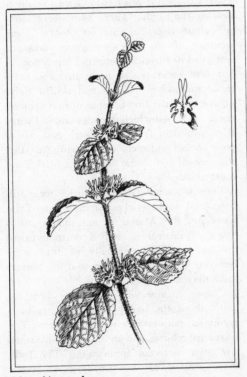

Marrubium vulgare

region, and was prescribed mainly for its diuretic, expectorant and bitter tonic effects. This aromatic bushy perennial with its erect and angular branching, leafy stems 30–80cm/ 11–31in. tall, has roundish or broadly heart-shaped, bluntly toothed, grey-green leaves, strongly wrinkled above but woolly below. From June to the autumn dense but inconspicuous whorls of whitish flowers are borne in the axils of the leaves. The whole herb has

a white or hoary appearance. Although native to most of Europe and northern Asia, the Horehound is now naturalized in many other countries, having escaped from cultivation. In the United States, where it was introduced by the settlers, it is now commonly found in dry sandy fields, on dry slopes, by the roadside and in waste places.

Marrubium, the Horehound's generic name, is believed to have evolved from *mara* or *marob*, a Hebrew word meaning a bitter juice, as this is one of the bitter herbs used by the Jews at the Feast of the Passover to commemorate the exodus of the Israelites from Egypt. Other authorities believe the name Marrubium is derived from Maria Urbs, an ancient Italian town, while the specific *vulgare* simply means common.

In medieval medicine the whole herb was administered internally in the treatment of chest complaints, either as 'decoctions of the dried leaves with the seed', the 'juice of the green herb with honey' or the 'whole of the plant in a syrup'. These were regarded as 'singular remedies' for 'the cough – persistent cough – whooping cough – phlegms' and 'similar afflictions of the chest'. Mattheolus, the sixteenth-century Dutch physician, advised the Horehound for those with 'hard livers' and for them that have 'itches and running tetters'. For the latter complaint the bruised leaves, or the extracted juice mixed with honey, was applied direct to the part affected, this also 'purging foul and stinking ulcers – and stays the running or creeping sores'. Culpeper wrote: 'The powder taken or the decoction, kills worms; the green leaves bruised, and boiled in hog's grease into an ointment, heals the bites of dogs, abates the swollen part and pains which come by pricking thorns . . . It is given to women to bring down their courses, to expel the afterbirth and to them that have sore and long travails as also to persons who have taken poison.'

The species was also prescribed in the United States during the nineteenth century in the form of a syrup, for 'all pulmonary affections'. Warm infusions were administered for producing perspiration 'and a flow of urine' and was 'used with great benefit in jaundice, asthma, hoarseness, amenorrhoea nd hysteria' while cold infusions were regarded as 'an excellent tonic in some forms of dyspepsia'. Joseph Taylor in his *Nature he Best Physician* of 1818 mentions its use or coughs.

The White Horehound is still grown in the erb garden, or on farms, for inclusion in medicines for relieving chronic coughs and olds, sore throats and asthmatic conditions. t is also added to confections and to the making of a pleasant tasting candy which is aid to be good for asthma. Herbalists usually prescribe the plant in teas and syrups for its onic and expectorant principles, mostly for he above complaints. Infusions of the plant aken at the rate of 1½ to 2 pints a day are aid to cause considerable loss of weight.

MARSDENIA

Asclepiadaceae, the Milkweed family
Condurango

The Marsdenias make up a genus of woody, wining, vine-like climbers with fragrant lowers, and are named after William Mars-en, an English Oriental scholar. The rincipal species, the Eagle or Condor Vine M. condurango, syn. *Gonolobus condurango* r *Condurango blanco*), a grape-like vine with warty bark and large, opposite, dark green eaves, became well known during the latter alf of the nineteenth century under the ame of Condurango as a 'cure' for cancer.

According to legend, the poisonous prin-iples of this plant, which is native to the Andes of South America and mainly to the outhern part of Ecuador, had been known to he Indians of that region for years. With this n mind, an Indian woman started giving ecoctions of its bark to her husband, hoping o kill him, as he was in great agony from a ainful growth. Instead of proving fatal the ine rapidly revived and cured him of his ancer. When this news reached the appro-riate authorities, the plant was introduced nto medicine by a Dr Eguiguren, who, ogether with his brother, the governor of the rovince of Loja in southern Ecuador, went n to successfully administer it as 'a cure'

for 'cancerous growths – syphilitic nodes and ulcers'.

Not long after, the bark began to be administered in the United States 'by pro-gressive physicians' where it 'at once asserted its value in cancerous, syphilitic and similar afflictions'.

The nineteenth-century herbalist, Professor Phelps Brown, wrote of the plant: 'An unequalled remedy for cancer, syphilis, ulcers, etc. In a short period, when taken, the typical symptoms subside, the pain

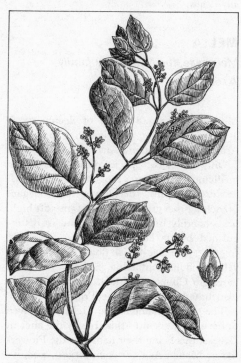

Marsdenia condurango

is diminished, the discharge thickens and becomes less offensive, the tumour becomes softer, the deposits lessen, the expression improves, and a cure is speedily effected. It has also diuretic and tonic powers, and cures many nervous diseases.'

Unfortunately, as with many other medi-cinal herbs when tested clinically over a period, the use of the Condurango proved to be of much less value than had been expected. It is still regarded as quite useful in the early stages of cancer, but possesses no active principles for stopping the progress of the disease. The bitter tasting bark, the most active part of the vine, contains a quantity of tannin, a glycoside, and an alkaloid similar to Strychnine in its action. It is still used in South America in the treatment of chronic syphilis and is also prescribed, usually in fluid extracts, for its alterative, diuretic and stomachic effects, and as a way of increasing the circulation. Overdoses cause vertigo and disturbed vision, often accompanied by convulsions followed with paralysis and occasionally death.

MELIA

Meliaceae, the Mahogany family
Azedaracha

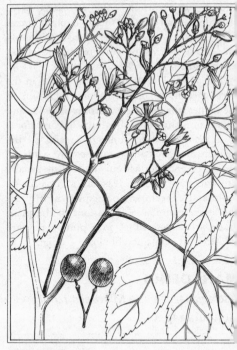

Melia azedarach

Most of this small genus of deciduous or evergreen flowering trees is native to tropical Asia, India, China and Australia.

Only one or two species were prescribed in medicine, including the Azedaracha (*M. azedarach*). This deciduous and elegant branching tree grows to about 15m/50ft high, has smoothly furrowed bark, and is distinguished by its large lax clusters of small, fragrant, pale lilac-bluish flowers, followed by yellow, stone-containing berries. Although native to China and India, it is now widely distributed throughout the Tropics.

The generic name of the Melia is believed to have been given to this tree by the ancient Greeks, this being their name for the Flowering or Manna Ash (*Fraxinus ornus*), a native of southern Europe, that had similar leaves. Azedarach is derived from the Persian *azaddirakht*, meaning noble tree. Another name, Bead Tree, refers to the stones or nuts in the fruits, which in Catholic countries are made into rosaries. Other names for the species include Nim, Margosa, Indian Lilac Tree, Holy Tree, Pride of China and Pride of India.

In Bengal and the surrounding region, the bark of the tree was and still is prescribed under the name of Neem in the treatment of stomach complaints, while an ointment made from the pulp of the berries was applied to destroy body lice. The oil from the seed was burnt in lamps and stoves, and applied direct as in North America, to treat obstinat ulcers, rheumatism and cramps.

In the United States during the nineteenth century, the bark was regarded as 'anthelmintic and in large doses as narcotic and emetic', and as 'useful in warm fevers and in infantile remittents' and 'for hysteria in women'.

A pulp made from the berries was prescribed to relieve 'scald head and other disease of the skin . . . lice and other ectozoa.'

The astringent and bitter tasting bark of the root and trunk is still given infused or in tinctures, in the southern parts of the United States for expelling worms, especially in children. The principle active constituents of the plant appear to be Tannic Acid and crystalline principle known as Margosin. A second Indian species, *Melia azadirachta*, smaller tree with bluish flowers, was sometimes substituted for the above.

MENISPERMUM
Menispermaceae, the Moonseed family
Yellow Parilla, Levant Nut, Pareira

Of the few species of Menispermum known, only the Yellow Parilla or common Moonseed (*M.canadense*) was prescribed to any extent in medicine. This deciduous climbing plant has soft woody stems and a long yellow root, and is a native of Canada and the United States.

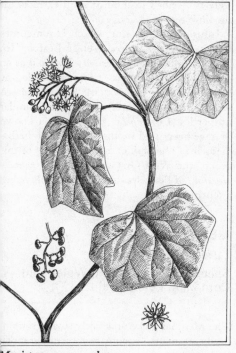

Menispermum canadense

It is found in moist woods and hedges and near streams, from Canada to Carolina and west to the Mississippi. It grows from 3–5m/ 0–16ft tall, has smooth, roundish, cordate leaves, and in summer bears small greenish-yellow flowers in axillary clusters, followed by small black fruits or drupes each containing one seed. These lunate or crescent-shaped seeds are referred to in the generic name, which is derived from the Greek *mene*, the moon, and *spermo*, seed, hence Moonseed, one of the plant's more common names.

Others include Vine Maple, Canadian Moonseed, Texas Moonseed, Moonseed Sarsaparilla, Yellow Sarsaparilla and American Sarsaparilla.

During the nineteenth century, the bitter-tasting, nearly inodorous powdered root of the Yellow Parilla was regarded as 'tonic, laxative, alterative and diuretic' and particularly so when prescribed for its 'anti-syphilitic, anti-scrofulous, anti-scorbutic and anti-mercurial' effects. As a purifier of the blood it was considered 'equal to Sarsaparilla' and its most active principle, the alkaloid Menispermin (it also contains Berberine), was prescribed with 'good effect in all diseases arising from either hereditary or acquired impurities of the system'. Decoctions of the powdered root were considered, taken internally, as a 'superior laxative' and very useful in the treatment of 'scrofula, rheumatics, syphilitic complaints, arthritis, cutaneous skin diseases, general debility and chronic inflammation of the intestines', large amounts 'causing vomiting, often accompanied with purging'.

The powdered root, liquid extracts and small amounts of Menispermin, are still prescribed for their laxative and alterative principles, in blood and skin disorders, as a tonic and nervine, and for relieving dyspepsia and general debility.

A closely allied but smaller species, known as *Menispermum dauricum*, which is native to parts of Siberia and eastern Asia, including north-east China, was occasionally administered there, too.

Several other closely related climbers belonging to the Natural Order *Menispermacea*, although very poisonous plants, had their medicinal uses. One, the Levant Nut (*Anamirta paniculata*), is found in India, Ceylon, the East Indies and the Malabar Coast. It has a corky bark, smooth, stalked heart-shaped leaves, panicles of pendulous flowers, the male and female on different plants, followed by roundish kidney-shaped berries, with a crescent-shaped very oily seed inside. Both berries and seed contain a bitter, poisonous crystalline compound known as Picrotoxin, which resembles Strychnine (*Nux vomica*) in action, and this when extracted

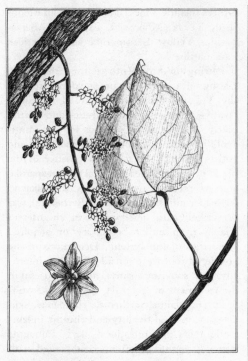

Anamirta paniculata

was similarly prescribed, as well as 'to check night sweats in wasting diseases' as in tuberculosis of the lungs. Picrotoxin itself, a very powerful convulsive poison, was at one time added as 'a bitter' to malt liquors and beers, and as a way of increasing their inebriating effects. It was also regarded as an antidote for morphine poisoning. The powdered berries in the form of an ointment were occasionally used in the treatment of obstinate skin diseases such as Barber's Itch, and to destroy body lice.

The herb is still prescribed as a stimulant and parasiticide, in ointments or fluid extracts. In countries where the plant grows, the seeds are sometimes thrown into rivers and ponds to stupefy the fish. Other names for this species include Fish Berries, Indian Berries, Levant Berries, Hockle Elderberry and *Cocculus indicus*.

The root, bark and the leaves of the Pareira (*Chondodendron tomentosum*, syn. *Cissampelos pareira*) also of the Moonseed family, were formerly prescribed for their tonic, diuretic and aperient principles. Native

to parts of Peru, Brazil and the West Indies this tall woody climbing vine has a deeply furrowed stem and large leaves up to 30cm, 11in. in length, and bears long racemes of dioecious flowers, followed by scarlet, then black, oval, grape-like berries. As an internal medicine, infusions 'stimulated the kidneys - relieved chronic inflammation and irritations of the urinary passages' and was also administered 'for the stone, rheumatism, leucorrhoea jaundice, dropsy and the gonorrhoea'. The roots (like the berries of the previous species) were exported to other countries, where they were prescribed in fluid or solid extracts for the illnesses listed above.

Infusions of the vine, which is sometimes listed as Pereira Brava, Velvet Leaf or Ice Plant, are still taken internally in Brazil as an antidote for poisonous snakebite, while the bruised leaves are externally applied. A second Brazilian species possessing similar properties, *Cissampelos glaberrima*, is known to have been used by the Indians as a herbal medicine. The bark of another species of this group, the Wild Grape (*Cissampelos convolulaceum*) of Peru, was and still is employed as a febrifuge.

MENTHA
Labiatae, the Mint family
Spearmint, Peppermint, Water Mint, Corn Mint, Pennyroyal

The Menthas make up a fairly small group of hardy aromatic, square stemmed perennial herbs, native to the northern temperate zone. As numerous natural hybrids occur and many intermediate forms are common, classification can prove very difficult.

The use of one of the more familiar species, the Common or Garden Spearmint (*M. spicata*, the *M. viridis* of trade lists), dates back at least to the time of the Romans. This hardy branched perennial 30–90cm/11–35in. tall has bright green lanceolate, sharply toothed opposite leaves, with a strong peppermint smell, and bears from July to October pink or lilac coloured flowers in rather slender cylindrical spikes. Although native to

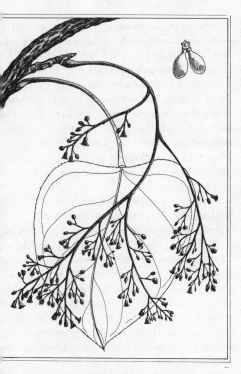

Chondodendron tomentosum

As a medicinal herb Dioscorides prescribed the juice mixed with vinegar to stay bleedings, for which it was widely prescribed during the medieval period, as 'for sores of the mouth and gums' and 'to amend an ill favoured breath' and as a wash for children's heads 'when the latter are inclined to sores'. Its leaves were used for whitening the teeth, certainly from the fourteenth century and its oil is still added as a flavouring to toothpastes, chewing gums, confections and soap. Gerard tells us: 'It is good against watering eies and all manner of breakings out on the head and sores' and 'is applied with salt to the bitings of mad dogs'.

Culpeper recommended the herb as it 'stays bleeding, stirs up venery, or bodily lust – stays the hiccough, vomiting, and allays the choler – dissolves imposthumes – is good to repress the milk in womens breasts – eases the pains of the ears – takes away the rough-

he Mediterranean region, it is now common o much of Europe and western Asia, where t is found in damp and waste places by track-ides and on mountains. It was probably ntroduced to North America by the Pilgrim athers, and was mentioned by John Josselyn n his seed list.

The use of the Spearmint dates back to the ime of the ancient Greeks, when it was melled as a restorative, added to bathwater nd used to scent the arms. Gerard tells us, quoting Pliny: 'It will not suffer milk to cruddle in the stomach' and is 'put in milk hat is drunke, lest those that drinke thereof hould be strangled'. It was probably the Romans who introduced the common Spear-mint to Britain and other countries within heir Empire. Chaucer referred to a little path of 'mintes' in his writings, and Gardiner, in he 1440s, described the cultivation of myntys'. In 1568 Turner recommended the eaves of the Spearmint 'for ye stomach' and hat it 'hath a singulare pleasantnes in sauces'. He says the garden Mint of his time was also known as the 'Spere Mynte'.

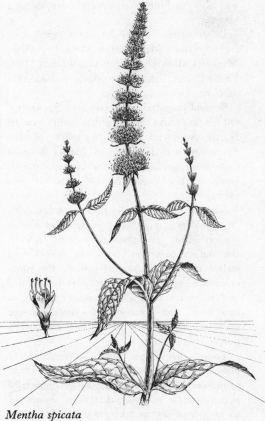

Mentha spicata

ness of the tongue, being rubbed thereupon – suffers not milk to curdle in the stomach – is very profitable to the stomach – will stay womens' courses' and is 'very profitable against the poison of venomous creatures'.

The herb, or the essential oil, is still medicinally used for its antispasmodic, carminative and stimulant principles, but is generally added, because of its carminative properties and pleasant taste, to other compounds. The distilled water relieves hiccough, flatulence and indigestion, while the sweetened infusion can be safely given in infantile complaints (its effects are less powerful than the Peppermint), such as vomiting, colic and nausea. In homoeopathic medicine a tincture from the fresh flowering plant is used for relieving strangury and gravel, and as a local application for painful haemorrhoids. In the kitchen the leaves of the Spearmint are added to many dishes, for example, new potatoes, peas, as a sauce to go with lamb and are also included in several drinks and beverages.

Other names for the Common Spearmint include Green Mint, Lamb Mint, Pea Mint, Mackerel Mint, Fish Mint, Our Ladies Mint, Yerba Buena, Erba Santa Marie and Menthe de Notre Dame.

Several essential oils known as Spearmint Oil are nowadays recognized in commerce. In North America, several varieties of the Spearmint are distilled; in Russia *Mentha verticellata*; in Germany the Horsemint (*M. longifolia*), the Water Mint (*M. aquatica*) or a variety of it.

Gerard describing the latter species says: 'Water Mint is a kinde of wilde Mint like to garden Mint: the leaves thereof are round, the stalkes cornered, both the leaves and stalkes are of a darke red colour; the roots creep far abroad, but every part is greater, and the herb it selfe is of a stronger smell: the flowers in the tops of the branches are gathered together into a round eare, of a purple colour.'

Today the Water Mint is regarded as possessing astringent, emetic and stimulant principles. The dried herb is generally prescribed for relieving diarrhoea, as an aid to menstruation, is taken warm to promote

perspiration in colds and influenza, and is sometimes combined with other remedies in the treatment of stomach complaints.

Some botanists consider the Hairy Mint (*M. sativa*) to be a variation of the Water Mint. The former, a rather coarse plant found throughout Europe, including Britain, and in parts of Russian Asia, is still prescribed sometimes under the name of Water Mint, Marsh Mint or Wild Mint, for its astringent, emetic and stimulant principles and as an emmenagogue.

One of the most fragrant Mints of all is perhaps the Peppermint (*Mentha x piperita*, a hybrid between *M. aquatica* and *M. spicata*), a hardy perennial common to much of Europe and parts of Asia, where it is found in such moist places as the banks of rivers and streams and in ditches, although now widely naturalized elsewhere. The branching stems reach 30–90cm/11–35in. in height, with lanceolate ovate short stalked opposite leaves and dense terminal spikes of reddish-lilac or purplish flowers.

The use of this plant, or perhaps a form of it, dates back to the time of the Greeks and

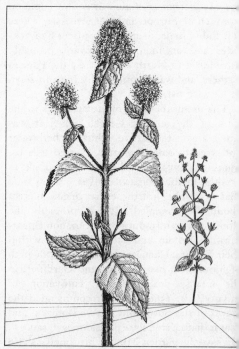

Mentha aquatica

Romans, when, according to Pliny, crowns of it were worn at feasts, sprays were placed on dining tables and cooks added its fragrance to sauces and wines. It is also believed to have been cultivated by the ancient Egyptians.

During the thirteenth century, the Peppermint was mentioned in the *Pharmacopoeias of Iceland*, but appears to have been little used in the rest of Europe at this time. Centuries later Culpeper tells us: 'It is useful for complaints of the stomach, such as wind, vomiting, etc., for which there are few remedies of greater efficacy. It is good in poultices and fomentations to disperse curdled milk in the breasts, and also to be used with milk diets.'

The herb was first included in the *London Pharmacopoeia* of 1721, under the name of *Mentha piperitis* 'sapore'. Its commercial cultivation started in England in about 1750 and has since been developed in many other countries, including France, Italy, Sicily, Germany, Morocco, Hungary, Bulgaria, Russia, East Africa, Australia, China and Japan. The largest amounts of Peppermint are now produced in the United States, in Michigan, Indiana, where the plant was first cultivated in the mid 1850s, and the north-western States. It is now also naturalized from Nova Scotia to Florida, west to Minnesota and Arkansas. The pungent aromatic, antiseptic oil, which is removed from the dried flower heads by steam distillation, is combined with other medicines in the treatment of coughs, colds, colic, flatulence and nausea, and is an important source of Menthol. Herbalists still prescribe the oil for its carminative, stimulant and stomachic effects, and as a cordial. As a flavouring agent, the Oil of Peppermint, which is derived from several types or forms of this species, is added to confectionery, toothpastes, perfumes, etc., and to the preparation of creme-de-menthe and other liqueurs. Other names for the Peppermint, a plant rats are said to detest, include Brandy Mint and Balm Mint.

Another common species, the Corn Mint (*M. arvensis*), is found as a very variable weed, often hybridizing with other species, in damp arable fields, pastures, ditches, thickets and marshes throughout most of Europe and parts of Asia. Its downy or hairy, rather weak leafy stems reach 10–60cm/3–23in., have stalked, oval- to lance-shaped toothed leaves and bear lilac to purple flowers in dense but rather distant clustered whorls in the axils of the upper leaves. In North America where the plant is now widely naturalized, it is sometimes known as the Field Mint.

The oil from the Corn Mint is used commercially in the preparation of herbal teas and syrups, in cosmetics and confectionery and is added as an ingredient to mouthwashes, toothpastes and liqueurs. As a simple remedy the bruised leaves (or the oil, both are very odorous) can be placed on the forehead for relieving nervous headaches. Two varieties of the species *Mentha arvensis* 'Piperascens' from Japan, and *Mentha arvensis* 'Glabrata' from China, are cultivated in those countries for the Menthol they contain, which is prescribed, amongst other things, for relieving rheumatic pains, neuralgia, toothache and laryngitis, bronchitis, etc. It can be inhaled or taken internally as a stimulant and carminative, and having an anaesthetic effect on the nerve endings of the stomach, is sometimes

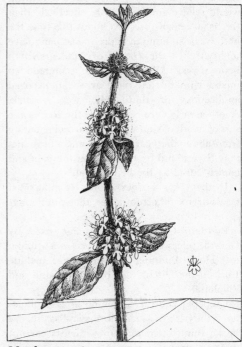

Mentha arvensis

used to help prevent sea-sickness. Even when diluted Menthol is able to kill certain bacteria.

The Pennyroyal (*M. pulegium*) has also been employed in medicine since ancient times. It is a variable, strong smelling downy plant, with stems 10–50cm/3–20in. long, but prostrate at the base. The leaves are small oval or oblong, shallowly toothed or entire, short-stalked and often drooping, and small whorls of lilac flowers appear from about July to October. It is native to the damp meadows and wet places of most of Europe and parts of temperate Asia, although now naturalized as a result of its cultivation in many other parts of the world, including North and South America. In the United States it is mentioned in one of the New World herbals as having been introduced by the Pilgrim Fathers.

This particular species was the Pulegium of the Romans, a Latin word now forming its specific name, which is derived from *pulex*, meaning flea, so-called because of its reputed power, especially if used as a strewing herb, to kill or keep these pests away. Both Pliny and Dioscorides write of its many virtues, the former even concluding that a wreath or chaplet of Pennyroyal worn about the head would relieve giddiness more effectively than the usual one of roses. At about this time the herb was also hung in bedrooms as conducive to health. In the *Herbal* of Apuleius, both Pennyroyal and Wormwood are recommended mixed with oil and vinegar as an external application for those who were seasick. Another early cure is found in the *Regimen*, a sort of handbook on domestic medicine dating from about the year 1100: 'Some affirm that they have found by trial – That the pain and gout is cured by the Pennyroyal.'

In the 1560s Turner wrote: 'If thou must needs drynk unholsum water, then put Pennyroyal in to it.'

Pudding Grass, another name used by Gerard, refers to its ancient use as a stuffing for 'Hog's Pudding'. Other names include Lurk-in-the-Ditch, Run-by-the-Ground and Piliolerial.

Culpeper and his contemporaries administered the herb in several forms and say its use 'make thin, tough phlegm – digests corrupt matter – provokes women's courses – expels

the dead child and afterbirth – stays the disposition to vomit – voids phlegm out of the lungs – purges by stool – is good for venomous bites – revives those who are faint and swoon – strengthens the gums – helps the gout – takes away spots or marks on the face – profits those who are splenetic or liver-grown – the leprosy – helps the toothache – the cold griefs of the joints – eases headache – pains of the breast and belly – helps cramps or convulsions of the sinews . . . helps the jaundice and dropsy – clears the eyesight . . . One spoonful of the juice sweetened with sugar-candy, is a cure for the hooping cough.'

The infused herb, the oil in pills, or fluid extracts, are still prescribed for their carminative, diaphoretic, emmenagogue and stimulant principles, as for obstructed menstruation especially if caused by sudden chills or colds, and for hysteria, flatulence and sickness. The Oil of Pennyroyal will also keep gnats and mosquitoes away.

Other species used in herbal medicine or as flavourings include the Horsemint (*M. longifolia*), an erect, strong-smelling perennial 30–100cm/11–40in. tall from Europe and parts of Asia, and now naturalized in North America; the Bergamot Mint (*M. citrata*, syn. *M. odorata*), regarded by some botanists as a variety of *Mentha aquatica*; the American Wild Mint (*M. canadensis*) a common plant, native to the low, marshy ground from New Brunswick to Virginia, then west to the Pacific Coast, the leaves of which were not only used in medicine, but were eaten as a nourishing food by the Maine Indians; and the English Horsemint (*M. sylvestris*).

The Apple Mint, Round Leaved or Apple Scented Mint (*M. rotundifolia*), a herb native to the ditches and similar damp places of most of Europe, was employed by the medieval monks and nuns to treat the 'languor' following fits, perhaps because its use was said to refresh the brain. The Large Apple Mint (*M. alopecuroides*) was similarly prescribed.

Another fragrant species, the Corsican Mint (*M. requienii*), is believed to be one of the smallest flowering plants in cultivation, bearing tiny individual lilac coloured flowers in summer, the stems rooting as they spread along to form a dense moss-like carpet of fresh green pinhead leaves.

The commonest and collective name of this genus, Mint, is derived from the Greek *mintha* or *minthe*, and the Latin *menta* or *mentha* – the last form being used by Theophrastus in 300 B.C. According to Parkinson: 'Aristotle and others in the ancient times forbade Mints to be used of souldiers in the time of warre, because they thought ... it tooke away, or at least abated their animosity or courage to fight.'

In Gerard's day many different sorts of Mint were cultivated, under such names as Crosse, Browne, Mackerel, Holy Heart, Horse and Brook Mint.

MITCHELLA
Rubiaceae, the Madder family
Partridge Berry

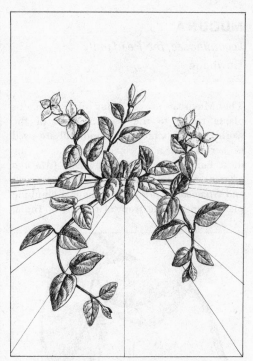

Mitchella repens

This hardy, slender, evergreen trailing herb, the Partridge Berry (*M. repens*), has creeping stems, small opposite rounded leaves, and bears in June and July pairs of white or pinkish fragrant flowers, followed by small, bright red, edible, but almost tasteless berries, which remain on the plants all winter. It is native to North America, where it is found in dry woods, especially pinewoods and in swampy places, from Nova Scotia to Minnesota, south to Florida and Texas. It was introduced into England in 1761, but is very rarely prescribed there.

The generic name of Mitchella was allocated to this plant in honour of Dr John Mitchell of Virginia, one of the first American botanists to correspond with Linnaeus, with *repens* its specific name referring to its creeping or trailing habit. As a medicinal herb it was certainly used well before his time, for the Indian women are known to have employed it for several weeks before a confinement in order to ensure a safe and easy birth. They also boiled down strong decoctions of the leaves into a thickish liquid, to apply to the sore or fissured breasts of nursing mothers. European immigrants arriving in America used the whole of the plant, not only for producing or promoting childbirth and labour, but also for its diuretic and astringent effects 'in dropsy – suppression of urine – and diarrhoea' for which the herb was prescribed decocted. The strong seeds were also taken 'for relief of dysentery'.

The herb is still given in fluid extracts, or is decocted for relieving diarrhoea, suppression of urine and in uterine complaints, such as amenorrhoea, dysmenorrhoea and menorrhagia.

Other names for this herb include Deerberry, Winter Clover, Checkerberry, Squaw-Herb, Squaw Vine, One Berry and Partridge Vine.

MUCUNA
Leguminosae, the Pea family
Cowhage

The Mucunas are a genus of leguminous plants native to the warmer parts of the world, two of which were and still are used in herbal and homoeopathic medicine, the most familiar being the Cowhage (*Mucuna pruriens*, syn. *M. prurita*, or *Dolichos pruriens* and *Stizolobium pruriens*). This is a climbing plant found in the tropical regions of India,

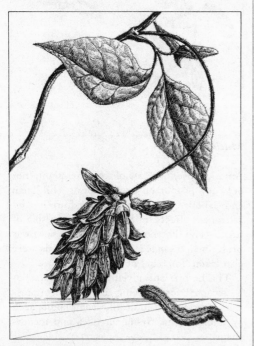

Mucuna pruriens

Asia, Africa, South America, the Fiji Islands and the West and East Indies. It has long slender branches with alternate lanceolate leaves and bears clusters of large white flowers, with purplish coloured butterfly shaped corollas, followed by leathery, dark brown pods about 10cm/4in. long, thickly covered with stiffish hair, each pod containing from four to six seeds.

The stinging hairs of these pods, which are easily shaken off, cause intense irritation in humans and in animal skin and therefore require great care in their handling, and it is these that form the medicinal portion. This is referred to in *pruriens*, the plant's specific name simply meaning 'itching'. Mucuna, now the generic name, was used by Marggraf in the 1650s for a Brazilian species. The common name of Cowhage is derived from the Hindustani *kawanch* or *koanch*, and is now met with in various forms, such as Cowitch, Couhage and Kiwach.

In India, the more tender immature pods are sometimes cooked and eaten as food, but before the hairs appear; or they were decocted, as were the roots, and taken as a diuretic in dropsy, while in some areas infusions were given to cholera victims. The main medicinal use of the plant, however, lay in the hairs of the pods which were given to expel intestinal worms. For this the hairs were mixed with honey or syrup and taken in doses of about a teaspoonful on two or three consecutive mornings. The idea was that the hairs passing through the body would pierce the worms, which would then loosen their hold on the intestinal walls of their host. A reliable cathartic was then administered to bring the parasites out of the body. Overdoses are known to have caused inflammation of the intestines, although it was generally regarded as a fairly safe remedy, but appears to have had little or no effect on the tape-worm (see *Kousso*). The seeds of the species are still eaten in certain areas as a stimulant and aphrodisiac.

The round seeds of the Florida Bean or Horse Eye Bean (*M. urens*, syn. *Dolichos urens*) from the East Indies, are occasionally used in homoeopathic medicine in the treatment of haemorrhoids and as substitutes for the Calabar Bean.

MYRISTICA
Myristicaceae, the Nutmeg family
Nutmeg

Although principally known for their modern use as a spice and flavouring, the fruits of the Nutmeg Tree (*M. fragrans*, syn. *M. officinalis*,

M. aromatica, or *Arillus myristicae*) were regarded during the sixteenth and seventeenth centuries as something of a cure-all in European medicine. They were obtained from an evergreen tree, also known as the *Nux Moschata*, which is native to the Banda, the Moluccas and other East Indian Islands, where it grows 15m/50ft or more in height. The tree has glossy, oblong, aromatic leaves, bears clusters of small, heavily scented yellow flowers, followed by fleshy peach-like pendulous fruits, which as they ripen, split open to reveal the brownish nutmegs inside, covered by a fleshy net-like crimson coloured aril. The latter when collected and dried is known as Mace, a delicate condiment. The fleshy husks of the seed are also used in the making of jellies and preserves.

The Nutmeg is believed to have been discovered by the Western world in 1512,

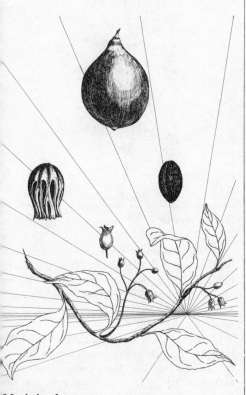

Myristica fragrans

when the Portuguese reached Banda or the Nutmeg Islands. From there the first seeds were sent back to Europe, where it was found that if a few of the kernels were eaten, they gave a feeling of buoyant vigour and health, sometimes accompanied by rather pleasant visions and other euphoric sensations, although this was generally followed by dizziness and nausea. As a result of the more pleasant effects, it was soon regarded in Europe as a valuable medicine and was prescribed for many illnesses, including the plague, putrid and intermittent fevers and the sweating sickness, in the majority of cases with little or no positive results. The Nutmeg's hallucinogenic effects is mentioned first by Lobelius in 1576, when writing of a 'pregnant English lady', who on eating ten or twelve of the fruits became 'deliriously inebriated'. Perhaps the lady concerned consumed this amount as a way of aborting her child, for at that time the seed was certainly credited with this power.

In 1722 Joseph Miller said of the seeds: 'They are heating, drying and carminative', and they 'strengthen the stomach and bowels, stop vomiting, help digestion, comfort the head and nerves, cure palpitation of the heart and prevent swooning, and are of service against vapors.'

In southern India, the Nutmeg, mixed with Betel (*Areca catechu*) and snuff, is taken as an intoxicant as also in certain parts of Indonesia, where it is powdered down and snuffed on its own.

The Oil of Nutmeg is now employed to mask the taste of unpleasant drugs and medicine to help prevent nausea and sickness, and is sometimes taken as a stimulant to the gastro-intestinal t.act. One of its active constituents is known as Myristicin, a tonic principle. The oil is occasionally added as a mild stimulant and carminative together with other ingredients to external plasters and to ointments for applying to piles. Nutmeg butter, an orange-yellow tallow-like fat is also used in medicinal ointments and in the making of candles.

The Oil of Mace possesses identical properties to that of the Nutmeg, and like the previous oil is used to correct the taste of other drugs in medicine for relieving flatulence, stomach weakness and to help digestion.

The Mace of another Nutmeg, *Myristica otoba*, when mixed with fat is still used in the treatment of rheumatism and gout. Two other sorts are occasionally seen on the markets. The first, the Macassar Mace (*M. argentea*), has a rather acrid taste and is rarely used in medicine, while that of the Bombay Mace (*M. malabarica*) lacks both fragrance and taste.

NEPETA
Labiatae, the Mint family
Catmint, Mauve Catmint

The Nepetas make up a fairly large group of hardy, herbaceous plants native principally to parts of Europe, Asia and the Himalayas.

The Catmint (*N. cataria*), has been cultivated from ancient times for its reputed medicinal uses. It is a strong smelling, erect and branching, downy perennial 40–100cm/ 15–40in. tall, having oval or heart-shaped leaves, and bearing broad whorls of white flowers, splashed with reddish spots, on leafy, branched spikes, from about June to September. It grows among rocks, on dry banks, by roadsides and on waste ground throughout Europe and much of Asia. It has also become naturalized in other temperate countries, as in Canada and the United States, where it is widely distributed, having escaped from cultivation. This species is generally regarded as being the true medicinal Catsmint (Kattes-minte). A more sprawling type, the Mauve Catmint (*N. mussinii*, sometimes listed as *N. faassenii*), which is indigenous to the Caucasus, occasionally escapes from cultivation and is then recorded as the medicinal sort. This attractive plant is probably a hybrid, and grows in hedges and along roads, where its slender, leafy stems, covered with fragrant greyish leaves, produce their lavender-blue or violet flowers in summer.

Pliny was one of the first to mention the uses of the Catmint, although both the Greeks and Romans cultivated the wild sort as its common name suggests for their cats,

who are supposed to be unable to resist its smell. This belief was echoed later by Gerard in his *Herbal*. On the other hand, rats are said to detest the herb and rarely if ever approach it. It was also regarded by the religious orders as a very good bee plant.

On the Continent, the Catsmint was grown during the early medieval period for its leaves and young shoots, much as they are in France today, for use as a seasoning in the kitchen. In England it had become a familiar herb of the kitchen garden by 1265, and appears to have been rubbed on meats before cooking.

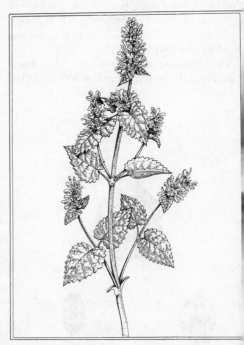

Nepeta cataria

Of its medicinal uses, Gerard writing 'Of Nep or Cat-Mint' tells us: 'It is a present helpe for them that be bursten inwardly by means of some fall received from an high place, and that are very much bruised, if the juice be given with wine or meade.'

Other writers of the period recommend the herb decocted, sweetened with honey 'for the cough' and for the 'barrenness of women'. Culpeper says: 'It is used in pains of the head coming of any cold cause, catarrhs, rheums and swimming and giddiness: and is of use in the stomach and belly. It is effectual for cramps or cold aches, and is used for colds, coughs, and shortness of breath ... The green herb bruised and applied eases the piles.'

Tournefort writes of a certain gentle hangman who was unable to perform his work until he had chewed on the root of the Catmint, which acted as a stimulant and gave him the courage to carry out his duties. Strong teas of the plant were prescribed for much the same thing 'for those that are meek and mild ... and would be forceful'.

The species is still prescribed for its carminative, diaphoretic, tonic and refrigerant principles. Infusions or teas are useful for inducing free perspiration in colds and fevers, for relieving pain and flatulence and for restlessness, nervousness and colicky complaints in children.

The dried leaves of the Catmint have also, from time to time, been smoked for the 'high' feeling they produce and for their hallucinogenic effects.

One of the most active principles found in the Oil of Catnip, known as Metatabilacetone, is also obtained from the pretty Chinese shrub *Actinidia polygama*. The young twigs and leaves of this plant have been used for centuries in Asia to tranquillize lions and tigers confined in zoos, while strong teas of its leaves give a feeling of well-being in humans, besides producing mild hallucinatory effects, and has been given since ancient times as a form of sedative.

(For the Ground Ivy, often listed as *Nepeta hederacea*, see *Glechoma*.)

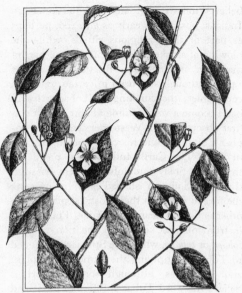

Actinidia polygama

NICOTIANA

Solanaceae, the Nightshade family

Tobacco

Most of the species belonging to this genus of half-hardy annual, perennial or shrubby plants are native to America, although one or two are found in Australasia and the Pacific Isles.

The custom of smoking Tobacco is

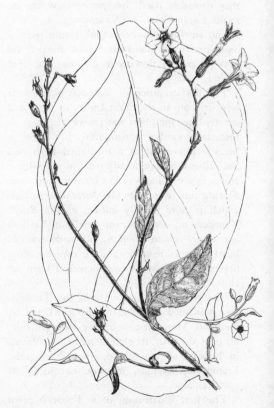

Nicotiana tabacum (front), *N. rustica* (back)

believed to have originated with the American Indians, possibly as early as A.D. 100, perhaps as part of their religious rituals, while the blowing of smoke on a patient formed part of many an ancient cure. By the end of the 1400s, although still used in certain religious ceremonies, the smoking of Tobacco leaves had become a very common habit, which was first observed by a Westerner when Christopher Columbus and his crew landed in Cuba in 1492. The Carib Indians also powdered the leaves finely and inhaled them as snuff through a hollow Y-shaped cane, by inserting the forked end into their nostrils, placing the other end in or near the powder. This simple instrument was known to the natives as a *tobaca* or *tobago*, which the Spaniards changed to Tobacco, applying the name to the plant and its leaves, although some authorities believe the word Tobacco refers to the island of Tobago. The local names for the leaves also included Picielt, Petun or Petum and they probably used the species now known as the Large Tobacco (*N. tabacum*), an erect, strong smelling, hairy annual, rising from a basal rosette of glandular leaves, bearing its pink or purple flowers in a dense terminal cluster.

The first commercial Tobacco plantations were laid out in the West Indies in 1535 and shortly after the plant was grown in Spain, at first as a garden ornamental, but soon it became important as a medicinal herb and heal-all and was generally used as a poultice. It was described as a recent introduction from Florida and was possibly *Nicotiana rustica*, which is now usually known as the Small Tobacco, an erect, strong-smelling, hairless annual 30–100cm/11–39in. tall, with oval- to heart-shaped leaves, and greenish-yellow flowers carried in a many-flowered terminal cluster.

One of the first accounts of the Tobacco was published in 1569, in a book written by Nicholas Monardes, a doctor from Seville. He gave the plant its generic name, Nicotiana, in honour of his friend, Jean Nicot, the French ambassador, *tabacum* becoming its specific name.

The first illustration of a Tobacco plant was published in 1577 in John Frampton's book, *Joyfull Newes Out of the Newe Founde Worlde*, an English translation of Monardes's original work. In this it was observed that the Negroes and Indians after inhaling the smoke 'doe remaine lightened without any wearinesse for to labour again . . .'

By tradition Sir Walter Raleigh introduced the Tobacco (*N. rustica* from Virginia) to England in 1586, bringing pipes, the 'weed' and an Indian with him. But John Hawkins, the English admiral, should really be credited with its introduction, having previously used it in England. There, as in other European countries, it soon caught on for 'drinking in pipes', although much controversy raged over its use, with various kings and popes bitterly denouncing it. Perhaps this is not to be wondered at when we read in Gerard's account *Of Tabaco, or Henbane of Peru*: 'The priests and Inchanters of the hot countries do take the fume thereof until they be drunke, that after they have lien for dead three or foure houres, they may tell the people what wonders, visions, or illusions they have seen, and so give them a prophetical direction or foretelling (if we may trust the Divell) of the successe of their businesse.' Of its medicinal uses he observed: 'Nicolaus Monardis saith, that the leaves hereof are a remedie for the pain of head called the Megram or Migram, that hath bin of long continuance . . . It is a present remedy for the fits of the mother, it mitigateth the paine of the gout, if it be rosted in hot embers, and applied to the grieved part . . . It is likewise a remedy for the toothache, if the teeth and gumbs be rubbed with a linnen cloth dipped in the juice, and afterward a round ball of the leaves laid unto the place . . . The weight of foure ounces of the juice hereof drunke procureth afterward a long and sound sleepe . . . Likewise there is an oile to be taken out of the leaves that healeth merri-galls, kibed heeles, and such like – It is good against poyson and taketh away the malignitie thereof, if the juice be given to drink, or the wounds made by venomous beasts be washed therewith.'

Such was the demand for Tobacco in Culpeper's time, that in 1640 over 7,000 shops sold the leaves in the London area alone, while its importation from the Americas ran to well over one million pounds' weight annually.

During the Plague of London in 1665, the chewing or smoking of Tobacco leaves became regarded as one of the most effective preventatives. Even small children joined in, taking their regular pipeful night and morning.

The leaves of both the species mentioned above are still reckoned as possessing emetic, narcotic and sedative principles, but are rarely prescribed in internal medicines, as they can cause, even in small amounts, emesis, depression and convulsions. An ointment made by simmering the leaves in lard is occasionally used as an application for old ulcers and painful tumours. The leaves, especially those of the Small Tobacco, contain a virulent alkaloid known as Nicotine, a colourless, acrid, oily liquid. In commerce this is extracted and employed in horticulture as an insecticide, but it is extremely poisonous and in humans is readily absorbed through the skin, and has proved fatal in the past.

The Large or Large Flowered Tobacco is still the principle species used for smoking, and this, together with its numerous forms and specially developed varieties, is grown commercially in many parts of the world, including North and South America, Cuba, China, Turkey, Greece and many subtropical countries. Generally speaking, the best quality leaves for smoking originate from the warmer countries.

Other species used as tobacco include the Persian Tobacco (*N. persica*) which as its name implies is cultivated in Iran; *Nicotiana fruticosa* from China; *Nicotiana quadrivalis*, from the United States, once smoked by the Indians of the Missouri and Columbia rivers, and *Nicotiana repanandu*, from North and Central America, now employed in making Havana cigars.

In Australia, with the arrival of the white man, the smoking of Tobacco became very popular among the natives, who used the leaves of three indigenous species – *Nicotiana suaveolens*, *N. gossei* and *N. escelsior*. Before this, the aborigines of some areas are known to have eaten the leaves, the flowering stalks and the flowers. The leaves of *N. escelsior*

were also dried in the sun, chewed into quid and rolled in the ashes of Red Gum, or certain other Acacia species. Small balls of this tacky mixture were then sucked or chewed as required.

OCIMUM
Labiatae, the Mint family
Sweet Basil, Bush Basil

This group of rather tender annual herbs is native to tropical Asia and Africa. It is now, however, widely cultivated in many other countries, such as Britain and much of

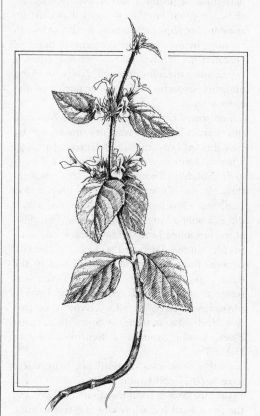

Ocimum basilicum

Europe, the Mediterranean region, the Pacific Islands and both North and South America, mainly for the sake of the aromatic, egg-shaped leaves, which are added as a flavouring to salads, soups, sauces and stews.

One of the most important species, indigenous to India and tropical Asia, is the Sweet Basil (*O. basilicum*). Known to have been grown by the ancient Greeks, its erect stems reach about 60cm/23in. tall, having ovate long stalked leaves, and bearing whorls of two-lipped greenish-white or purple tinged flowers, in terminal racemes in summer. The specific name of the plant, *basilicum*, is derived from the Greek words *basilika* or *basilikos*, meaning royal, or *basileus*, king. Unfortunately *basilicum* appears to have become confused with the Latin *basiliscus*, a basilisk, the mythical lizard-like monster, said to have a fatal glance and breath. The herb thus acquired a rather evil reputation, although often employed in medicine as an antidote for poison. Mattioli, in the sixteenth century, mentioned that the generic name of Ocimum or 'Ocymum' is derived from a Greek word meaning to smell, referring to the pungent aromatic scent the majority of the species emit.

For many centuries, however, the use of this particular herb was overshadowed by thoughts of venomous creatures. In 1579 Thomas Lupton wrote in his book *A Thousand Notable Things*, that: 'An Italian, through the oft smelling of an herb called Basil had a scorpion bred in his brain, which did not only a long time grieve him, but also at the last killed him.' Gerard observed, some people 'shunne Basil and will not eat thereof, because that if it be chewed and laid in the sunne, it ingendreth worms'. Tournefort recounts that Dr. Raymond, an English physician in Italy 'found by Experience that this Herb, if put under a Stone in a moist Place, would produce a Scorpion in two Day's Time'.

Only two species of Basil are believed to have been in cultivation in Britain up to the 1550s: the Sweet Basil mentioned above, and the Bush Basil (*O. minimum*) also from India. This is a much smaller, compact plant reaching 15–30cm/6–11in. tall, with oval leaves and terminal spikes of white flowers in summer. However, the number of species and their varieties gradually began to increase, and in 1726 Richard Bradley was presented with over fifty sorts in a year. This fresh interest in the genus was probably due to the species losing much of their evil reputation by the 1650s, leaving them more or less free of superstition. In Parkinson's time the leaves were made into 'snuffing powders' and if laid about the house 'banisheth flies from indoors'. The 'Physicall Properties' of the seed taken in a powder, would also 'procure a cheerful and merry hearte', the bruised leaves were applied to 'snakebites, insect bites and stings', while 'Basile Tea' taken hot 'relieves suppressed menses in women' and 'helps to expel the afterbirth'. The same was frequently administered to women suffering from the 'milder nervous diseases – vertigo – langor – and migraine'.

At present, the two Basils mentioned are little employed in herbal medicine, although the juice of the Sweet Basil, which has a clover-like fragrance, is occasionally used as a vermifuge in South America. Both, however, together with several other species, are much used as seasoning herbs in the kitchen and are often mixed with others to add flavour to vinegars, vegetables, soups and butter dishes and to most of the meats. In London, the famous seventeenth-century Fetter Lane sausage owed its distinctive taste to Basil, while the *soupe au pistou* of Nice and the *pesto* sauce of Genoa, still rely on this aromatic genus. Another variety, *Ocimum gratissimum*, is cultivated in India and China for its use as a culinary herb and is prescribed in the treatment of colds. In India, the native habitat of several Ocimums, the Holy Basil (*O. sanctum*) is held sacred to both Krishna and Vishnu, and is still grown there as a guide to heaven, and near the temples as a protection.

In Japan the leaves of the sweetly scented *Ocimum crispum* were used for relieving colds, as was *Ocimum canum* in India. The leaves of this last plant are still given in homoeopathic medicine in the form of a tincture. Other species still used include the Fever Plant (*O. viride*) from West Africa, the leaves of which are taken as a febrifuge in the form of a tea; *Ocimum teniflorum*, from Java, as a stimulant; and *Ocimum guineense*, once a popular remedy of the Negroes for relieving fevers. From the

West Indies comes *Ocimum americanum*, and this was prescribed for relieving dysentery and various chest complaints. An essential oil is extracted from this plant.

OPHIOGLOSSUM

Filices (or Ophioglossaceae) the Fern family
Adder's Tongue Fern

Only one species of this small genus of hardy deciduous ferns was prescribed in herbal medicine, the Adder's Tongue (*O. vulgatum*). The plant is native to various parts of Europe, including the British Isles and other temperate countries, where it grows in

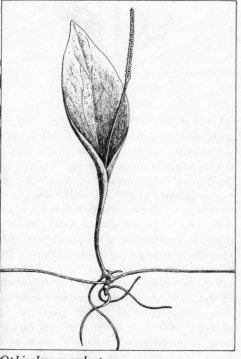

Ophioglossum vulgatum

grassy meadows and similar places. The plant itself grows up to 30cm/11in. high depending on moisture and position, and consists of a small underground rhizome, producing in spring a smooth, undivided, leathery 'leaf' or frond, borne on a slender leaf-stalk. The

fertile part, the spore cases, although often absent, are produced in a double row on a long plantain-like unbranched spike. The tongue-shaped sporophylla is referred to in Ophioglossum, the generic name, and is derived from the Greek *ophis*, a serpent, and *glossa*, a tongue, hence Adder's Tongue, one of its commonest names.

During the medieval period the juice of the Adder's Tongue, or Christ's Spear as it was sometimes known, was highly valued for the treatment of wounds. The roots and leaves were generally 'boyled in olive oil', or made into 'salves and oyntments' and externally applied. As an inward medicine the juice was often mixed with 'the water distilled from the Horsetail' and this was taken for the 'wounds of the breast, bowel, gut and other parts of the body' and by those troubled 'with casting, vomiting or bleeding from the mouth and nose, or otherwise downwards'. Gerard says 'the leaves stamped in a stone mortar and boiled in oil, then strained, will yield a most excellent green oyle or rather a balsame for greene wounds ...'. This and similar preparations were sometimes known as the 'Green Oyls of Charity'.

The fresh leaves, which Culpeper tells us are 'to be found in May or April' for they 'quickly perisheth with a little heat', are still regarded as possessing antiscrofulous, emollient and emetic principles, and are occasionally prescribed infused as an internal remedy, and as a poultice for applying to scrofulous ulcers, tumours, chilblains, cuts and sores. Infusions taken in wineglassful doses are said to be good for relieving the hiccough and vomiting.

ORIGANUM

Labiatae, the Mint family
Wild Marjoram, Sweet Marjoram, Dittany of Crete

The Marjorams are mostly hardy herbaceous or semi-shrubby plants with aromatic leaves, native mostly to the Mediterranean region, although now widely cultivated as garden ornamentals elsewhere. Their generic name is derived from the Greek *oras* meaning mountain and *ganos*, splendid or joy, thus Joy of the Mountain, referring to the colour and scent of their flowers and leaves, and to the hills they originally came from.

One of the commonest species, the Wild Marjoram (*O. vulgare*), is found throughout Europe, including the British Isles, Asia and North Africa, although now naturalized in many other countries, such as the United States, where it is sometimes found as an abundant weed, especially in the region of the Catskill Mountains. It is an aromatic, very variable hairy perennial 30–80cm/11–31in. tall, with stalked, oval, often slightly toothed leaves, and loose clusters of two-lipped flowers with purple bracts from July to September. A plant common to grassy places, such as dry meadows, screes, scrub and the edges of cornfields, it particularly likes chalky soils.

In England this species is known to have been cultivated by the monks in their herbariums from at least the thirteenth century onwards. The extracted acid-tasting oil was applied to hollow or aching teeth to ease the pain. Infusions of the powdered tops were taken for headaches, and used fresh or dried were applied in hot fomentations to various aches and pains, swellings, rheumatism and colic.

During the Tudor period, the Common or Wild Marjoram was often mentioned as an aromatic strewing herb and was used as such until the end of the seventeenth century, and bunches of it were hung up in dairies, or placed between the pails to keep the milk fresh, especially in warm or stormy weather. The flowering tops were sometimes used to dye wool a purplish colour, or linen a reddish-brown.

In the sixteenth and seventeenth centuries, the plant had become widely used and was regularly prescribed to 'strengthen the stomach and head – relieve the sourness of the stomach – cleanse the body of choler – remove loss of appetite – coughs and consumption of the lungs – expel poison – help the bite of mad dogges – and other venemous creatures – provoke urine and terms in women – remedy infirmities of the spleen –

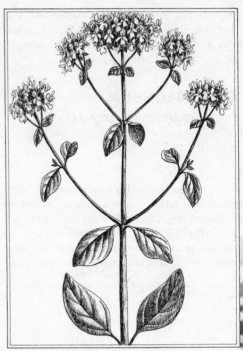

Origanum vulgare

help the dropsy and yellow jaundice – relieve scurvies, scabs – the running itch and tetters'.

The whole of the herb, which contains a strong, bitter tasting volatile oil, obtained by distillation, is still prescribed, mostly for its emmenagogue, stimulant, mild tonic and carminative effects. Warm infusions when taken produce perspiration and this will help promote menstruation if suppressed by cold. Herbalists still prescribe the infusion for relieving spasmodic complaints, such as asthma and coughs, or the fresh or dried tops in the form of a tea for nervous headache. The leaves (put into muslin bags) add a pleasant smell to bath water and are said to be good for easing aches and stiff joints, as is the oil if applied direct. This oil however is not to be confused with the 'Red Oil of Thyme', which is extracted from *Thymus vulgaris* and also sold under the name of 'Oil of Origanum'.

The Sweet or Knotted Marjoram (*O. majorana*, syn. *Majorana hortensis*), like the previous species, was administered medicinally by the ancient Greeks, and although native to North Africa, is now widely cultivated elsewhere. It is a very aromatic shrubby perennial up to 50cm/20in. tall, having small, opposite, oval- to lance-shaped greyish hairy leaves, and bearing small globular clusters of purplish, or occasionally white flowers in summer.

Both the Sweet and Wild Marjoram were extensively used by the Greeks, internally and externally in the treatment of dropsy, convulsions or spasms, and as an antidote for poison. They also planted the herbs on the graves of their dead, believing it would help them to sleep in peace.

Parkinson notes the many domestic uses of the 'swete margerome' while Culpeper writes of its medicinal qualities: 'Our Common Sweet Marjoram is warming and comforting in cold diseases of the head, stomach, sinews and other parts, taken inwardly or outwardly applied.' He advised it to help 'diseases of the chest, obstructions of the liver and spleen, old griefs of the womb, and the windiness thereof, and the loss of

speech, by resolution of the tongue ... It provokes womens' courses if put up as a pessary. Made into powder, and mixed with honey, it takes away the marks of blows and bruises; it takes away the inflammation and watering of the eyes, if mixed with fine flour and laid into them ... It is profitably put into ointments and salves that are warm, and comforts the outward parts, as the joints and sinews, for swellings also, and places out of joint. The powder snuffed up the nose provokes sneezing, and thereby purges the brain; chewed in the mouth it draws forth much phlegm ...'

The extracted oil of the herb, known as 'Oleum Majoranae', is still regarded as a useful external application for bruises and sprains, but although possessing certain stimulant, emmenagogue and mildly tonic principles, it appears to be little administered as an internal medicine.

As a culinary herb, the leaves add a delightful flavour to soups, stews and stuffings. Chopped up fresh or dried, they make a tasty garnish if sprinkled over cabbage, Brussel sprouts, carrots, marrow and salads. The leaves of both the above and the species mentioned below, retain their taste and fragrance when dried. For this the young shoots are best gathered when spindling for flower, tied in bundles and hung up in a shady place to dry. The leaves are then snipped from the shoots and are generally stored in jars for winter use.

By the end of the sixteenth century, several other Origanums had been introduced into British gardens from the Continent, where they were mostly cultivated as culinary herbs. For instance, sometime before 1568 Turner mentioned the Dittany of Crete (*O. dictamnus*), a native of southern Europe, which he had seen 'growynge in England in Maister Riches gardin'. This little plant, with its downy oval-roundish leaves, reaches about 30cm/11in. tall, and bears pinkish flowers in drooping spikes. The Pot Marjoram (*O. onites*) from Sicily, a hardier and more shrubby species, was certainly grown in England before 1597. The Marum Syriacum or Assyrian Masticke (*O. syriacum*) was to become a valued pot plant during the seven-

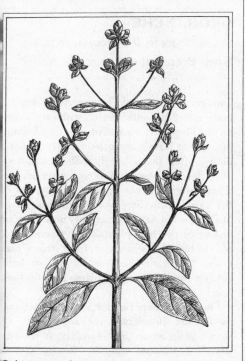

Origanum majorana

teenth century. Gerard says that in England, this herb was 'maintained with great care and diligence from the iniurie of our cold climate', while Evelyn warns it must be protected from cats, 'therefore guard it with a Furs or Holly branch'. Other species employed in cooking and as a flavouring include the Winter Marjoram (*O. heracleoticum*) from Greece, and the Marjoram of Candy.

A brownish-red powder known as 'Iodide of Carvacrol' or 'Cypress Origanum Oil' is extracted from the Cyprus Origanum (*O. dubium*) and sometimes used as an antiseptic in certain skin diseases, such as eczema.

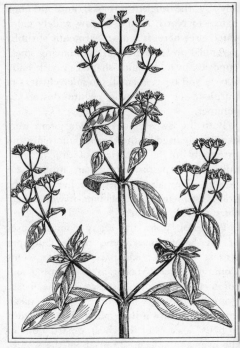

Origanum onites

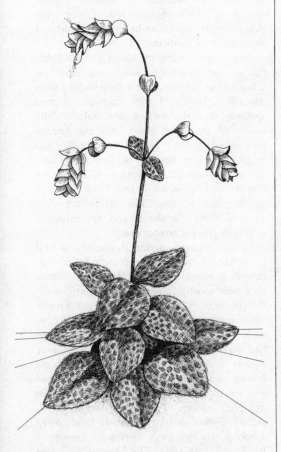

Origanum dictamnus

OROBANCHE

Orobanchaceae, the Broomrape family
Great Broomrape, Cancer Root

This genus consists of a large group of downy, unbranched parasitic herbs, without chlorophyll. They have succulent stems and scales in place of leaves, the colour varying from a dingy, often flushed, yellowish-brown, reddish-violet to purple, blue and even orange. There are numerous species in all parts of the world, including North America, much of Europe and Asia, the majority only growing on one or two host plants. The generic name of Orobanche is derived from the Greek *orobos*, a vetch, and *ancho*, to strangle, referring to the effect the plants have on their hosts.

One of the more familiar species, the Great or Greater Broomrape (*O. major*, syn. *O. rapum-genistae*), which is native to various parts of Europe and the Soviet Union, generally attaches itself to the roots of the

Gorse or Broom, and was once prescribed for its diuretic effects, although rarely used nowadays. This stout, honey-brown, leafless, club-like perennial reaches 70–100cm/ 27–40in. tall, the stem bears tapering scales, which become bracts towards the top. From May to July each stem bears a dense spike of yellowish, purple-tinged flowers.

As a medicinal herb the Greater Broomrape was prescribed throughout most of Europe during the sixteenth and seventeenth centuries 'as a remover of stone in the bladder and kidneys – and as a provoker of lusty urine' (as was the Broom itself) and was usually administered decocted in wine, as a bitter tasting, very astringent internal medicine. The juice externally applied was regarded as 'a singular remedy' in the treatment of 'old green wounds – the runnings of ulcers and sores – malignant and scabby ulcers, those that be hollow also' and 'for fretting sores'. For 'cleansing the skin' and for freckles, black or blue spots or pushes thereof' the flowering tops decocted were used as a wash.

A second species of Broomrape, known as

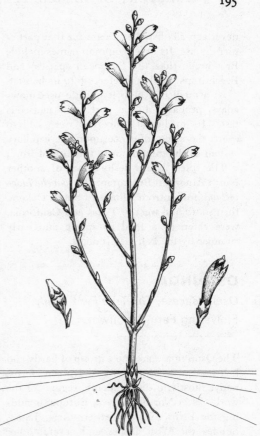

Orobanche virginiana

the Cancer Root (*O. virginiana*, syn. *Epifagus virginiana*), a native of eastern North America, where it is found from Wisconsin, south to Florida and Louisiana, was prescribed there during the nineteenth century as 'an eminent astringent'. This dull reddish inconspicious herb attaches itself to the root of the Beech (*Fagus sylvatica*), its smooth slender branched, leafless stem reaches 30–50cm/11–19in. tall and bears small clusters of whitish or whitish-purple flowers in August and September.

The whole of this plant, with its disagreeable taste, after 'yielding its virtues' to water or alcohol, was administered 'with benefit in fluxes and diarrhoea – erysipelas – and certain afflictions of the bowel', and as a useful 'application to obstinate ulcers, aphthous ulcerations', while locally 'applied to wounds it prevents or arrests the process of mortification' and 'arrests gangrenes'. Although known as the Cancer Root the species was

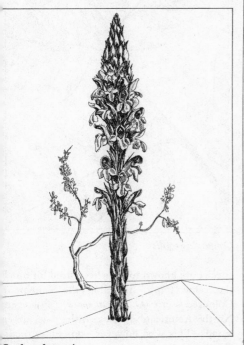

Orobanche major

never actually listed as a cure for that partic-
ular disease. Its other common names include
Broomrape (like the European species) and
Beechdrops, the latter referring to its habitat.

As a medicinal herb it is little used nowadays, probably due in part to its nauseous
taste. Its medicinal properties were said to
exert 'the same influence upon the capillary
system as the mineral drug tincture of iron'.

The thick, white fleshy bases of another
North American Broomrape, *Orobanche ludo-
viciana*, found from Illinois to South Dakota,
then south and west to Texas and California,
were eaten as a food in spring and early
summer by the Pah Ute Indians.

OSMUNDA

Osmundaceae, The True Fern family
Flowering Fern, Moonwort

The Osmundas make up a group of hardy and
half-hardy deciduous or evergreen ferns,
native mostly to the temperate regions of the
world, as in North America, Europe, including the British Isles, northern Asia, Japan,
besides the West Indies and several other
warmer countries. The different sorts vary in
height from about 30cm/11in. to over 2m/
6ft; they have feathery fronds, and the spores
are borne on separate leafless spikes, or on
spikes which develop from the ends of the
fronds, which gives rise to Flowering Ferns,
their common collective name. Their generic
name, Osmunda, is believed to be derived
from either 'Osmunder' one of the names of
Thor, the Norse god of thunder and war, or
from *os*, a bone, and *mundare*, to cleanse,
probably referring to some medicinal use.

One of the better known species formerly
prescribed in medicine was the King's Fern
or Royal Fern (*O. regalis*), a graceful plant
found throughout the United States and in
much of Europe, including parts of the
British Isles and other temperate countries.
It grows in watery and swampy places, forming a mass of rootstocks on the ground,
producing in summer several bright green
fronds up to and sometimes over 2m/6ft in
height. In the United States, this particular

species is commonly known as the Buckshorn
Brake, which alludes to the shape of its main
root or caudex, the part used in medicine.
These roots were generally dug up in August
and dried with great care and stored until
required for their 'abundance of mucilage',
which was extracted by boiling in water,
sweetened, and administered for 'coughs,
diarrhoea and dysentery' and as a tonic
'during convalescence from exhausting diseases'. Just one root infused in a pint of hot
water for half an hour 'will convert the whole
into a thick jelly' and this was considered
'very valuable in leucorrhoea and other
female weaknesses', while: 'The mucilage
mixed with brandy is a popular remedy as an
external application for subluxations and
debility of the muscles of the back.' Other

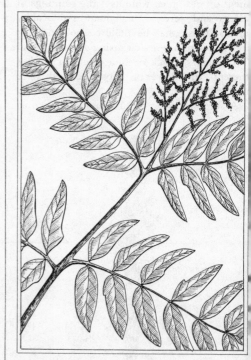

Osmunda regalis

species are known to have been used for much
the same thing, including the Cinnamon
Coloured Fern (*O. cinnamomea*), an elegant
North American species with pale green
fronds. This was, however, sometimes medicinally listed as a 'rather inferior plant'.

A fern of a different sort, the Moonwort (*O. lunaria*), although now botanically known as *Botrychium lunaria* (Natural Order Ophioglossacea) was formerly classified as a species of Osmunda, as listed by Culpeper in his *Herbal* and by other apothecaries of that time. The common name of this curious little herb, which is native to Britain and various parts of Europe, refers to the shape of its leaves which reach up to 30cm/11in., and are described by Culpeper as having 'one dark, green thick and flat leaf, standing upon a short footstalk, two fingers in breadth'. This is 'divided on both sides into five or seven parts, each part is small like the middle rib, broader forwards, pointed and round resembling a half moon . . .'

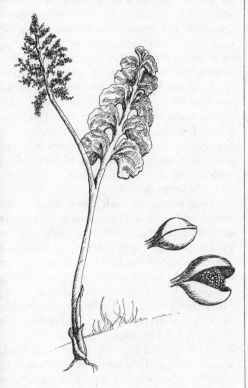

Osmunda lunaria

Only the leaves of this plant were prescribed in medicine, first 'boiled in any convenient red wine' which when drank 'stays immoderate fluxes – vomitings – bleedings – the whites – helps blows and bruises – is good for ruptures and similar burstings – and consoli-

dates all fractures and dislocations'. The leaves in oils, ointments and balsams, were also applied 'to heal fresh or green wounds'.

Today, neither the leaves of the Moonwort or the roots of the Flowering Ferns appear to be prescribed to any extent in herbal medicine.

The roots of several Osmunda species are nowadays exported from such countries as Canada, the United States and Japan, and these when cut and shredded become the Osminda fibre used in the potting of orchids.

PAPAVER
Papaveraceae, the Poppy family
White Poppy, Field Poppy

This genus is made up of a large number of hardy annual, biennial and perennial plants, native mainly to Europe, Asia and North America. Their generic name, Papaver, is believed to be derived from 'pap' referring to the milk-like juice found in the stems of some kinds.

The use of several species dates back to ancient times. The Egyptians made garlands of the stems and flowers, as well as adding the seed as a condiment to their food. The Greeks and Romans also added the seeds to cakes and bread as a flavouring, and according to Dioscorides, took them medicinally as a means of 'softening the belly'.

When Homer wrote that the Poppy was a well-known plant, common in gardens, he was probably referring to the White or Opium Poppy (*P. somniferum*). This erect, waxy, grey green annual 50–150cm/19–60in. tall, has large, deeply lobed or toothed clasping leaves, and bears from about May to July large whitish, lilac or purple flowers, followed by large hemispherical shaped capsules filled with brownish seeds. Probably native to the fields, waste ground and the waysides of Central Europe or the Middle East, it is now naturalized throughout Europe. It is also widely cultivated for the various alkaloids it contains in such countries as the United States, Egypt, Iran, Turkey, China and India.

This particular species has been valued for

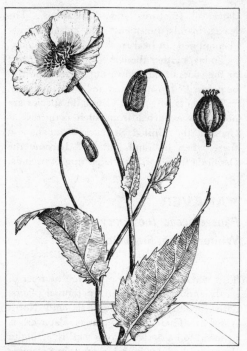

Papaver somniferum

centuries for the crude opium yielded by the seed pods, which has been prescribed since before the birth of Christ as a narcotic pain-killer and inducer of sleep. The plant had several other uses and was grown by the ancient Greeks for its edible non-narcotic seeds which, mixed with honey or wine, were regularly eaten by athletes especially those training for the Olympic Games. The Romans also sprinkled the top of their bread with White Poppy seed, a custom still observed throughout much of Europe and Britain today, and it was probably their soldiers who introduced the plant to several of these countries.

During the late medieval period, strong decoctions of the 'seed vessels' taken internally were regarded 'as of a gentle narcotic nature' and were administered 'to ease pain and cause sleep'.

The main reason for the plant's continued cultivation was, however, its opium content. Culpeper writes: 'Opium is nothing more than the milky juice of this plant, concreted into a solid form. It is procured by wounding the heads [the seed pods], when they are almost ripe, with a five-edged instrument, which makes as many parallel incisions from top to bottom; and the juice which flows from these wounds is the next day scraped off, and the other side of the head wounded in like manner. When a quantity of this juice is collected, it is worked together with a little water, till it acquires the consistence of pitch, when it is fit for use.'

According to Gerard: 'It mitigateth all kinds of paines, but it leaveth behinde it oftentimes a mischiefe woorse than the disease itself.' Culpeper prescribed it for various complaints: 'It relaxes the nerves, abates cramps, and spasmodic complaints – but it increases the paralytic disorders, and such as proceed from weakness of the nervous system. It incrassates thin serous acrid humours, and thus proves a speedy cure for catarrhs and tickling coughs, but must never be given in phthisical or inflammatory complaints; for it dangerously checks perspiration, unless its effects are counteracted by the addition of ammoniac or squills ... An overdose causes immoderate mirth or stupidity, redness of the face, swelling of the lips, relaxation of the joints, giddiness of the head, deep sleep, accompanied with turbulent dreams and convulsive starting, cold sweats and frequently death.'

Crude opium by itself has a disagreeable smell, and a hot biting taste, making it difficult to stomach. This was overcome by Paracelsus (1493–1541), the Swiss alchemist and physician, who made up a solution of opium in alcohol, to which over the following centuries numerous people became completely enslaved. This deadly mixture, known as Tincture of Opium, or Laudanum, was readily available from the nearest apothecary's shop until Victorian times in England, where it was frequently administered to teething or upset babies, simply to make them sleep. Professor Phelps Brown, writing of the plant's medicinal uses in the United States during the late nineteenth century, concurred: 'Opium is a narcotic and stimulant, acting under various circumstances as a sedative, antispasmodic, febrifuge and diaphoretic. It is anodyne, and extensively used for that purpose. There is no herbal medicine more extensively used, as well as abused, than Opium, and though a valuable remedy ... it is capable of doing great harm. Laudanum and paregoric are the forms mostly used in domestic practice, but the 'soothing syrups' and 'carminatives' found in nearly every nursery and household all contain Opium in some form, and work a great deal of mischief.' Paregoric was a camphorated Tincture of Opium and was prescribed not only to soothe and lessen pain, but was added in cough mixtures, and to relieve diarrhoea.

At least twenty-one different alkaloids are known to have been extracted from the White Poppy. Among the most important are the painkilling drugs Morphine (named after Morpheus the god of sleep), Codeine, Heroin, Narceine, Codamine and Papaverine. The latter is a non-addictive substance employed by doctors when they want to increase the flow of blood in a patient.

The crushed capsules or flowers are still prescribed in syrups for their anodyne and narcotic principles, or are added as ingredients to cough medicines. As a poultice, the crushed capsules can be combined with Chamomile flowers. In certain countries, including Britain, the law forbids the cultivation of any species or variety of Poppy from which opium can be extracted, that is unless a permit is first obtained. Even so, several decorative varieties of the Opium Poppy are still found in gardens, where they produce in summer, showy flowers of salmon and crimson to purple.

The species is still occasionally grown as a commercial crop in Britain, as it is in other parts of Europe and the countries previously mentioned, usually for its opium content. A variety with grey seeds is sold as a bird food under the name of 'Maw Seed'.

In the kitchen the seed of this plant is used as a topping on bread, rolls, cakes and pastries, and to give certain types of bread a better flavour. In India, they are an ingredient in the making of the native pancakes known as chupatties. The seeds have a nutty taste and contain a high percentage of oil.

Another species commonly prescribed in medicine was the Field or Corn Poppy (*P. rhoeas*) an erect, stiff-haired, branched, very

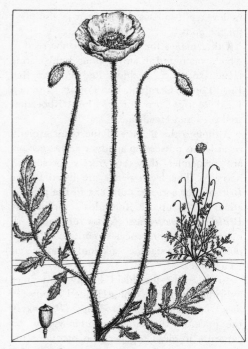

Papaver rhoeas

variable, wiry annual 25–90cm/10–35in. tall, with pinnate leaves and bearing single, deep scarlet flowers, often with a dark patch at the base, on long stalks, from about June to August. Although probably native to the Near East, it is now widely found in fields, cultivated ground and in waste places throughout Europe, Asia, North America, and the majority of temperate countries of the world.

Both Gerard and Parkinson recommended this odorous plant in the treatment of pleurisy. Culpeper elaborated: 'A syrup is made of the seed and flowers, which is useful to give sleep and rest to invalids, and to stay catarrhs and defluxions of rheums from the head into the stomach and lungs, which causes a continual cough, the forerunner of consumption – it helps hoarseness of the throat, and loss of voice, which the oil of the seed does likewise. The black seed boiled in wine, and drank, stays the flux of the belly and womens' courses. The poppy heads are usually boiled in water, and given to procure rest and sleep; so do the leaves in the same manner ... It cools inflammations, and agues. It is put in hollow teeth to ease the pain; it is also good for the gout.'

Other names for the species, some seed of which was found in an Egyptian tomb dating from 2500 B.C., include Red Poppy, Red Field Poppy, Common Red Poppy, Common Field Poppy, Corn Poppy, Flores Rhoeados, Redweed and Headache.

Although the flowers of the plant are still regarded as possessing anodyne and expectorant principles they are rarely prescribed herbally. The fresh petals are listed in the *British Pharmocopoeia* of 1885 in the preparation of 'Syrup of Rhoeados', and in the *British Pharmaceutical Codex* of 1949. All members of the species contain a non-poisonous crystalline alkaloid known as Rhoeadine.

In the wild the Field Poppy sometimes hybridizes with the Long Headed Poppy (*P. dubium*) and Babington's Poppy (*P. lecoqii*), the juice of the latter turning yellow on exposure to air. Culpeper also mentions the Welsh Poppy (*P. cambrica*, now known as *Meconopsis cambrica*) and the Black Poppy (*P. nigrum*). He writes that the flowers of the latter 'are of a gentle sudorific nature, and are peculiarly good in pleurisies, quinsies, and all disorders of the breast.'

PARIS

Liliaceae, the Lily family
(Sometimes listed under Trilliaceae)

Herb Paris

Only one or two species make up this genus of hardy herbaceous perennials, and only one was widely prescribed in herbal medicine, the Herb or Herba Paris (*P. quadrifolia*) which is native to much of Europe, including Britain and Russian Asia. It grows in damp, shady woods and similar places, its unbranched stems reach 15–40cm/6–15in. tall, and produce near the top a whorl of four large pointed stalkless leaves. From the centre of these rises a solitary, foetid-smelling, greenish-yellow flower, followed by a purple-black globular fruit containing the seed, which splits open when ripe.

The generic name of the plant is derived from the Latin *par* meaning equal, referring to the regularity of the leaves, as does the specific *quadrifolia*, four leaved. Its commonest name, Herba Paris, alludes to the same thing, meaning herb of equality. That of Herbe True-love could also point to the seeds and berries, which during the medieval period were crushed and taken in wine as aphrodisiacs throughout Europe and much of Russian Asia. These however are potentially dangerous and contain a glucoside known as Paradin which if taken even in small amounts can cause nausea, accompanied by violent sickness, convulsions, severe dizziness and 'a great sweating and dryness in the throat'. Poisonous as the plant is, Culpeper wrote: 'the leaves or berries are good as antidotes against all kinds of poison, especially that of aconites, and pestilential disorders.' Gerard

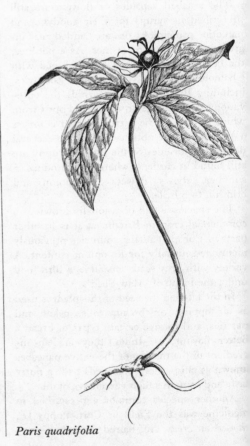

Paris quadrifolia

vas of the same opinion, adding: 'The same s ministered with great successe unto such s are become peevish.' The leaves were also used in Russia for treating madness. This ould have worked to a certain degree by ubduing or drugging the patient, for the plant has a narcotic action similar to that of opium.

In small doses, the roots, leaves and berries were prescribed for 'the pains of the colic – ramps – coughs – bronchitis – other rackings f the chest – and palpitations of the heart' while the juices of the seeds or leaves outwardly applied in a cooling ointment, were thought to be 'effectual for green wounds – ilthy sores and ulcers – tumours and swellings in the privy parts or groin – in other oarts' and 'will allay inflammations'. The xtracted juice of the berries was sometimes pplied as a cure for inflammation of the yes.

At present the herb is rarely if ever used by erbalists because of its poisonous effects, the oots probably being the least virulent part. Occasionally tincture of the fresh herb has been prescribed as an antidote for arsenic or mercurial poisoning. Other names previously used for this plant include *Aconitum pardali-inches* and *Solanum quadrifolium*.

A similar species, *Paris polyphylla*, is believed to have been used in the medicine of the Himalayas. This little herb bears flowers of much the same colour as the previous plant, but produces more leaves.

PHYSOSTIGMA
Leguminosae, the Pea family
Calabar Bean

The Calabar Bean (*Physostigma venenosum*) is a strong, twining perennial creeper, native to the Gulf of Guinea and the west coast of Africa. It reaches a height of some 45–50m/ 147–164ft has pinnately trifoliate leaves, and bears pendulous racemes of purplish flowers, followed by dark brown pods about 15cm/6in. long, containing dark brown or blackish-brown kidney-shaped seeds.

These extremely poisonous seeds, or beans,

which ripen throughout the year, although generally found during the rainy season, were used by the tribes of western Africa, as a simple method of determining by ordeal whether a person accused of a crime or witchcraft was guilty. The prisoner had to eat a certain amount of the seed. Should he vomit within a specified period, thus ridding himself of the poison, he was acquitted as innocent. Alternatively, if the seeds were retained, thus violently poisoning the person concerned, he or she was accounted 'guilty'. Certain types of crime were also punishable by forcing the guilty to drink an infusion of the crushed seed, which usually resulted in death within the hour.

The most active constituent of these beans, a colourless or pinkish crystalline alkaloid known as Physostigmine, is nowadays used medicinally as a way of stimulating the intestinal muscles, especially in chronic constipation, and externally in the treatment of eye disease, where it rapidly contracts the pupils. Taken internally, it raises the blood pressure, slows the pulse and depresses the

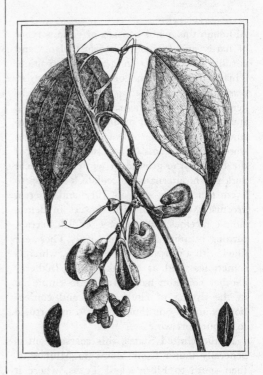

central nervous system, and was sometimes prescribed with the Deadly Nightshade (Atropa) in the treatment of epilepsy, nervous irritation, cholera and even acute tetanus.

One of the known antidotes for Calabar Bean poisoning is Atropine, itself a powerful alkaloid derived from the Deadly Nightshade. Poisoning by Physostigmine can also be counteracted by Strychnine, which has to be injected. Both methods are very dangerous, and are administered after the stomach has been evacuated.

Although native to the countries above, the Calabar Bean has since been introduced into several other regions, such as India and Brazil. The word Calabar itself probably refers to the river, town and district of that name in southern Nigeria. Other names for the species include Esere, Ordeal Bean and Chop Nut.

PHYTOLACCA

Phytolaccaceae, the Pokeweed family
Pokeweed

Although this genus consists of various types of hardy and tender herbaceous plants and shrubs, only one is in general cultivation. This is the Virginian Poke or Pokeweed (*P. americana*, syn. *P. decandra*), which is indigenous to North America and the principal species once used in medicine. This strong-smelling hardy herbaceous perennial, has smooth fleshy stems up to 3½m/11ft tall, that die back to the ground in winter, they bear dark green, alternate, lanceolate leaves up to 25cm/10in. long, and in July and August greenish-white or pinkish flowers in dense, simple racemes, followed by reddish berries, turning purplish black when ripe. These are filled with a purplish-crimson juice, which is sometimes used as an ink, hence Inkberry another common name. It is also employed in the dyeing of cloth, paper and confectionery and at one time was used in Portugal to colour port wine.

In the United States, this coarse plant is generally found from Maine to Minnesota, then south to Florida and Texas, where it grows by roadsides, on hills, in clearings, barnyards and in uncultivated soils, especially in rich, moist loams. Since its introduction to parts of North Africa and southern Europe, it has become naturalized besides being cultivated as a showy ornamental in several other countries including France, Germany and the British Isles.

The Delaware Indians are believed to have been the first to use the herb in medicine, prescribing it as a form of cardiac stimulant, and tribes in Virginia used it as a strong body purger. All these tribes also removed the more succulent growths in spring, cooking them in the way spinach or asparagus is today, taking care not to include any part of the poisonous root. These young shoots are still found on some American markets, under the name of 'sprouts'.

The stout, fleshy, perennial tap root of the Pokeweed formed the principal medicinal part, and was prescribed in small amounts, generally from one to five grains, for its emetic, cathartic, alterative and slightly

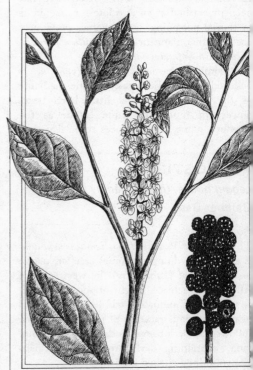

Phytolacca americana

narcotic principles. During the nineteenth century it was employed to excite the 'whole glandular system, and is very useful in syphilitic, scrofulous, rheumatic and cutaneous diseases'. The fully ripe berries were given for much the same thing, but were said to be milder in action, although several children are known to have died after eating them. The most active principle found in the herb is an alkaloid known as Phytolaccin, but several other constituents are yet to be identified.

The powdered root, or liquid extracts of the roots and berries are still administered for their emetic, cathartic and alterative effects, mainly for chronic rheumatism, as a remedy for dyspepsia, dysmenorrhoea, scabies, ulcers and ringworm. It has also been experimentally prescribed of late in the treatment of certain kinds of cancer.

Other names for the Pokeweed include Pigeon Berry, Garget, Skoke, Phytolaccae Radix, Phytolacca Americana, Blitum Americum, Bear's Grape, Branching Phytolacca, American Spinach, Jalap, Cokon, Crowberry, Cancer Root, American Nightshade and Chongras. Phytolacca, the generic name, is derived from *phyto*, a plant and *lacca*, a Latinized form of *lac* referring to the crimson-coloured juice of the berries. The commonest names of Poke and Pokeweed are derived from the Indian *Pocon*, alluding to any plant containing a red or yellow dye.

In Chile, the species known as *Phytolacca drastica* was and still is, as its specific name suggests, prescribed as a violent purgative.

PLANTAGO
Plantaginaceae, the Plantain family

Common Plantain, Buck's Horn Plantain, Ribwort Plantain, Psyllium Plantain

Most of the Plantains used in herbal medicine are native to various parts of Europe and Asia. This genus consists of annual or perennial herbs with their leaves arranged in basal rosettes near the ground, bearing small but numerous inconspicuous flowers on

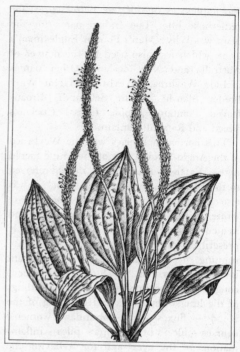

Plantago major

terminal heads or spikes, usually on long unbranched stems. Their generic name, Plantago, is derived from the Latin *planta* referring to the sole of the foot, to which the leaves of several kinds were likened. One or two of the species appear to have rated very highly in ancient medicine for Dioscorides, Pliny and Galen all praised their many uses, recommending them mainly as astringents and vulneraries in the treatment of bleeding and mad dog bites, for inflammation, asthma and fevers, and as a general remedy for eye disorders.

One such plant, the Common or Greater Plantain (*P. major*), is a low-growing perennial 10-60cm/4-23in. tall, with broad oval leaves, and bears, mostly during the summer months, greenish-yellow flowers on long spikes. Although native to Europe and parts of Asia, where it is found in lawns and similar grassy places, as well as in farmyards and well trodden ground, it is now widely naturalized elsewhere. On its introduction to North America it became known as Snakeweed, because a mixture of its juice and salt was applied as one of the 'better cures' for rattlesnake bite. The Indian name for the plant was White Man's Foot or Englishman's Foot, which was also used by the natives of Australia and New Zealand. Other names include Waybread, Weybroad, Great Way-brede, Slan-lus (from Scotland), Broad-leaved Plantain, Ripple Grass, Cuckoo's Bread and Ratstail Plantain.

This particular species was the Weybroed of the Anglo-Saxons, one of their nine sacred herbs. Later, Gower in the 1390s, referred to the Plantain as a 'herbe sovereine'; it was also mentioned by Chaucer; Shakespeare wrote of it as excellent for broken shins and as a cure for sores. Besides this, it was widely prescribed for 'inflammations of the skin – running or spreading sores – malignant ulcers – ulcers of the lungs – vehement coughs – and rackings of the chest – bleedings of the lungs – spittings and breeding of the blood – fluxes – too abundant womens' courses – ulcers in the reins – piles – inflammations of the eyes' and for 'relieving the making of foul and bloody water'.

Culpeper recommended the juice mixed with the Oil of Roses for easing 'the pains of the head proceeding from heat. The same also is profitably applied to all hot gouts in the hands and feet ... One part of the herb water and two parts of the brine of powdered beef, boiled together and clarified, is a remedy for all scabs and itch in the head and body, all manner of tetters, ringworms, the shingles, and all other running and fretting sores.' Salmon in his *Herbal* (1710) recommended the Essence of Plantain, Houseleeks (Sempervivum) and lemon juice as a good cosmetic.

The fresh leaves are still prescribed for their cooling, alterative and diuretic principles. If bruised and rubbed on, or applied in the form of a poultice, they will stay the bleeding of minor wounds, and bring relief to burns, insect and nettle stings, etc. Infusions of the bitterish, astringent tasting leaves are sometimes taken for relieving diarrhoea and piles. In China the leaves of this plant were once eaten as a pot-herb or as spring greens.

The Hoary Plantain (*P. media*), like the previous species, is found throughout Europe in meadows and by the wayside, and is now naturalized elsewhere, and was prescribed for much the same things. This downy, greyish-looking perennial has longer but narrower, oval to elliptic leaves, bearing rather shorter stalked spikes of greyish flowers with pinkish-lilac stamens. Gerard writes: 'The juice dropped in the eies cooles the heate and inflammation thereof.' The seeds boiled 'in any convenient decoction' were also given

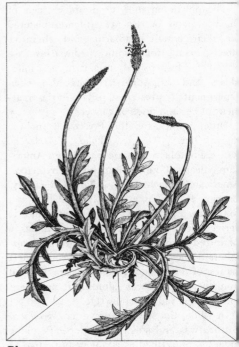

Plantago coronopus

for their laxative and demulcent principles at least to the end of the nineteenth century.

The Buck's Horn Plantain (*P. coronopus*) is usually a downy, prostrate growing annual or biennial, with variable, but generally pinnately lobed, rosette forming dark green leaves (occasionally linear and hardly toothed) with a single vein. From April to October yellowish flowers are borne in slender cylindrical spikes on hairy stems 5–40cm, 2–15in. tall. The plant is found throughout Europe in dry sandy places, on paths and bare ground, especially near the sea.

Salmon notes that the name 'Common

Buck's Horn Plantain' refers to the shape of its leaves, these 'resembling the snaggs of a Buck's Horn', adding that 'the leaves lie round about the root on the ground, resembling the form of a star' from which it took another name, Herba Stella.

Of its medicinal uses he writes: 'The qualities, specification and virtues are the very same as those of Plantage major . . . The decoction in wine, if it is long drank, cureth the stranguary, and is profitable for such as are troubled with sand, gravel, stones, etc. . . . The cataplasm of leaves and roots with bay salt applied to both wrists and bound on pretty hard . . . cures agues admirably.' In Gerard's time one of the cures for the ague was to wear the entire plant, root included, around the neck. He says if a drink made from the boiled leaves were taken night and morning 'for certain days together', it helps 'most wonderfully those that have sore eyes, watery or blasted, and most of the griefs that happen unto the eyes'.

Medicinally, the Ribwort Plantain (*P. lanceolata*) was sometimes substituted for the Common Plantain. It is a hairless or finely haired perennial 5–70cm/2–27in. tall, with narrow lance-shaped, finely toothed, three to seven veined leaves, and bears from about April to October yellow anthered brownish flowers on wiry furrowed stalks. Although native to all Europe and parts of Asia, it is now naturalized throughout the world, growing in lawns, meadows, pastures, in ditches, by roadsides and on wasteland.

Its seeds, like several other Plantago species, have absorbent coats, which after rain become mucilaginous. To obtain this gelatinous substance, the seeds were collected and soaked for a time in hot water, and the resulting mixture was then used to stiffen muslin and certain other fabrics. The juice extracted from the fresh green leaves was medicinally used to promote the healing of wounds, and according to Culpeper, the same as 'commended for the ague, to lessen it.'

Other names for the plant include Cocks, Hemps, Hen Plant, Lamb's Tongue, Jackstraw, Black Jack, Soldiers Ribwort, Ribble Grass, Snake Plantain, Black Plantain and Long Plantain.

The shiny dark brown, tasteless, but mucilaginous seeds of the Psyllium Plantain (*P. psyllium*) also yield a large amount of mucilage and were prescribed internally and externally for their demulcent and emollient principles, as were the leaves, much as for the Common Plantain. This species is found in the southern parts of Europe, North Africa and southern Asia, although now naturalized elsewhere. It is known by several other names, such as Psyllium Seed, Fleaseed, Fleawort,

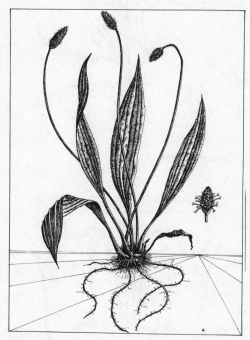

Plantago lanceolata

Psyllion and Psyllios. Gerard writes of it: 'Fleawort is called in English, Fleawort; not because it killeth fleas, but because the seeds are like fleas.' He continues: 'The seed of Fleawort boiled in water or infused, and the decoction or infusion drunke, cooleth the heate of the inward parts, and quencheth drowth and thirst . . . The seeds stamped and boiled in water to the form of a plaister, and applied, takes away all swellings of the joints, especially if you boile the same with vinegar and oil of roses, and apply it as aforesaid.' He warns: 'To much Fleawort seed taken

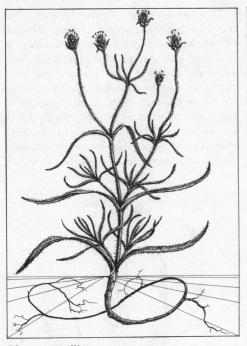

Plantago psyllium

inwardly is hurtfull, to mans nature . . .'

Gerard also prescribed the plant now identified as the Shrubby Plantain (*P. semper-virens*, syn. *P. suffruticosa* or *P. cynops*), a much branched, woody based, tufted shrublet 5–40cm/2–15in. tall, which he had 'growing in my garden'.

The dried seed of the Ispaghul Plantain (*P. ovata*, syn. *P. ispaghula*, or *P. decumbens*), which is found in such countries as the Canary Islands, Spain, Iran and India, were some-times mixed with sugar and prescribed in chronic diarrhoea and dysentery, and for relieving the inflamed membranes of the intestinal canal. As an astringent in childrens' diarrhoea, the seed was usually roasted first. Like certain other species, the mucilage contained in the seed coat of this plant was used to stiffen linen. Other names for the Ispaghul Plantain include Ispaghula and Spogel Seed. The seeds of the Indian species *Plantago amplexicaulis*, are also sold as Ispaghula, and these are administered as a demulcent for dysentery and intestinal complaints.

POLYGONATUM
Liliaceae, the Lily family
Solomon's Seal

About 30 species of this genus of mostly hardy, herbaceous perennials are known. The majority are found in the northern temperate regions, for example North America, Europe including the British Isles, North Africa, Asia and the Himalayas.

The most popular kind to be used in herbal medicine was the common Solomon's Seal (*P. multiflorum*, syn. *Convallaria multiflora*) a hairless perennial, native to much of Europe, extending to Siberia and Japan although often grown elsewhere. It has a thick creeping rootstock and graceful arching stems 30–60cm/11–24in. high, with elliptical alternate leaves and bearing in early summer white drooping bell-like flowers, tipped with green, on slender pendulous stalks, followed by bluish-black spherical berries. In the wild this plant grows in woods or similar shade

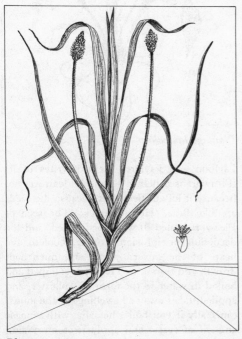

Plantago ovata

laces, and is also found locally in Canada
nd the United States, generally in beech
woods and on damp calcareous soils.

The most familiar name of the species,
Solomon's Seal, also refers to several other
plants of the genus, and probably alludes to
their rootstocks, which if cut through reveal

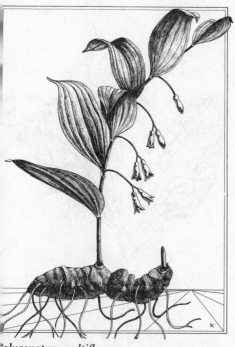

Polygonatum multiflorum

markings once likened to certain Hebrew
characters, but which are, in fact, the round
seal-like scars left by the previous stems. The
generic name, Polygonatum, is derived from
the Greek words *poly*, meaning many, and
ony or *gonatos*, knee, referring either to the
knotted roots, or to the jointed stems, while
multiflorum, the specific name of the plant
mentioned here, means 'many flowered'. Its
other names include Scala Coely, Sigillum
Salomonis, Lady's Seal, St Mary's Seal,
Job's Tears, Jacob's Ladder, White-Wort,
White-Root, David's Harp, David's Seal and
Ladder to Heaven.

Dioscorides prescribed the Solomon's
Seal for the healing of wounds and the
setting of broken bones, although Galen
warned that neither the root nor the leaves

should be taken as an internal medicine. (The
sweet rather pleasant tasting berries have
since been found to contain a poisonous
constituent known as Anthraquinone, which
can cause vomiting and diarrhoea.) During
the medieval period the crushed root was still
prescribed in Europe and Asia as an external
application to broken bones and fractures. In
England, where it was sometimes called
Scalacely, it had become a cultivated herb by
the 1450s, although it had been used medicinally for many years before that. Gerard in the
late 1500s recommended it for mending
broken bones both in humans and cattle. He
also advised: 'The root of Solomon's seale
stamped while it is fresh and greene, and
applied, taketh away in one night, or two at
the most, any bruise, blacke or blew spots
gotten by fals, or womens wilfulnesse, in
stumbling upon their hasty husbands fists,
or such like.' Culpeper adds: 'The distilled
water of the whole plant takes away morphew,
freckles, etc., from any part of the body.'

In the United States during the nineteenth
century, the roots of this species were
regarded as tonic, astringent and mucilaginous and were prescribed for 'the whites',
pectoral infections, menorrhagia, female debility, inflammations of the stomach and
intestines, erysipelas, neuralgia, the itch and
local inflammations, etc. A North American
species of Solomon's Seal (*P. biflorum*) was
sometimes used as a substitute in herbal
medicine there. The starchy roots of the plant,
which is known in America as the True
Solomon's Seal, were at one time eaten as a
food by the Indians.

One or two other species possessing similar
medicinal properties were prescribed to a
lesser degree, including the Sweet Scented or
Angular Solomon's Seal (*P. odoratum*, syn.
P. officinale) which is locally found in the
woods and rocky places of Europe, parts of
Asia and China. This plant is similar in
appearance to the Common Solomon's Seal,
has angular stems and fragrant flowers – as
odoratum, its specific name, suggests. In
Turkey, the tender young shoots are still
boiled and eaten, much like asparagus.

The roots and the rhizomes of the common
Solomon's Seal are prescribed nowadays

generally infused for their astringent, demulcent and tonic principles, and are sometimes combined with other remedies in the treatment of pulmonary infections, dysentery, piles and certain womens' complaints. The powdered roots can be usefully applied as a poultice to piles, inflammations, tumours and bruises.

PRIMULA
Primulaceae, the Primrose family
Cowslip, Primrose, Auricula

The Primulas are mostly low-growing, perennial flowering herbs, native mainly to the northern temperate zone, including North America, Europe, China, the Himalayas and Japan. Their generic name, Primula, is derived from the Latin word *primus*, meaning first, referring to the early flowering of some kinds.

One of the most popular species prescribed in the medicine of medieval Europe and Asia was the Cowslip (*P. veris*, syn. *P. officinalis*), a downy perennial found in open woods, meadows and pasture land. Its bright green wrinkled leaves narrow at the base to form a rosette on the ground. From April to May nodding clusters of sweetly scented drooping yellow flowers, with orange spots in the throat, are borne on leafless stems rising 10–30cm/4–15in. above the leaves.

The actual meaning of Cowslip, the commonest present-day name of this plant is rather obscure, although it could be derived from the Old English *Cusloppe*, referring to its liking for fields and pastures where cattle are kept (it was once believed to have sprung from cow dung). Other names of this sort include the Anglo-Saxon *Cuy lippe*, Cooslip and Cowflop. Other common names include Fairies Basins, Fairies Cups, Saint Peter's Keys, Virgin's Keys, Herb Peter, Paigle, Drelip, Peagles and Peggle.

Two other names, Palseywort and Herba paralysis, point to the medicinal uses of the herb in the treatment of 'palsey, convulsions, spasms, giddiness and cramps'. Gerard mentions its use for the palsy, and says it is

'good against the paines of the joint and sinews'. He adds: 'An unguent made with the juice of Cowslips and oil of Linseed, cureth all scaldings or burnings with fire, water, or otherwise.'

Culpeper tells us: 'An ointment made with

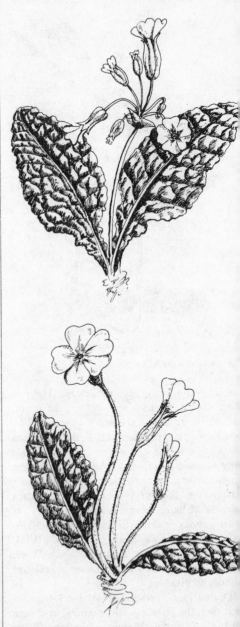

Primula veris (top) and *Primula vulgaris* (below)

em (the leaves), taketh away spots and
rinkles of the skin, sun burnings and
eckles, and adds beauty exceedingly; they
medy all infirmities of the head coming of
eat and wind, as vertigo, ephialtes, false
paritions, frenzies, falling sickness, palsies,
nvulsions, cramps, pains in the nerves . . .
e roots ease pains in the back and bladder,
d open the passages of the urine. The leaves
e good in wounds, and the flowers take
vay trembling.' The use of the root in
eating pains of the back and muscular
eumatism is also referred to in another old
me – *Radix Arthritica*. Hill, in the 1750s,
ys the powdered root boiled in ale, or the
rup made from the flowers, were taken by
untry folk – for giddiness, wakefulness and
milar troubles.

At one time the flowers of this plant, in the
rm of Cowslip Wine, made a very popular
untry drink, taken not only for pleasure,
it as a nervine and sedative. This is still
ade, as are conserves of the flowers, which
ere formerly eaten with sweetmeats, added
salads, or used with other herbs to stuff
rtain kinds of meat.

The flowers are still prescribed in teas and
anes for their antispasmodic, nervine and
dative principles, to help relieve nervous
ain, cramps, convulsions, spasms and
rious other pains.

The Primrose (*P. vulgaris*) is a low-
owing, hairy perennial, with crinkly lance-
ate rosette-forming leaves tapering to the
lk. It bears from March to May, solitary,
ft pale yellow flowers on long shaggy stalks
ing from the rootstock. Like the previous
ecies it had several medicinal uses. It is
und in the woods, meadows, orchards and
the banks of ditches and streams in most
Europe and parts of Asia, although now
dely cultivated as a garden ornamental
ewhere. In the wild it often hybridizes
th the Cowslip and the True Oxlip (*P.
tior*).

Culpeper says the roots of the Primrose
re 'used as a sternutory to the head – the
st way of using them is to bruise them, and
press the juice, which being snuffed up the
se, occasions violent sneezing, and brings
ay a great deal of water, but without being

productive of any bad effect . . . Dried and
reduced to powder it will produce the same
effect, but not so powerfully. In this state it is
good for nervous disorders, but the dose
must be small.' He adds: 'A dram and a half
of the dried roots taken in autumn, is a strong,
but safe emetic.' Parkinson was of the opinion
the plant was good for headaches. During the
nineteenth century, in North America, the
Primrose was administered internally for
paralysis, rheumatism and gouty infections,
much as recommended by Pliny so many
centuries earlier.

The dried rootstocks, or the whole of the
herb in flower, is still given infused or in
tinctures, for its vermifuge, antispasmodic
and sedative principles. Both the flowers and
the root contain a fragrant oil known as
Primulin, the acrid taste of which is due to
Saponin. Other names for the plant include
Butter Rose, Pimrose, Easter Rose, Simmerin,
Lent Rose and, like the previous species,
Herba paralysis.

The Auricula (*P. auricula*), a variable
perennial with a lax rosette of basal, generally

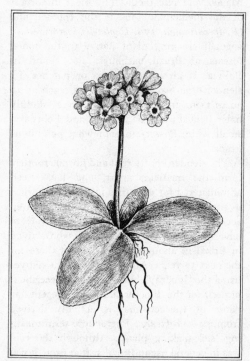

Primula auricula

entire, hairless fleshy leaves, bears from May to July umbels of sweetly scented flowers on stems 5–25cm/2–10in. high, was formerly used in the Alps in the treatment of coughs. This showy perennial, often listed as Bear's Ear or Mountain Cowslip, is native to the mountains of Central Europe, but is now widely grown as an ornamental in many other countries. A tincture made from the Chinese species, *Primula obconica*, is employed in homoeopathic medicine.

PSYCHOTRIA
Rubiaceae, the Madder family
Ipecacuanha

This genus consists of a number of flowering shrubs, which have smooth leathery or hairy leaves, bear small clusters of pendulous though insignificant white or greenish flowers, followed by small inedible, roundish, blue or red berries. They are native to the warmer parts of the world, such as tropical America, Malaya and Nicaragua. The most important of the medicinal kinds is the Ipecacuanha (*P. ipecacuanha*, syn. *Cephaelis ipecacuanha*), a small creeping plant native to the moist forests of Brazil, although also found in Bolivia. It grows in clumps or patches, its slender often woody-based stems reach up to 30cm/11in. and bear oblong leaves, slightly hairy beneath and in January and February, small white flowers in somewhat pendulous heads.

The slender knotty root and fibrous rootlets form the medicinal part, and have been administered for centuries in South America, in small doses as an emetic. The first written account of the plant appears, however, to have been by a Portuguese friar who arrived in Brazil in about 1570, and lived there for the next 30 years. After observing the natives using the 'Igpecayla' he started to prescribe it himself for the 'bloody flux'. The present day name of Ipecacuanha, is actually derived from *ipe-kaa-guene*, a Portuguese term meaning 'sick-making plant'. Although the root was in general use in Brazil at that time, it was not until 1672 that it was first brought to

Europe. In 1680 some reached the physician Helvetius, who immediately set out t[o] discover their medicinal uses. After severa[l] trials he produced a remedy for the treatmen[t] of dysentery, for which he was granted th[e] sole right of vending by Louis XIV, late[r] selling the formula to the French governmen[t]

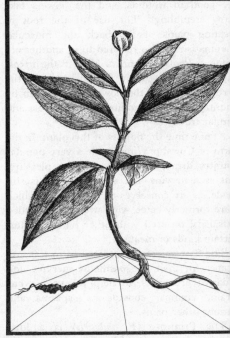

Psychotria ipecacuanha

who made it public in 1688.

The greyish or reddish-brown roots, know[n] in commerce as Brazilian or Rio Ipecacuanh[a] are still valued, when deprived of the[ir] alkaloids, for their diaphoretic, emetic an[d] expectorant principles. Small doses a[re] prescribed for relieving coughs and colds, [to] promote perspiration, as a stimulant for th[e] stomach, liver and intestines, for relievin[g] dysentery, and is an old remedy for croup [in] babies. The most active principle extract[ed] from the root is an alkaloid known as Emetin[e] which if injected subcutaneously rapid[ly] eases tropical or amoebic dysentery, althoug[h] its toxic action on the heart has to be careful[ly] watched. Large doses of the root generally a[...]

as emetic, but can, like the alkaloid, cause gastro-enteritis, dilation of the blood vessels, heart failure and pulmonary inflammation.

The roots of similar species employed in medicine include the Cartagena Ipecacuanha (*P. acuminata*) from Colombia, and the Black or Peruvian Ipecacuanha (*P. emetica*) from Peru and Bolivia, which in commerce is known as Striated Ipecacuanha.

The generic name of these plants, Psychotria, is derived from *psyche*, meaning soul or life, probably referring to their medicinal uses. A number of the species are also used as dye plants.

Several other plants containing certain emetic principles are also known as Ipecacuanha, including the American Ipecacuanha (*Gillenia stipulacea*); the Wild Ipecacuanha (*Euphorbia ipecacuanha*); the Guinea Ipecacuanha (*Boerhavia decumbens*); the Venezuela Ipecacuanha (*Sarcostemma glaucum*) and the Ipecacuanha de Allemands (*Vincetoxicum officinale*).

PULMONARIA
Boraginaceae, the Borage family
Lungwort

The Lungworts make up a small genus of hardy, low-growing perennial herbs, with about six species native to various parts of Europe, where they are mostly found in thickets and damp open woods. Their generic name, Pulmonaria, is derived from the Latin *pulmo* or *pulmonis*, meaning a lung, and this with their collective name of Lungwort refers to the use of some of the genus in treating a range of chest complaints.

The species generally prescribed in medicine, *Pulmonaria officinalis*, is found in most of Europe, including the British Isles, and is a hairy, weak-stemmed perennial up to 30cm/12in. tall, with alternate, mostly spotted, oval or heart shaped leaves, the lower ones stalked, and bearing from March to June, a succession of pinkish or reddish flowers, which on maturing turn to violet-blue.

The use of this plant in medicine probably originated from the appearance of its leaves,

which are green, blotched or speckled with white. These were likened to unhealthy lungs under the Doctrine of Signatures which taught that the various herbs carried evidence of their healing virtues on them, or else gave a sign, as in this case, of the ailment or illness for which they could be prescribed. As William Coles, a contemporary of Culpeper, explained, God gave such herbs 'for the use of Men and hath given them particular signatures whereby a Man may read even in legible characters the use of them.' Therefore the leaves of the Pulmonaria became widely employed throughout Europe, especially during the sixteenth and seventeenth cen-

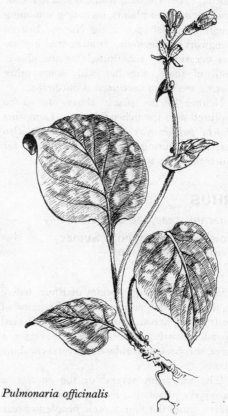

Pulmonaria officinalis

turies, for 'all disorders and diseases of the breast'.

The herb's other common names include Jerusalem Cowslip, Cowsloppus of Jerusalem, Jerusalem Sage, Bethlehem Sage, Joseph and Mary, Adam and Eve, Soldiers and Sailors, Joseph's Coat, Sage of Bethlehem, William and Mary, Hundreds and Thousands, Beggar's Basket and Spotted Dog.

During the nineteenth century, this particular species of Lungwort was 'freely cultivated' in the United States, where it is now occasionally found in the wild. It was prescribed there for its demulcent and mucilaginous principles, and in decoctions was considered 'very useful in bleeding from the lungs' in 'bronchial and catarrhal affections and other affections of the respiratory organs'.

The Lungwort is nowadays regarded as having little medicinal use, although its leaves are still prescribed in herbalism for the mucilage they contain, which is said to soothe various chest complaints, including whooping cough. A similar species, the Narrow Leaved Lungwort (*P. longifolia*), from central Europe was occasionally substituted for the above. Both of these, together with some other species, were also once used as pot herbs.

Neither of the plants above are to be confused with the lichen known as Lungwort (*Sticta pulmonaria*) although this was also prescribed during the medieval period for much the same things.

RHUS

Anacardiaceae, the Cashew family

Poison Oak, Staghorn Sumac, Wig or Smoke Tree

There are about 150 species of Rhus, native to the temperate and sub-tropical regions of both hemispheres. It is a rather complicated genus, consisting of deciduous and evergreen trees, shrubs, sub-shrubs and several climbing plants.

The sap from several of the species is extremely poisonous. Even contact with the leaves causes the skin of some people to break out in a distressing rash, often accompanied by painful swellings or inflammation, and in severe cases ulceration. One such plant that can cause an eczema-like eruption if touched, is the Poison Oak or Poison Vine (*R. toxicodendron*), a low-growing shrub native to North America, where it is found in dry

woodland from New Jersey to Georgia and Texas. A similar plant, the Common Poison Ivy (*R. radicans*), a low straggling shrub, sometimes seen as a stout woody vine climbing over trees, is found from Nova Scotia to British Columbia, then south to Florida and Mexico. The Western or Californian Poison Oak (*R. diversiloba*) an erect, occasionally climbing shrub up to 2½m/8ft high, is found from Washington through California to Mexico. All three are generally known, depending on area, as Poison Ivy, Poison Oak or Poison Sumach. The first two, and occasionally the third, are classed by some botanists as varieties of one species, because all three have leaves divided into three ovate leaflets, variously indented and lobed and downy beneath, and bear in June slender clusters or panicles of inconspicuous greenish-white flowers in the axils of the leaves, followed by clusters of small globular greyish-white waxy berry-like fruits.

The acrid tasting juice from the fresh leaves of *Rhus toxicodendron* was formerly prescribed in the medicine of North America for its

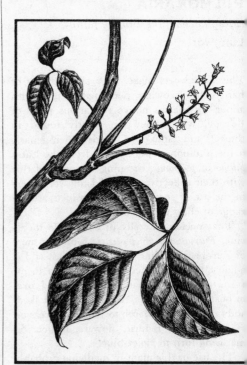

Rhus toxicodendron

irritant, rubefacient, stimulant and narcotic' principles 'in palsies, paralysis, drowsiness, stupours, delirium, rheumatism, stiffness, herpetic troubles [and] certain other eruptive diseases' as a 'vesicant for producing blisters', and at one time was officially listed in the *Pharmacopoeia* of the United States. Although the plant was introduced into England in the 1640s, it was not employed in medicine there until the end of the eighteenth century when it was first used in the treatment of obstinate herpetic eruptions.

The juice from the leaves is still regarded as possessing irritant, narcotic and stimulant principles, and is prescribed for obstinate skin diseases, in small doses as a sedative for the nervous system, and incontinence. A tincture of it is used in homoeopathic medicine for relieving nettle stings, ringworm, eczema and for rheumatism.

The Poison Sumach (*R. vernix*), as its common name implies, is also poisonous to the touch, and is found in swampy ground, growing up to 7m/23ft tall, from Quebec and Minnesota, south to Florida and Texas. The milky juice from this species was also used as a vesicant, and for marking linen. It is still added as an ingredient to liquid dressings (or varnishes) for finishing boots and shoes. Its other names include Poison Elder, Poison Dogweed and Poison Ash.

The root bark of the Fragrant or Sweet Scented Sumach (*R. canadensis* syn. *Rhus aromatica* or *Schmaltzia crenata*), a smaller species only reaching about 1½m/5ft high, found in rocky situations from Vermont, Ontario and Minnesota to Florida and Texas, was and still is occasionally prescribed infused or in liquid extracts for its astringent and diuretic principles in diabetes, leucorrhoea, diarrhoea and discharges of the bladder and kidneys. The acrid-tasting red fruits of this plant were used by the Indians to make refreshing drinks, as were those of the Squaw Bush or Ill Scented Sumach (*R. trilobata* syn. *Schmaltzia trilobata*), which some botanists consider to be a variety of the Fragrant Sumach. The stems of both these plants were split and used in basket making by the Indians of California, Arizona and New Mexico.

The pleasant acid-tasting fruits of the Sour Berry or Lemonade Tree (*R. integrifolia*) from southern California were also used by the Indians to flavour cooling drinks. This shrub grows about the sand dunes along the coastal cliffs, has leathery evergreen leaves and bears small pink flowers in crowded clusters. A similar drink is made from the red fruits of the Dwarf or Mountain Sumach (*R. copallina*), a glossy looking shrub indigenous to the dry soils from Maine to Minnesota, down to Florida and Texas. It is this species that provides 'Copal Resin' and 'Copal Varnish' when mixed with Oil of Turpentine.

The sour, crimson haired berries of the Smooth or Scarlet Sumac (*R. glabra*) another shrubby species, reaching 2–4m/6–13ft high, were infused and taken for their refrigerant and diuretic principles in the treatment of febrile diseases and bowel complaints, or were simply used in the making of 'Indian Lemonade'. In the late nineteenth century it was said that: 'The bark of the root has sometimes been used with success in decoction or syrup as a palliative of gonorrhoea, leucorrhoea, diarrhoea, hectic fever, dysentery and scrofula. Combined with the barks of white pine (*Pinus strobus*, syn. *P. albus*) and slippery elm in certain particular doses of decoction, it will, with other very simple treatment, cure syphilis.' Infusions of the berries were regularly taken for diabetes, gargled for quinsy and ulcers of the throat, and used 'as a wash for ulcers, running tetters, ringworm – and other foul skin diseases'. The milky fluid or sap that oozed from the bark 'on being dried and powdered', was sometimes mixed with lard or linseed oil and applied to haemorrhoids.

The powdered berries, liquid extracts of the berries, or of the bark, or of the active principle known as Rhusin, are still prescribed in herbal medicine for some of these complaints. A medicinal wine is also made from the berries, as is a black dye.

The leaves and bark of this species (and others) are employed in industry for dyeing wool and in the tanning of leather, and are sometimes cultivated for this purpose, for example in Virginia.

The Staghorn Sumach or Lemonade Tree (*R. typhina*, syn. *Rhus hirta*), is a common species native to rocky or dry, gravelly soils from Nova Scotia to South Dakota, then south to Georgia, Indiana and Iowa. It grows in thickets, by the borders of woods, alongside fences and in neglected fields and was frequently substituted in medicine for the previous plant. A smooth barked shrub, which is now naturalized in southern Europe, it reaches about 7m/23ft in height, has pinnate leaves with oblong-lanceolate, sharp pointed leaflets, dark green above and pale beneath, and bears in June, or sometimes a little later, dense terminal panicles of small greenish-yellow flowers, followed in early autumn by small, crimson-haired berries, which remain on the tree all winter. Its common names of Staghorn Sumach and Velvet Sumach refer to the young branches and twigs, which are covered by a dense, velvety hair like the horns of a stag. Another name, Vinegar Tree, refers to its sour tasting fruits, again a major ingredient in the making of Indian Lemonade. The Sugarbush (*R. ovata*), from the dry hills and mountains of southern California, is a glossy evergreen bearing stiff panicles of flowers. These turn into red berries, which were eaten by some Indian tribes as a form of sugar.

Only one species from the Old World appears to have been used in medicine, the Wig or Smoke Tree (*R. cotinus*, syn. *Cotinus coggygria*). This dense, spreading shrub up to 3m/10ft in height, has rounded to obovate aromatic leaves, and bears from May to July lax spreading pyramidal clusters of yellowish or purplish flowers. These lengthen to become plume-like with spreading hairs, and resemble a wig when seen from a distance which, together with its blue-green leaves, gave rise to its common names. It is native to certain parts of southern Europe, where it is found on dry hills, rocky places and open woods.

Of its medicinal uses Culpeper says: 'The seeds dried, reduced to powder and taken in small doses, stop purgings and hemorrhages, the young shoots have great efficacy in strengthening the stomach and bowels, if taken in a strong infusion. The bark of the

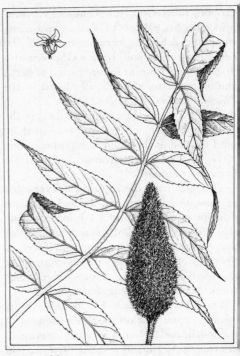

Rhus typhina

roots has the same virtues, but in an inferior degree.' Its wood, known as 'young fustic', yields a yellow dye, and is used in the tanning of leather. Other names for the shrub include Venetian Sumach and Hungarian Sumach.

A second species native to the dry thickets and stony places of the Mediterranean parts of Europe, the Sicilian Sumach (*R. coriaria*), is cultivated there, as it is in Cyprus as a field crop for its bark, which yields both yellow and red dyes. Its young branches are dried and powdered, and employed for tanning Moroccan leather. Although regarded as potentially poisonous, its fruits and leaves have been prescribed in medicine as a styptic and astringent.

Several other species are used in commerce, including the Lacquer or Varnish Tree (*R. verniciflua*) from China and Japan, the sap of which is used to tan different kinds of leather, and is the source of the varnish used in Japanese lacquerware; and the Japanese Wax or Wax Tree (*R. succedanea*) from the eastern parts of Asia, the Himalayas and Japan. The wax-like substance from the berries of this species is made into candles, is added as an adulterant to white beeswax, and was similarly used in the making of pomades. The roots of the Tizra or Tizara (*R. pentaphylla*) from North Africa are also used in tanning.

ROSMARINUS
Labiatae, the Mint family
Rosemary

Only two or three species of Rosmarinus are known, and only one, the Rosemary (*R. officinalis*) a native of the Mediterranean region and Asia Minor, was used in medicine. A variable, much branched, dense evergreen shrub 1–3m/3–10ft high, with linear leathery leaves, glossy green above, but covered with whitish hairs beneath, it bears, usually in April and May, although found at all seasons, pale whitish to lilac flowers in small axillary leafy clusters. In the wild it is found in bushy places among rocks and on dry hills.

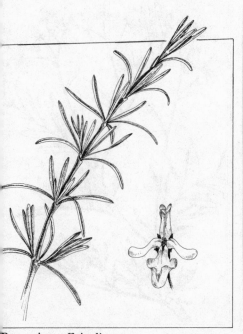

Rosmarinus officinalis

The generic name of this herb, Rosmarinus, is derived from the Latin *ros*, meaning dew, and *marinus*, sea, referring to its habit of growing near the coast. Its cultivation inland can be traced back to the classical period, when it was mentioned by the ancient Greeks as having a stimulant effect on the mind and as a useful aid to the memory. Students at their books entwined Rosemary sprigs in the hair, and consequently the herb became known as a symbol of remembrance.

The Romans probably introduced this species into Britain, as they did in other parts of their Empire, although nothing is recorded of this. It was mentioned in the *Herbal of Apuleius* and the *Leech Book of Bald*, but, traditionally, the first plants were sent to England by the Countess of Hainault, to her daughter Philippa, the Queen of Edward III (1327–77) together with a manuscript extolling the plant's virtues.

Several Plague Tracts of the fourteenth and fifteenth centuries recommend the burning of Rosemary branches indoors, as a preventative against the Black Death, for its aromatic vapours were valued highly as a fumigant which would dispel this and similar contagious diseases. The leaves were regularly burnt in sick rooms and occasionally in churches, as a cheap substitute for incense. Rosemary and Juniper berries (*Juniperus communis*) were also burnt in hospitals to purify the air.

From the fifteenth to seventeenth centuries, the Rosemary appears to have been extremely common. Gerard observes that in Languedoc it was so plentiful 'the inhabitants burne scarce anie other fuel', while Evelyn says the flowers 'are credibly reported to give their scent above thirty leages off at sea, upon the coast of Spain'. Parkinson recorded that where the wood grew large enough 'being cloven out into thin boards' it was employed in the making of lutes, carpenter's rules 'or such like instruments'.

The herb's medicinal uses seemed endless, with Banckes' *Herbal* of 1525 giving an authoritative list: 'Take the flowers thereof and boyle them in fayre water and drinke that water for it is much worthe against all manner of evils in the body. – Take the flowers thereof and make powder thereof and binde it to thy right arme in a linnen cloath and it shall make thee lighte and merrie. – Take the flowers and put them in thy chest among thy clothes or among thy Bookes and Mothes shall not destroy them. – Boyle the leaves in white wine and washe thy face therewith and thy browes and thou shalt have a faire face. Also put the leaves under thy bedde and thou shalt be delivered of all evill dreames. – Take the leaves and put them into wine and it shall keepe the Wine from all sournes and evill savours and if thou wilt sell thy wine thou shall have goode speede. – Also if thou be feeble boyle the leaves in clene water and washe thyself and thou shalt wax shiny. – Also if thou have lost appetite of eating boyle well these leaves in cleane water and when the water is colde put thereunto as much of white wine and then make sops, eat them thereof wel and thou shalt restore thy appetite againe.' He also recommended it for gout, coughs and toothache.

Culpeper advised: 'The dried leaves shred small, and smoked as tobacco, helps those that have any cough, phthisis, or consumption ... The leaves are much used in bathings; and made into ointments or oil, are good to help cold benumbed joints, sinews, or members. ...'

Other apothecaries of Culpeper's period administered the herb in the treatment of 'nervous headaches – tremblings – and female complaints' often finely powdering the leaves into snuffs for use as sneezing powders, and adding the oil to various hair preparations, as this had been found to possess 'wonderful properties for encouraging growth'.

Rosemary was also prescribed throughout the United States during the nineteenth century as a 'stimulant, antispasmodic and emmenagogue', while its oil was 'principally employed as a perfume for ointments, linaments and embrocations'.

The oil, infusions or teas of the herb, are nowadays prescribed for their tonic, astringent and diaphoretic principles, and these make an excellent nervine or stomachic, and are said to be good for relieving headache. The oil, mainly from the flowering tops, is still added to liniments, embrocations, hair lotions, shampoos and similar preparations as a preventative for dandruff, and is used in the preparation of Eau-de-Cologne.

In the kitchen the leaves can be used as a flavouring, and added to soups, sauces and stews, etc., much as they were during the fifteenth century, when John le Philip de Liguamine tells us the Rosemary was the normal condiment for salted meats.

Other names for the Rosemary include Polar Plant, Incensier, Compass Weed, Compass Plant and Rosmarinus coronarium.

RUTA
Rutaceae, the Rue family
Common Rue

The Ruta genus consists of a group of aromatic perennial herbs and sub-shrubs, native mainly to the Mediterranean region and the Canary Islands. Only one, the Common Rue (*R. graveolens*), appears to have been

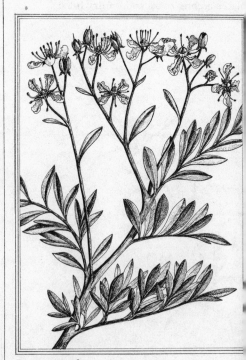

Ruta graveolens

prescribed in medicine. This strong smelling, woody based, shrubby branching perennial grows up to 80cm/31in. tall, has pinnate blue-grey usually glaucous leaves, and bears from May to July terminal clusters of small yellowish flowers. It is native to south-east Europe, where it is found on dry hills and among rocks, although now widely grown elsewhere in gardens, as in the rest of Europe, including the British Isles, and North America.

The ancient Greeks valued Rue as a seasoning herb in cooking. They also regarded it as a cure for the plague. Mithridates used it as a major ingredient in his antidote for poisons. In Pliny's time the herb was regarded as beneficial for at least eighty-four maladies. He considered a potion of Rue to be much more effective if drunk in the open air, and recorded that engravers, carvers and painters of his day ate Rue alone to preserve their sight, for which it is still occasionally prescribed, on the basis that it strengthens the ocular muscles. Dioscorides, and much later Gerard, claimed weasels ate Rue before fighting snakes and so the herb became used as a cure for snakebite.

This is another herb probably introduced into several parts of Europe, including the British Isles, by the Romans, because of its medicinal importance, although little is recorded of it in Britain until after the Norman Conquest. Then it became extensively cultivated and used.

Medicinally it was prescribed chiefly 'against poysons and dangerous medicines', much as in classical times. The seed could be crushed or taken in wine, or the leaves decocted and mixed with the flowers of Dill. When drunk, this would 'expel all pain and torments' and the same if externally applied 'relieves the painful area also', besides 'inflammations of the lungs – cough – hardness of breathing – all pains of the chest and the side – and the shaking fits of agues', while the juice of the leaf applied 'removeth the warts'. Turner mentions the herb in 1562, followed by Gerard, who recommended it pickled with Samphire (*Crithmum maritimum*) to 'quicken the sight'.

Culpeper prescribed Rue in several forms:

'It provokes urine and women's courses – is good to help the wind colic – hardness and windiness of the mother – and frees women from the strangling or suffocation thereof, if the parts be anointed with it – it kills and drives forth the worms of the belly – it helps the gout or pains in the joints, hands, feet or knees, applied thereto – being bruised and put into the nostrils, it stays the bleeding – it helps the testicles, if bathed with the decoction and bay leaves [Laurus nobilis] – It takes away wheals and pimples, if bruised with a few myrtle leaves [Myrtus communis] if it be made up with wax and applied. It cures morphew, and takes away all sorts of warts, if boiled in wine with some pepper and nitre, and the place rubbed therewith; and with almond [Prunis communis] and honey helps the dry scabs, or any tetter or ringworm.'

The twiggy branches of the herb made into simple brushes were used in churches to sprinkle holy water before High Mass and in exorcisms. As an esteemed 'antipestilential' even the Law Courts were strewn with the herb, a practice which continued into the eighteenth century, while posies, or nosegays, of it were carried by the judges at the assizes and courts as a protection against 'jail fever' and to keep the fleas at bay.

The whole of the plant is still prescribed in powders or fluid extracts for its antispasmodic, emmenagogue and stimulant principles, obtained from either the fresh or dried herb. The best parts to use are the young shoots removed before flowering. The dried leaves taken in the form of a tea help to promote menstruation, and are of use in hysterical conditions, and for relieving coughs, croup, flatulence and amenorrhoea, although excessive doses act as a poison and can cause nervous derangement. A volatile oil, Oil of Rue, is distilled from the fresh herb, and is still prescribed for some of these illnesses.

As a culinary herb, the bitter and rather disagreeable leaves are sometimes added in small amounts, finely chopped, to salads, for example, in parts of Italy. Many farmers regard Rue as one of the better tonic herbs for hens and use the leaves to help cure croup and other poultry ailments.

SALVIA

Labiatae, the Mint family

Common Sage, Clary, Wild Clary,
Red Topped Sage, Chia

This large genus consists of both hardy and tender annuals, shrubs and herbaceous perennials, with tubular two lipped flowers, ranging in colour from white to blue, to scarlet and purple. They are native to many countries, including North and South America, Mexico, southern Europe, the Mediterranean region, North Africa and the Himalayas. Their generic name, Salvia, is derived from the Latin *salvare* or *salveo*, meaning to save, and refers to the medicinal properties of some kinds.

The species mostly prescribed in the medicine of the ancient Greeks was the Common Sage (*S. officinalis*), an aromatic sub-shrub 20–70cm/7–27in. tall, bearing thick grey, oblong-oval or lance-shaped, stalked wrinkled leaves, and from May to July, lax whorls of violet-blue flowers in terminal spikes. It is native to the northern shores of the Mediterranean, where it is found on dry banks and in stony places.

The use of this plant dates back to well before the birth of Christ, with Theophrastus, Dioscorides and Pliny all recounting its uses at length. The Romans used it, particularly as an aid to conception.

By the seventeenth century the 'Sawge', as it was known, was regarded in England as an essential plant for the garden, and was medicinally prescribed, much as in previous times, as an insurer of long life, for which it was considered to be most potent just before flowering:

> He that would live for aye,
> Must eat Sage in May.

Gerard, who was cultivating several varieties of the herb in his garden by 1597, tells us it 'is singularly good for the head and brain, it quicknethe the senses and memory, strengtheneth the sinews, restoreth health to those that have the palsy, and taketh away shaky trembling of the members.'

Culpeper used the leaves and flowers in several forms and tells us 'it is good for the liver and to breed blood. A decoction of the leaves and branches made and drank provokes urine, expels the dead child, brings down womens' courses, and causes the hair to become black. It stays the bleedings of wounds, and cleanses foul ulcers and sores. – Three spoonfuls of the juice taken fasting, with a little honey, stays the spitting or casting of blood of those in consumptions. .... It is profitable for all kinds of pains in the head coming of cold and rheumatic humours – all pains of the joints, whether inwardly or outwardly – falling sickness – lowness of spirits – the palsy – diseases of the chest or breast – hoarseness – bloody flux – plague – and cramp – It also helps the memory, warming and quickening the senses ...'

Even as late as the eighteenth century extravagant claims were made for the herb. Hill writes: 'Sage will retard that rapid progress of decay that treads upon our heels so fast in the latter years of life, will preserve the faculties and memory, more valuable to

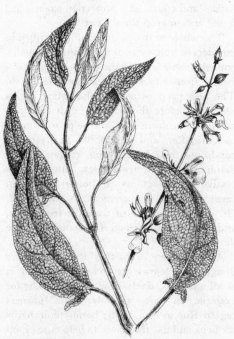

Salvia officinalis

the rational mind than life itself without them.' Such were its alleged powers, the species became commonly known as Salvia salvatrix – Sage the Saviour. Before the days of toothpaste, its leaves were used to rub the teeth to whiten them and strengthen the gums.

In the United States in the nineteenth century, Sage was much valued 'in cases of gastric debility' and for 'checking flatulency with speed and certainty. The infusion is much used as a gargle for inflammation and ulceration of the throat and relaxed uvula, either alone or combined with vinegar, honey or sumach,' and 'the leaves are smoked for asthma'.

The leaves are nowadays prescribed for their aromatic and astringent principles, as in gargles for relaxed throats, quinsy, tonsillitis and laryngitis, and infused for weak digestions, loss of appetitite, nervous headaches, colds, biliousness and upset livers. At one time the leaves were officially listed in the London Pharmacopoeia, and in those of the United States, Austria and other countries.

In the kitchen, the pungent, slightly acrid tasting leaves can be cooked and added to a range of dishes as a flavouring. One of its oldest culinary uses is as a flavouring for cottage cheese. The essential oil, extracted from crops grown commercially, is added not only to foods, but also to soaps and perfumes.

The Clary (S. sclarea) was also formerly regarded as a very important medicinal herb. This is a robust, sticky, strong smelling biennial 30–120cm/11–47in. tall, with greyish, velvety haired, wrinkled, oblong heart-shaped leaves, irregularly toothed at the margins. From May to September, it bears whorls of whitish flowers flushed with violet, with conspicuous membraneous bracts of violet or pink, which although native to the Mediterranean region, where it is found on dry banks, among rocks and along tracksides, is now naturalized and cultivated elsewhere.

Ettmueller recorded that this herb was used by German wine merchants, infused with Elder flowers, as an adulterant, adding it to their Rhenish wines, thus converting them into a form of Muscatel. Hence Muskateller Salbei (or Muscatel Sage) one of the plant's familiar German names. In England, where it was brought into general cultivation in the early 1560s, it was sometimes employed in brewing instead of the hop. Lobel says its use in ales and beers makes it more heady and fit to please drunkards who thereby 'become either dead drunke, or foolish drunke, or madde drunke'.

The commonest English name for this species, Clary, is derived from the specific sclarea, a Latin word evolved from clarus – clear, which with Clear Eye, See Bright and Eyebright points to one of its medicinal uses 'for the clearing of the eyes – and dimness of sight'. Hill, in the early 1760s, explains the herb's value in opthalmic disorders: 'As soon as the seed is put in the warmth and moistures of the eye, operating upon its own substance' it becomes covered 'with a thick and tough mucilage; as it continues moving in the eye this entangles the little substances which had got in by accident and occasioned the pain; and brings them out with it.'

Culpeper advises that: 'The mucilage of the seed made with water, and applied to tumours or swellings, disperseth and taketh them away. It also draweth forth splinters, thorns, or other things got into the flesh. The leaves used with vinegar, either by itself or with a little honey, doth help boils, felons, and the hot inflammations that are gathered by their pains, if applied before it be grown too great.' He also recommended the dried root in a powder to 'provoketh sneezing', which he says 'purgeth the head and brain of much rheum and corruption'.

Culpeper, like several other contemporary apothecaries and herbalists, prescribed the herb 'both for men and women that have bad backs' and 'to strengthen the reins'. For this the fresh leaves were dipped in a batter of flour, eggs and a little milk, fried in butter and served at the table.

The leaves of the Clary are still prescribed infused for their antispasmodic, balsamic and carminative principles, generally as a stomachic for the digestion, and occasionally in the treatment of kidney disorders. In commerce the plant is valued for its oil, known as Clary Oil or Muscatel Sage, and this with its distinctive lavender odour is employed as a fixative in perfumes.

On the herb's introduction to Jamaica and the West Indies, it was soon used to clean and cool ulcers, relieve inflammations of the eyes, and when decocted in Coconut oil as an ointment for insect stings.

Other names for the Clary include Clarry, Garden Clary, Common Garden Clary, Herb Clary, Toute-bonne and Orvale.

The Wild Clary (*S. horminoides*) is an erect, little branched, hairy perennial 30–80cm/ 11–31in. tall, with variable oblong-oval, generally jaggedly, sometimes almost pinnately lobed leaves, and bears from May to September whorled spikes of violet-blue flowers, white spotted along the lower lip. It is found in dry meadows and similar grassy places in much of the Mediterranean and western parts of Europe.

Like the Clary, the smooth seeds of this species when moistened produce a soft tasteless mucilage and these were also used for eye irritations, thus earning the name Oculus Christi or Christ's Eye, a term which Culpeper thought blasphemous. He did, however, regard it as useful in ophthalmic afflctions.

A similar species, the Vervain Sage (*S. verbenaca*), also from the Mediterranean parts of Europe, was prescribed in medicine much as the Wild Clary. This latter variety has larger flowers, but without the white spots at the base of the lower lip. The Meadow Clary or the Meadow Sage (*S. pratensis*), a less common plant, was occasionally substituted for both the above.

Several other Salvias native to Europe and the Mediterranean region had their various uses. One such was the Red Topped Sage (*S. horminum*), an erect hairy annual 10–40cm/4–15in. tall, with oval or oblong, finely toothed, wrinkled, hairy stalked leaves, and from April to June violet-purple or pinkish flowers, with purplish or reddish bracts. The seed of this plant was formerly added to vats of fermenting alcoholic liquors to increase their potency. The infused leaves were usually gargled 'for the soreness of the gums and mouth', while the powdered leaves made a good sneezing powder.

The infused leaves of the aromatic Apple Bearing Sage (*S. pomifera*) from Crete and the

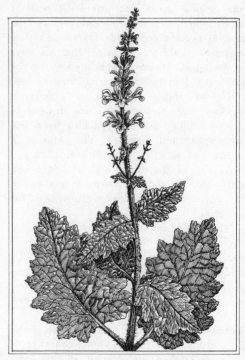

Salvia horminoides

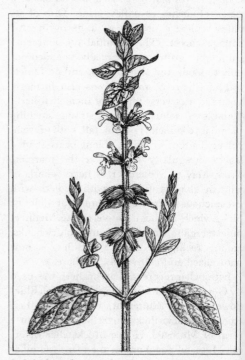

Salvia horminum

islands of Greece, were taken there as a means of promoting copious perspiration, although excessive doses are recorded as having caused lethargy and feebleness, sometimes accompanied by fainting. The common name of this species refers to the semitransparent galls or swellings that form on the plant, caused by the insect known as *Cynips salviae*. These 'Sage Apples' as they are known, are still collected, generally on 1 May, and are candied with sugar into a medicinal sweetmeat or conserve, a favourite delicacy of the Greeks.

Other species yielding aromatic oils used in commerce include the Three Lobed Sage (*S. triloba*) (the origin of Spanish Sage Oil), the leaves of which are also used in Greece and Italy in the making of a tea; and *Salvia cypria*, from the Cypress region, which contains a high proportion of Eucalyptol. The very strong-smelling leaves of the Jupiter's Distaff (*S. glutinosa*), native to the southeastern and central parts of Europe, but now found elsewhere, were once widely employed, especially in Holland, to improve the flavour of country wines.

An American Salvia, the Chia (*S. columbariae*), is native to the plains and hills of California and northern Mexico. A low growing annual, generally producing stalks up to 50cm/20in. tall, it has dark green, deeply cut, rough or hairy, mostly basal leaves, and bears from about March to May dense whorls of blue flowers near the top of the stalks, followed by dark brown, slightly flattened seeds. Once it was used by the Indians of those areas as a food plant. They either used the seed to make little flat cakes or loaves, or mixed it with wheat flour for the same, giving the bread a nutty flavour, besides adding the crushed seed with ground wheat or corn meal to their soups and gruels. The Indians also made a nutritious beverage from the herb by steeping the crushed or ground seed in water. The first white settlers in California used the mucilaginous grounddown seed as a poultice in the treatment of gunshot and other wounds.

The seeds are still considered a valuable food and are sold in the Spanish markets in Mexico. The seeds of the White Sage (*S.*

apiana), together with that of several other species, were also made into *pinole* or meal by the Indians. The Black Sage (*S. mellifer*, syn. *Ramona stachyoides*), from southern California, with several other species yields a useful aromatic oil, sometimes used as a flavouring.

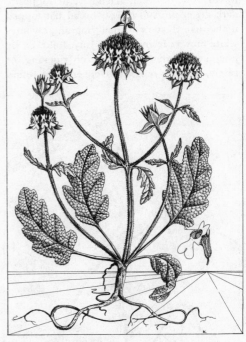

Salvia columbariae

SAMBUCUS

Caprifoliaceae, the Honeysuckle family

Common Elderberry, Dwarf Elder, American Elder

Most of the Sambucus genus consists of hardy, berry-bearing, deciduous shrubs or small trees, although one or two are of a herbaceous habit; all are native mainly to Europe, including the British Isles, Africa, North America and Australia. Their generic name, Sambucus, dates back to the time of the ancient Greeks and may refer to the musical instrument known as a *sambuke* which is believed to have been made from the wood of one of its species. Even today, the Italians carve the sampogna, a simple musical instrument, from the Elder's branches.

The most familiar species, the Common Elderberry (*S. nigra*), is a shrub or small tree up to 10m/32ft tall, having fetid, opposite dark green pinnate leaves, broad flat-topped umbel-like clusters of small fragrant, creamy-white flowers from June to July, followed by juicy berries that turn black on ripening, or rarely, whitish, pinkish or cream. It is found

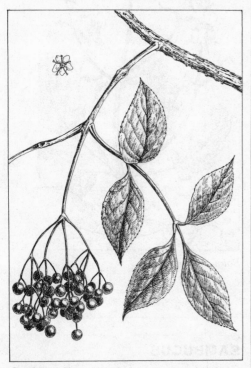

Sambucus nigra

throughout most of Europe and parts of Asia, in woods, hedges and waste places, although now introduced elsewhere, including North America.

The Romans, so Pliny tells us, employed the Elderberry in medicine and used the juice of the berries as a hair dye. The plant was later mentioned at the famous Italian medical school of Salerno, and in the western parts of Europe was used by 'leeches' in England and Wales. Its present-day name of Elder is probably derived from the Anglo-Saxon *aeld* or *ellarn*, meaning fire or kindle, for the hollow stems were used for blowing up fires. Hence Pipe Tree, Bore Tree and Bour Tree, with its other names including Burtre (another Anglo-Saxon form), Bourtree, Bottry, Scaw, Ellhorn, Black Elder, Eldrum, Borral, Eller, Tea Tree, Trammon and Devil's Wood.

The wood was used in the making of shoe-maker's pegs, butcher's skewers; and needles which were used in weaving. The bark and root with other ingredients yielded a blackish dye, the leaves a green one and the berries or juice, a blue-lilac, violet or purple colour, depending on the other ingredients. The juice and berries were not only used for making Elderberry wines, cordials, preserves and jellies, but were regularly added as an adulterant to other English and foreign wines and to turn cheap port into tawny.

The parts of the Elder used in medicine were the bark, leaves, flowers and berries. In a wide variety of forms, they were prescribed both 'inward and outwardly' for all manner of complaints. John Evelyn writes: 'If the medicinal properties of its leaves, bark and berries were fully known, I cannot tell what our countryman could ail for which he might not fetch a remedy from every hedge, either for sickness or wound.' A treatise on the species, *The Anatomie of the Elder*, written by Martin Blockwich or Blockwitzius in 1644 ran to over 200 pages, and listed about seventy different diseases for which the plant was prescribed.

Gerard says the seeds contained within the berries 'are good for such as have the dropsie, and such as are too fat, and would faine to be leaner, if they be taken in a morning to the quantity of a dram with wine for a certain space.' He goes on to recommend the green leaves pounded with 'Deeres suet or Bulls tallowe' as good for hot swellings and tumours and to assuage the pain of the gout.

Culpeper writes: 'The first shoots of the Common Elder boiled like asparagus, and the young leaves and stalks boiled in fat broth, do mightily carry forth phlegm and choler ... the bark of the root boiled in wine, or the juice thereof drank, works the same effects [for dropsie], but more powerfully than either the leaves or fruit . . . It mollifies the hardness of the mother, if women sit thereon, and opens their veins, and brings down their courses: the berries boiled in wine, performs the same effects: and the hair of the head washed therewith, is made black . . . The leaves or flowers distilled in the month of May, and the legs often washed with the said distilled water, takes away the ulcers and sores of them. The eyes washed therewith, it takes away the redness and blood-shot; and the hands washed morning and evening therewith, helps the palsy, and shaking of them.' The flowers infused in lard as *Unguentum Sambuci* were also considered very useful for applying to wounds, burns and scalds, and was regularly added to face creams, cosmetics, pomades and other household preparations. For 'the pain of the piles' decoctions of Elder flowers and those of the Honeysuckle (*Lonicera caprifolium*) were applied in a warm fomentation with milk 'which greatly abateth them'.

The juice of the berries, or even Elderberry wine taken hot, is still said to be good for relieving colds, while infusions of the flowers and peppermint helps influenza. The leaves have since been found to contain an alkaloid known as Sambucine and the glycoside Sambunigrin, and a purgative resin. In homoeopathic medicine the Elder is prescribed mainly for glottal spasm. The bruised leaves of the Elder, which give off an unpleasant smell, are sometimes used to keep flies and insects away.

The Dwarf Elder (*S. ebulus*), unlike the Common Elder, is a coarse, patch-forming herbaceous plant, with stout, erect, foetid, leafy green stems ½–2m/1½–6½ft tall, pinnate leaves and oblong-lance shaped, pointed, sharply toothed leaflets; from June to August the plant bears broad flat-topped clusters of small white flowers. It is found in thickets, clearings and by the roadsides throughout most of Europe.

The plant's medicinal effects were much more drastic than the Elderberry. Culpeper remarks, it 'is more powerful than the Common Elder in opening and purging choler, phlegm, and water, in helping the gout, piles and womens' diseases' and that it 'colours the

hair black, helps the inflammation of the eyes, and pains in the ears, the bite of serpents, or mad dogs, burnings and scaldings, the wind colic, colic and stone, the difficulty of urine, the cure of old sores, and fistulous ulcers.'

The decocted leaves are still prescribed for their diaphoretic, diuretic, expectorant and purgative principles in dropsy, and for relieving the suppression of urine. In France the bruised leaves boiled in wine are applied as a poultice to boils, swellings and contusions. Tinctures made from the unpleasant tasting roots, or fluid extracts of them, are also employed in homoeopathic medicine. (The Dwarf Elder mentioned here is not to be

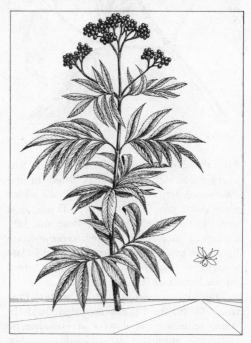

Sambucus ebulus

confused with the Dwarf Elder or Wild Elder (*Aralia hispida*) of the United States, also used in the treatment of kidney complaints, dropsy, gravel, and various urinary diseases.)

A North American species, the American or Sweet Elder (*S. canadensis*), is a very common plant found in thickets, waste places, alongside roads and near habitation from Nova Scotia to Manitoba, south to Florida and Texas and now grown in other countries.

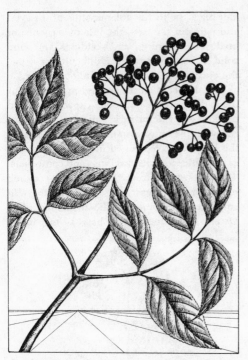

Sambucus canadensis

Like the Common European Elder, it had many medicinal uses and is listed in the *Pharmacopeoia* of the United States. This pithy shrub grows about 3½m/11½ft high, has opposite leaves, and bears in June and July numerous pleasantly scented creamy-white flowers in broad flat clusters, followed in late summer and early autumn by round, deep purple berries or fruits.

The late nineteenth-century writer, Professor O. Phelps Brown, recorded that: 'In warm infusions the flowers are diaphoretic and gently stimulant. In cold infusions they are diuretic, alterative and cooling and may be used in all diseases requiring such action, as in hepatic derangements of children, erysipelas, erysipelatous diseases, etc. . . . The expressed juice of the berries, evaporated to the consistence of a syrup, is a valuable aperient and alterative; one ounce of it will purge . . . The flowers and expressed juice of the berries have been beneficially employed in scrofula, cutaneous diseases, syphilis, rheumatism, etc. . . .'

The parts still used in official medicine are the flowers, berries and the inner bark. The fresh root of the shrub does however appear to contain a virulent alkaloid and this in the past has caused the deaths of several children, producing symptoms similar to Hemlock (*Conium*) poisoning.

The bluish-black berries of the Blue Elder or the Blue Berried Elder (*S. glauca*), another North American species and found from Montana and Vancouver, south to Utah and California, were once an important food for the American Indians. They are still added, generally mixed with other fruits, to jellies and pies. The berries of a South American species, *Sambucus australis*, are also made into preserves, and infusions of its leaves are prescribed for indigestion and as a diuretic in Argentina and Brazil. In Peru a syrup from *Sambucus peruviana* is administered for relieving sore throats and ulcers. The bitter berries of the Red or Alpine Elder (*S. racemosa*), an erect, much-branched shrub 1–4m/3–13ft high, native to the shady woods of central Europe, were used in wine making. In Australia, the fruits of two species, that of *Sambucus gaudichaudiana* and *S. xanthocarpa* are eaten as food by the aborigines.

SANICULA
Umbelliferae, the Parsley family
Sanicle

About 40 members of this genus of rather weedy biennial and perennial herbs are found in the temperate regions of the world, particularly in areas of thickets and open woods. The most familiar of the European species is the Sanicle or Wood Sanicle (*S. europaea*). This smooth, little-branched perennial 20–60cm/7–23in. tall, with long stalked palmately lobed leaves, bears from May to July whitish or pale pink flowers in dense globular umbels at the top of long slender stalks, followed by ovoid fruits with numerous hooked bristles. During the medieval period, it was regarded as a valuable 'vulnary herbs' and as a cure in the treatment of wounds, bleedings, spitting of blood and the like. This use is referred to in Sanicula, its generic name, which is derived from the Latin *sano* or *sanus*, meaning sound, healthy or cure. The specific name *europaea* simply refers to its natural habitat, which includes not only the whole of Europe (except Iceland) but Asia Minor, Syria, Iran and parts of Africa. In these areas it grows in moist woodlands and similar shady places.

The parts of the plant generally prescribed in medicine were the flowering tops and the fresh green leaves which were collected on a fine morning as soon as the sun had dried the dew, and when decocted were prescribed to speedily heal 'green wounds – imposthumes – inward bleedings – chronic coughs – tumours on any part of the body – ulcers of the stomach – contusions – varicose ulcers and other ulcerous conditions.' Culpeper commended it for these afflictions and also 'laxes of the belly; the ulcerations of the kidneys also, the pains in the bowels, and gonorrhoea, or running of the reins, being boiled in wine or water, and drunk.'

Culpeper's contemporary, Parkinson, tells us: 'The country people who live where it

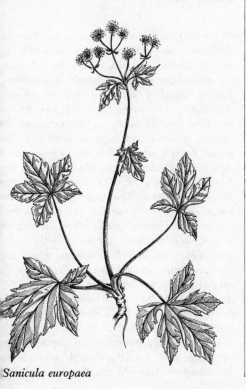

Sanicula europaea

groweth, do use it to annoint their hands when they are chapt by the winde ...' The country people also fed the fresh leaves to their cows who had just calved, to promote the expulsion of the afterbirth and to stop any bleeding.

The leaves of the Sanicle, which is also known as Pool Root, Butterwort and Self-Heal, are still prescribed infused for their alterative, astringent, antiseptic and haemostatic principles in the treatment of dysentery, diarrhoea, stomach ulcers, sores, leucorrhoea, haemorrhoids, varicose veins and various blood disorders.

The fibrous root of an American species, the Black Snake Root (*S. marilandica*), was once used in powder form or decocted in the treatment of intermittent fever and chorea, for which it was said to be very efficacious.

SAPONARIA
Caryophyllaceae, the Pink family
Soapwort

The Saponarias make up a group of hardy annual and perennial free-flowering plants, most of which are native to Europe. Of these only one, the common Soapwort (*S. officinalis*), appears to have been widely used in medicine. A stout, hairless perennial with erect branching stems 30–90cm/11–35in. tall, it has broadly elliptic-oval opposite leaves and bears terminal clusters of large pinkish flowers of various shades from about June to October. Although probably native to the hedges and damp waste ground of central and southern Europe, it is now extensively naturalized elsewhere, having escaped from cultivation, for example, the British Isles, northern Europe, parts of Asia and North America.

The roots of this plant, when soaked in warm water, produce a soap-sud like substance which has been employed in the home at least from the time of Dioscorides. The generic name Saponaria refers to this use and comes from the Latin *sapo*, meaning soap. Several of its later names also allude to its cleansing properties, such as Soaproot, Crow

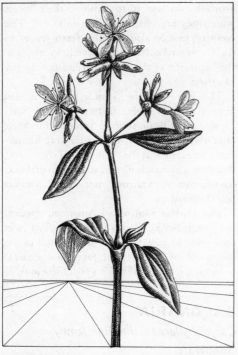

Saponaria officinalis

Soap, Crowther Soap, Latherwort and Fuller's Herb. Gerard, at the end of the sixteenth century, wrote 'of the great scouring qualitie the leaves have; for they yield out of themselves a certain iuice when they are bruised, which scoureth almost as well as soap.' This when 'mixed with the water from springs' was used to clean tapestries, hangings and carpets, and, according to Parkinson, 'wild sopewort' was used 'to scour the country-Women's treen [wooden] and pewter vessels'.

In the medicine of the medieval period, the decocted roots and leaves were usually prescribed in irritating skin diseases and for 'the jaundice and other visceral obstructions'. For 'the sufferers of syphilis and the gonorrhoea' the dose was extremely large, being 'half an ounce daily of the inspissated juice', but as a tonic 'weaker infusions will suffice'. The dried root was also 'snuffed' to cause violent sneezing.

During the nineteenth century the herb was administered in both Canada and the United States as a valuable remedy 'in the treatment of diseases of the liver, scrofulous, syphilitic and cutaneous afflictions of a severe character' and in 'catarrh, rheumatism, gonorrhoea, whites, and green sickness'.

The bitter leaves and dried roots are still given for their alterative and detergent effects, generally in the form of a liquid extract in the treatment of scrofula and general skin diseases. It should be taken with care, owing to the Saponin content (Saponin glycoside) for even in moderate amounts this can cause gastro-enteritis, followed by depression of the central nervous system.

In homes and museums, extracts are still employed for cleaning wall hangings and tapestries, etc., and for producing a 'head' on beers.

Other names for the common Soapwort include Bouncing Bet, Sweet Betty, Bruisewort, Hedge Pink and Wild Sweet William.

SASSAFRAS
Lauraceae, the Laurel family
Sassafras

Only two species make up this genus of hardy deciduous aromatic trees, one is native to central China, and the other, the Sassafras (*S. variifolium*, syn. *S. officinale, S. sassafras, Laurus sassafras* and others), to North America. This latter, a handsome spicy-smelling tree reaching about 15m/49ft in height, is generally found in dryish, sandy loams, tucked into the borders of woods and alongside roads, from Massachusetts to Michigan, Iowa and Kansas, south to Florida and Texas. The bright green alternate leaves are extremely variable and may be oval and entire, or three lobed; others are mitten shaped, and all three may form on the same tree. The greenish-yellow flowers, which are produced in umbelled racemes, appear with or just before the leaves, to be followed by dark blue fruits (or drupes) on pinkish fruiting stalks. The tree's roots often send up thicket-forming suckers.

It is generally believed that the Sassafras or Ague Tree was discovered in 1602 by Bartholemew Gosnold the English explorer, who found it growing wild on one of the Elizabeth Islands off the coast of southern Massachusetts. Before long regular shipments of Sassafras root were exported to London and various other European cities, where they were used as tea, as a flavouring for soups, or simply as a condiment.

In medicine the agreeably flavoured aromatic root and the bark of the roots were regarded as alterative, stimulant, diaphoretic and diuretic, and were prescribed decocted as an external wash 'for skin eruptions – diseases and inflammations of the eyes – as in opthalmia', while infusions of the crushed bark taken frequently in wineglassful doses

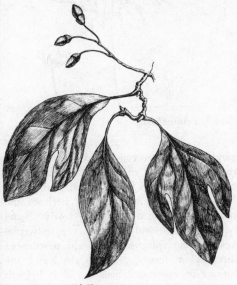

Sassafras variifolium

'relieves rheumatism and the gout'. The bark of the rust-brown coloured root was also taken in the form of a tea as 'a springtime renovator of the blood'. The mucilaginous young leaves are still used in the southern states of America after being dried and powdered, for thickening and flavouring soups or as a condiment.

The rootstocks are still used in commerce, generally in the form of brownish-white chips which are distilled in large quantities for the fragrant oil they contain. This Oil of Sassafras is mainly employed for flavouring and for scenting cheap soaps and perfumes. Once it

was used to mask the bitterness of opium medicines, and was taken in larger amounts to cause abortions, a very risky procedure as it can produce narcotic poisoning and even death.

The root and the bark of the root is still administered, usually combined with other medicines, for its diaphoretic, diuretic and stimulant principles and was once commonly prescribed for rheumatism and malaria, although little used today, or it can be taken in the form of a medicinal beverage. The oil used in perfumes can be extracted from the fruits, while the bark and wood of the tree yield a yellow dye.

The name Sassafras is also applied to several other medicinal plants including the Californian Sassafras (*Umbellularia californica*), the leaves of which are taken decocted for headaches, colic and diarrhoea; the Swamp Sassafras (*Magnolia glauca*, syn. *M. virginiana*) of which the bark and seed cones were prescribed for their aromatic, diaphoretic and bitter tonic principles, and the Australian Sassafras (*Atherosperma moschatum*), a poisonous plant prescribed for relieving rheumatism, syphilis and bronchitis.

SCABIOSA
Dipsacaceae, the Teasel family
Devil's Bit, Small Scabious

The Scabiosas make up a genus of hardy annual, biennial and perennial plants with terminal heads of pincushion-like flowers, (hence Pincushion Flower, their collective vernacular name). They are native mainly to Europe, Asia, North Africa and the Mediterranean region. Their generic name, Scabiosa, is derived from the Latin *scabere*, to scratch or itch, referring to the medicinal properties of some kinds, which under the name of *Skabiosa* or *Scabyas*, were supposed to be able to cure irritations and 'scabby eruptions' of the skin, including scabies.

The principal species used in the medicine of medieval Europe was generally known as the Devil's Bit (*S. succisa*, syn. *Succisa pratensis*). An erect or spreading, sparsely branched perennial 15–100cm/6–39in. tall, it

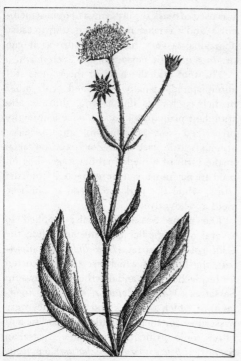

Scabiosa succisa

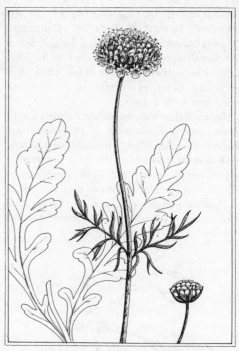

Scabiosa columbaria

has elliptic leaves, a very short rootstock and rounded heads of bluish-purple, rarely white or pink, flowers appearing from about June to October. It is found in dampish meadows, woods, marshes and fens throughout much of Europe and in parts of Asia.

The name Devil's Bit refers to its root, which in its first year of growth looks something like a carrot or radish. This gradually becomes woody, and the bottom part decays away, leaving the top part looking as if it had been broken off, although it sends out lateral growths as compensation. According to the *Grete Herball* of 1526 the herb derived its name of Devil's Bit 'bycause the rote is blacke and semeth that it is iagged with bytynge, and some say that the devyll had envy at the vertue thereof and bete the rote so far to have destroyed it.'

The Devil's Bit was considered a very valuable plant. Outwardly applied it took away 'blackness or other markings from the skin – is used as a wash in cutaneous eruptions – and for sores and scurf of the head – will ease swellings and inveterate tumours – often

gargled it relieves soreness and swellings of the throat' and 'as an internal medicine it promotes sweat in fevers – and purifies the blood'. Culpeper wrote: 'The herb or the root (all that the devil hath left of it) being boiled in wine and drank, is very powerful against the plague, and all pestilential diseases or fevers, poisons also, and the bitings of venomous beasts. ... It helpeth also to procure women's courses, and easeth all pains of the mother, and to break and discuss wind therein, and in the bowels. The powder of the root taken in drink, driveth forth the worms in the body. The juice or distilled water of the herb, is very effectual for green wounds or old sores, and cleanseth the body inwardly and the seed outwardly, from sores, scurf, itch, pimples, freckles, morphew, or other deformities thereof, especially if a little vitriol be dissolved therein.'

The whole of the herb is still prescribed for its demulcent, diaphoretic and febrifugal principles, and is taken as a tea for relieving coughs, fevers and internal inflammations, and is sometimes combined with other remedies. Other names for the plant include Ofbit, Devil's Bit Scabious, Premorse Scabious and the Blue Devil's Bit.

The Small Scabious or the Lesser Field Scabious (*S. columbaria*) was frequently substituted for the above, and is a very variable erect, little branched perennial 15–70cm/6–27in. tall. It has obovate, pinnately lobed leaves bears bluish-lilac, or rarely pink or whitish flowers from about June to October, is common to much of Europe except the north, and grows in grassy places, in cornfields, on dry banks and among rocks.

Culpeper writes of it: 'It is effectual for all sorts of coughs, shortness of breath, and all other diseases of the breasts and lungs, ripening and digesting cold phlegm, and other tough humour, voiding them forth by coughing and spitting – it ripens all sorts of inward ulcers and imposthumes; pleurisy also, if the decoction of the herb dry or green be made in wine, and drank for some time together. The green herb bruised and applied to any carbuncle or plague sore, will dissolve and break it in three hours. The same decoction drunk, helps the pains and stitches in the side. The decoction of the roots taken for forty days together, or a dram of the powder of them taken at a time in whey, helps those that are troubled with running or spreading ulcers, tetters or ringworms . . .'

The Field Scabious (*S. arvensis*, syn. *Knautia arvensis*) possesses similar medicinal properties to the species described above, and is a little branched and very variable perennial 30–150cm/11–59in. tall. The leaves are mostly pinnately lobed and the long stalked bluish-lilac flowers appear from May to October. It grows throughout Europe, the Caucasus and western Siberia, in dry fields, cornfields, pastures, heaths and bushy places.

SCOPOLIA
Solanaceae, the Nightshade family
Scopola

This small genus of herbaceous perennials is the link between the Deadly Nightshade (Atropa) and the Henbane (Hyoscyamus) and like those plants it contains a powerful poison. Scopola (*S. carniolica*, syn. *S. atropoides* or *Belladonna scopola*) was the member of the genus principally used in medicine. This leafy, branched perennial up to 60cm/23in. tall, bears in spring, solitary, short-stalked and drooping, brownish-purple to yellow flowers. It is native to the woods and damp hilly places of central and eastern Europe, although occasionally found further west, for example, Germany, generally as an escape from cultivation.

The dried, knotty rhizomes of this plant provided the medicinal part and were administered for their narcotic effects, as a mydriatic for dilating the pupils of the eyes. Since it had a similar action to both the Deadly Nightshade and the Henbane, it was generally prescribed in the same way as those herbs. The root of the Scopola, however, is somewhat richer in alkaloids, including Scopolamine (or Hyoscine), which is used in North America in the manufacture of Belladonna plasters. Extracts and fluid extracts of the plant are mentioned in the Pharma-

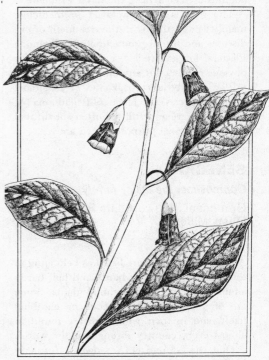

Scopolia carniolica

copoeias of the United States.

As an internal medicine the Scopola had to be carefully prescribed in very small amounts and was administered during the nineteenth century in the United States as a cerebral sedative, for 'all convulsive diseases – the fit – hysteric fits – hysteria – mania – madness' even for 'insomnia' and as 'a way of subduing those people suffering from continuous sexual excitement'. At one time the extracted alkaloid, Scopolamine, was combined with morphine and administered to patients as a form of anaesthetic. This 'twilight sleep' as it was known was first administered in 1899 or 1900 and was given either on its own or before chloroform or ether. Unfortunately, it not only deadened pain, but often caused loss of memory; numerous deaths were recorded through its improper use. Taken in small amounts the root dilates the pupils of the eyes, the mouth dries, the pulse rate accelerates and the patient appears drowsy or weary. Larger amounts lead to confusion, often to delirium and occasionally to great difficulty in breathing. Apparently Strychnine was once administered to relieve the latter problem.

The root is still employed in medicine, mainly as a mydriatic in the treatment of eye diseases and in the production of Belladonna Plasters for external use, but rarely, for obvious reasons, for anything else.

The slightly larger rhizomes of an almost identical species, the Japanese Belladonna (*S. japonica*), were and still are often substituted for the medicinal purposes listed above.

SENECIO

Compositae, the Daisy family
Groundsel, Ragwort, Life Root, Dusty Miller

About 1,000 species are listed as belonging to this extensive genus of hardy and half-hardy annual, biennial and perennial plants. Some are of a shrubby, herbaceous or climbing habit, and in their wild state are found in almost every country throughout the world.

One, the Groundsel (*S. vulgaris*), formerly had several medicinal uses. An erect, variable

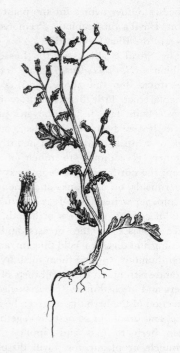

Senecio vulgaris

sometimes downy annual or biennial up to 45cm/17in. tall, it has slightly fleshy, narrow pinnately lobed leaves, and bears for much of the year small yellow usually rayless flowers. Found throughout Europe and Russian Asia, in cultivated soils, gardens and waste places, it is now naturalized in numerous other countries.

Pliny believed that the Groundsel was a useful remedy for toothache and says if the sufferer uprooted the plant with his hands, touched the tooth concerned three times, spat on the ground each time, then reset the plant in the ground – should it root and grow again, the pain would go.

As a healing herb the Groundsel was known to the Anglo-Saxons as *gundeswele* or *grundeswylige* meaning, perhaps, ground eater or swallower, referring to its invasive habit. This developed to *growdyswyli* in the fifteenth century, when it was highly regarded as a medicinal plant and was cultivated as such in monastic gardens. The familiar name Groundsel had evolved by Gerard's time. He tells us: 'The leaves stamped and strained into milke nd drunke, helpe the red gums and frets in Children . . . Dioscorides saith, That with the fine pouder of Frankincense it healeth wounds n the sinues.'

According to Culpeper it had many virtues, and 'is cooling in inflammations' and 'is an easy emetic when made like tea. Taken in ale, t acts against the pains of the stomach, strangury and jaundice – it destroys worms, and is useful in scrofulous tumours and inflammations of the breast and scald head.' He recommends it, outwardly or inwardly 'as a good purgative – for the gripes and colics of infants – the sore breasts of women – to provoke urine – for gravel in the reins and kidneys – knots and kernals in any part of the body . . .' He adds: 'An infusion of it taken inwardly cures staggers and bot-worms in horses.'

The whole of the fresh or dried herb is nowadays prescribed for its anthelmintic, diuretic and diaphoretic principles, and in the form of a tea is taken for biliousness and sickness, or in slightly stronger infusions where a laxative is required. It is sometimes included in lotions for the eyes, and in applications for smoothing rough or chapped hands. In homoeopathic medicine it is administered for suppressed or delayed menstruation, and for painful or irregular menstruation in young girls. Other names for the Groundsel include Grundy, Swallow, Simson, Sention and Ground Glutton.

The Ragwort (*S. jacobaea*), like the previous species, was widely prescribed in medieval medicine. An erect, robust, branched biennial or perennial 30–150cm/11–59in. tall, with deeply dissected leaves, it bears from June to November, numerous bright golden yellow flowers in dense, flat-topped compound clusters. It is found in dry grassy places, in poor pasture, on dunes and by the wayside in most of Europe and parts of Asia, including Siberia, but is now extensively naturalized elsewhere, for example, north-west India, South Africa, Canada and New Zealand.

Gerard tells us that this species was known in Latin as 'Herba St. Jacobi: in English, St. James his Wort: the countrey people doe call it Stagger-wort, and Staner-wort, and also Rag-wort, and Rag-weed.' The name Stagger-wort alludes to its use as a remedy for 'staggers', a disease affecting horses. The plant's other names including Flos Sancti Jacobi, or St James Wort, Benweed, Curly Doddies, Stammerwort (it was prescribed for speech impediments), Stinking Nanny, Dog Standard and Cankerwort. This last name refers to its use in the treatment 'of running sores – cankers – and cancerous ulcers'.

Gerard also noted: 'It is much commended, and not without cause, to helpe old aches and paines in the armes, hips, and legs, boiled in hog's grease to the forme of an ointment. Moreover, the decoction hereof gargarised is much set by as a remedy against swellings and

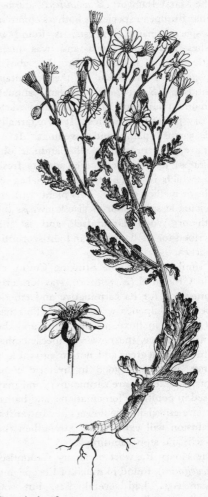

Senecio jacobaea

impostumations of the throat, which it wasteth away and thoroughly healeth . . .'

Decoctions of the herb, or liquid extracts of it, are nowadays prescribed for their detergent and diaphoretic effects, in the treatment of coughs, colds, catarrh, to relieve the pain of sciatica, rheumatism and similar gouty pains. They are also used as a gargle for relaxed throat and added to applications for ulcers, sores and wounds.

Farmers dislike this plant on their land as it contains various alkaloids that can prove toxic to cattle. A similar alkaloid contained in *Senecio latifolius* has been found in South Africa to be responsible for Malteno Disease, an illness affecting cattle and horses.

The Marsh Ragwort (*S. aquaticus*), another familiar European species as both its common and specific name suggests, is found in marshes and damp soils and was often substituted in medicine for the above. Culpeper also made use of the Mountain Groundsel (*S. sylvaticus*) – 'an annual, common on our ditch banks, and other waste and dry places'. He writes: 'It is externally good against pains and swellings. It is detersive, and proper in all glandular obstructions; it is antiscorbutic, and its fresh juice, which is the best, may be taken in broths or medicinal ales.' This plant, with its rather unpleasant odour, is also known as the Heath or Wood Groundsel, and is still prescribed for its detergent and antiscorbutic properties.

A similar species, the Stinking Cotton or Viscid Groundsel (*S. viscosus*), was formerly administered for its carminative and emetic properties. Culpeper writes of it: 'This has been praised in fluxes of the belly, and the dysentery; it has the power of ipecacuanha, but in a less degree, and not so agreeable a manner, it is very good in hysteric complaints. The leaves are carminative, and may be used in poultices, fomentations, and baths, but more especially the flowers . . . Inwardly, an infusion will expel wind, strengthen the stomach, and stop vomiting.'

The Hoary Ragwort or Hoary Groundsel (*S. erucifolius*), found in much of Europe and Russian Asia, had several uses, but was generally prescribed 'as an external medicine'.

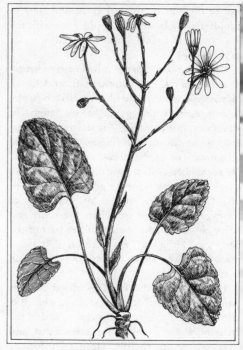

Senecio aureus

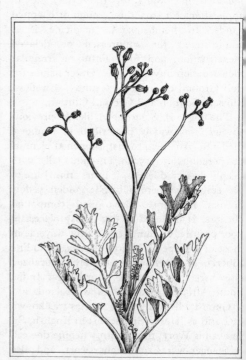

Senecio maritimus

Culpeper says: 'Its virtues are similar to the others of its kind, and it resembles them in its taste and smell.'

A North American species known as the Life Root (*S. aureus*), which also grows in the northern and western parts of Europe and in Asia, was once prescribed for its 'astringent, emulcent, diuretic, emmenagogue, pectoral and tonic principles'. It is a perennial plant found in low marshy ground, and by the banks of creeks and streams, where its slender erect, fluted cottony unbranched stems may reach 30–60cm/11–23in. in height. The radical leaves are roundish or kidney-shaped, and the golden yellow flowers are borne in spring and summer.

Professor O. Phelps Brown, writing in the late nineteenth century, informs us: 'There are several varieties of this plant, but all possess the same medicinal properties . . . [it] exerts a very powerful and peculiar influence upon the reproductive organs of females. This has given it the name of Female Regulator. Combined with the Lily, and other native and foreign plants, it is one of the most certain cures in the world for aggravated cases of leucorrhoea; also in cases of menstrual suppression. It will operate excellently in gravel, and other urinary affections.'

Solid or liquid extracts of the powdered root, or of its most active constituent, senecin, are still administered for some women's complaints and pulmonary troubles and diarrhoea. Other names for the species include Squaw Weed, Ragwort, False Valerian and Golden Senecio.

A West Indian Senecio, commonly known as Dusty Miller (*S. maritimus*, syn. *Cineraria maritima*), was at one time used in the treatment of eye disease. It is a shrubby species with large lanceolate, deeply divided, silvery leaves, covered with soft white downy hair, and bears in summer terminal clusters of small bright yellow flowers. The juice was once regarded as a very useful means for removing capsular and lenticular cataracts of the eyes.

The generic name of these plants, Senecio, is derived from the Latin *senex*, meaning old, referring to the white or greyish hair-like pappus of the seed heads that give them the vernacular name of Old Man.

SIEGESBECKIA
Compositae, the Daisy family
Holy Herb

The Holy Herb (*S. orientalis*) is a shrubby composite plant from Mauritius in the Indian Ocean. It has hairy branching stems about 60cm/23in. tall, with coarsely toothed, broadly triangular leaves, and bears small leafy panicled flower heads. The bracts, when ripe, become covered with sticky glandular hairs.

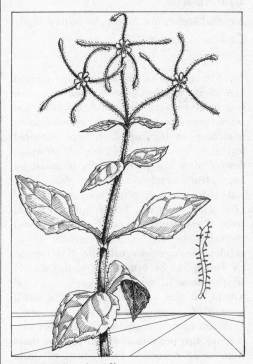

Siegesbeckia orientalis

The whole of this herb was formerly used by the inhabitants of Mauritius and the surrounding islands, in the treatment of leprosy and for other near-incurable skin diseases and ulcers, such as those resulting from syphilis. The juice was extracted and applied direct to the affected part, covering it as it dried with a sort of elastic film, that was also found useful for protecting burns and wounds from infection. In Britain and other parts of Europe, the juice was often mixed with glycerine for painting on ring-worm. In China, where the species is a common weed, the juice was administered internally in the treatment of agues, rheumatism and stone of the kidneys. As an alterative, liquid extracts are still prescribed there. The juice contains a white crystalline substance resembling Salicyclic Acid, and this in the form of salts is prescribed as a mild antiseptic, and in the treatment of rheumatism and for relieving pain.

SIMABA

Simarubaceae, the Simaruba family
Cedron

The principal species of this genus prescribed in medicine was the Cedron (*S. cedron*) a small tree indigenous to Colombia, Ecuador and central America. From an erect growing stem, branching at the top, with large pinnated leaves, it bears large panicles of brownish flowers often 1m/3ft in length, followed by large fruits each containing one hard, yellowish, intensely bitter seed about 4cm/1½in. long, 3cm/1in. broad and 1½cm/¾in. thick. These have been employed for several centuries now, in central America, as an antidote for poisonous snakebite. If unfortunate enough to be bitten, the victim simply scraped some of the seed directly on to the wound, at the same time taking a small amount of it powdered in water. The seeds were also carried around by the Indians who believed this precaution would prevent them from being poisoned. The natives of Costa Rica and Trinidad also used the seed to treat intermittent fevers.

During the nineteenth century in both Britain and the United States, the Cedron Seed was regarded as an important and 'excellent antispasmodic' and as 'one of the most valuable articles of the kind known to the educated herbalist'. It was administered 'in all nervous affections' and as 'the cure for hydrophobia' as well as an 'antidote for the majority of acro-narcotic poisons'.

The seed is still prescribed for its antispasmodic, sedative, tonic, febrifuge and bitter principles and is generally infused and administered in the treatment of dyspepsia and malarial complaints. The powdered and bitter-tasting bark is also used to kill vermin

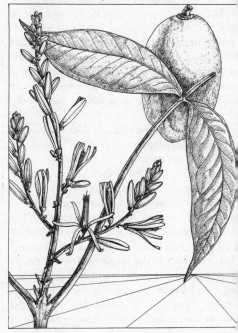

Simaba cedron

SOLANUM

Solanaceae, the Nightshade family
Bittersweet, Black Nightshade,
Horsenettle, Potato

This very extensive genus of both hardy and half-hardy, flowering berry-bearing, herbaceous, shrubby or climbing plants, is indigenous to many parts of the world including North America, Mexico, Chile Costa Rica, tropical Africa, Europe and part of Asia.

One of the most important of these was the Bittersweet or Woody Nightshade (*S. dul camara*), a shrubby, woody based perennial with long trailing or climbing straggling stems 2m/6½ft or more in length. The upper leaves are variable, pointed oval to heart shaped, the lower ones lobed and sometime covered with downy velvety hair. Drooping clusters of purple flowers with yellow anthers, are borne from June to September, followed by egg-shaped berries, first green then orange and finally a bright red, which generally remain for some time after the leaves have fallen. It is found in woods, hedges, thickets and damp waste places throughout Europe (except Iceland) and parts of Asia, although now naturalized elsewhere.

The use of this species dates back at least

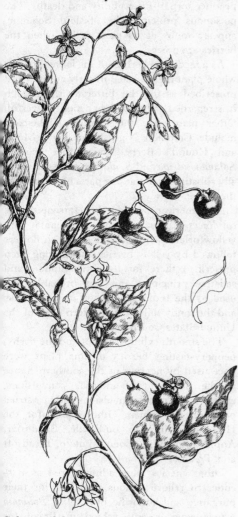

Solanum dulcamara (top), *Solanum nigrum* (below)

to the time of Theophrastus, when it is believed to have been employed in the treat-

ment of skin diseases. The medieval name of Amarodulcis, literally Bitter-sweet, refers to the taste of the roots and stems, which when chewed are bitter, then sweet. Its other popular names include Mortal, Violet Bloom, Scarlet Berry, and Amara Dulcis.

Gerard observed: 'The juice is good for those that have fallen from high places, and have been thereby bruised, or dry beaten – for it is thought to dissolve blood congealed or cluttered anywhere in the entrals and to heal the hurt places.' Culpeper reports: 'It is good to remove witchcraft both in men and beast, as all sudden diseases whatsoever. Being tied about the neck, it is a remedy for the vertigo or dizziness of the head, and that is the reason the Germans hang it about their cattle's necks, when they fear any such evil hath betided them.' The 'country people commonly used to take the berries of it, and having bruised them, they applied them to felons, and thereby soon rid their fingers of such troublesome guests.' From the latter use, the treatment of whitlows, the herb derived its names of Felonwort and Felonwood. Boerhaave, the Dutch physician, also employed the young shoots as a restorative, while Linnaeus regarded the plant as a valuable remedy in the treatment of inflammatory diseases, fever and rheumatism.

The Bittersweet is also common to parts of North America, where it was widely prescribed during the latter half of the nineteenth century for its narcotic, diuretic, alterative, diaphoretic and discutient principles. Professor O. Phelps Brown observed: 'It is serviceable in cutaneous diseases, syphilitic diseases, rheumatic and cachectic effections, ill-conditioned ulcers, scrofula, indurations, sores, glandular swellings, etc. In obstructed menstruation it serves a good purpose. It is of benefit in leprosy, tetter and all skin disease.'

Although once included in the British Pharmacopoeia, the Bittersweet is not widely used today. Its root, bark and shoots, generally collected from two- to three-year old plants, are still prescribed, however, in decoctions or liquid extracts for their alterative, resolvent and narcotic principles, in rheumatism, ulcers and obstinate skin eruptions. The whole of the herb is listed as potentially poisonous (but is less so than its relative the Deadly Nightshade), containing the alkaloid Solanine, and Dulcamarine, a glycoside. In large doses Solanine will lessen sensibility, slow the heart, reduce the temperature, causing vertigo, delirium, convulsions and possibly death. Fortunately the juicy looking berries rarely prove fatal if eaten, and children who have been poisoned by them have generally recovered within twenty-four hours, although their effects can be very unpleasant, causing gastro-enteritis and various nervous symptoms, such as apathy, paralysis and unconsciousness.

An annual species, the Black or Garden Nightshade (*S. nigrum*), an erect, branched, very variable leafy plant 20–60cm/7–23in. tall, has oval entire shallowy lobed leaves, and bears from about May to October, whitish flowers with projecting cones of yellow anthers, followed by green berries turning black. Native to most of Europe (except Iceland) and to parts of Asia, it is found on waste ground, arable fields, vineyards, on rubbish dumps, and has since naturalized itself elsewhere. It was once commonly administered in the treatment of skin disease.

As an inward medicine, the distilled water from the whole herb was employed 'to cool hot inflammations', while the juice of it or of the berries, sometimes with Oil of Roses, ceruse (white lead) or vinegar added, was applied as a wash to 'the shingles – all running, fretting or corroding ulcers – scurvy sores – and to swellings in the private parts'. Without the ceruse it was frequently gargled 'for inflammations of the mouth and throat'. Culpeper tells us: 'A pessary dipped in the juice, and dropped into the matrix, stays the immoderate flow of the courses; a wet cloth therein, and applied to the testicles, upon any swelling therein, gives ease, also to the gout, if it comes of hot and sharp humours. The juice dropped in the ears, eases pains that arise from heat or inflammation: it is good for hot swellings under the throat.' In Asia Minor and the Arab countries, the fresh bruised leaves were applied to burns and ulcers, and in other countries the leaves were placed at the head of infants' cradles to make them sleep quickly and soundly.

This species is also found wild in various parts of North America, where it was prescribed during the late nineteenth century 'as a narcotic and sedative, producing when given in large doses, sickness and vertigo'. Professor O. Phelps Brown writes of it: '[The leaves] have been freely used in cancer, scurvy and scrofulous affections, in the form of an ointment. Very small doses are taken internally. The berries are poisonous, and will produce torpor, insensibility and death.' The poisonous principle, the alkaloid Solanine, appears to be at its most active when the berries are green.

As a medicinal herb both the leaves and the whole plant are collected in early autumn and prescribed as for the Bittersweet, although it is regarded as being rather more powerful. Other names for the Garden Nightshade include Common Nightshade, Petty Morel and Hound's Berry. Two other species, *Solanum luteum* and *S. alatum*, were occasionally substituted in various parts of Europe for the above.

An American species, the Horsenettle (*S. carolinense*), a coarse-growing perennial with yellow prickles, bears white or bluish flowers followed by yellow berries. It has long been prescribed there for its antispasmodic and sedative principles and was probably first used by the Indians. It grows in waste areas and the sandy soils of the eastern parts of the United States, south to Florida.

The smooth cylindrical root and the fleshy, peppery-tasting berries of this plant were once used by negroes of the southern States in the treatment of infantile convulsions, epilepsy, hysterical convulsions and menstrual problems in women. Other names for the Horsenettle include Bullnettle, Sandbrier, Apple of Sodom, Poisonous Potato, Treadsoft and Treadsaf.

Other species were administered as narcotics to relieve various pains, or for their purgative and sudorific principles; *Solanum pseudo-quina* is still valued in Brazil for reducing fevers, while *S. toxicarium* is used by the natives of French Guiana as a reliable source of poison. Other Solanums provide edible fruits, which were and still are eaten as

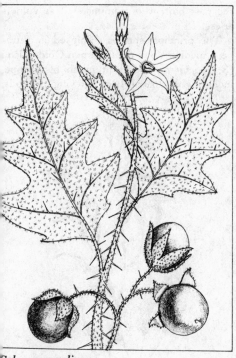

Solanum carolinense

The Spaniards introduced this species into Europe in the early sixteenth century, having noticed that the South American Indians rooted out its tubers and cooked them as food. From Spain it was introduced into Italy, from there to Belgium, subsequently finding its way into Germany and France. It was first introduced to Britain, or rather Ireland, by the colonists sent out by Sir Walter Raleigh, who brought some tubers back from Virginia in 1586, which were planted on Sir Walter's estate at Youghall near Cork. In England the first potatoes were cultivated in Lancashire 'for the epicure' and not as a food for 'the common people' until the 1750s. The Puritans opposed their use as no mention of them could be found in the Bible. As the food value of Potatoes became better known, so their cultivation was encouraged by the Royal Society and in 1725 they were introduced to Scottish gardens. By the 1760s they were being grown there as a

food, these include: *S. anguivi* from Madagascar, *S. quitoense* and *S. muricatum* from Peru, *S. aethiopicum* and *S. album* from China and Japan, *S. ramosum* from the West Indies, the Kangaroo Apple (*S. laciniatum*) from Tasmania, *S. vescum* from Australia, the Garden Huckleberry (*S. intrusum*), probably native to Africa, and the Aubergine or Egg plant (*S. melongena*), from tropical Asia. The leaves of certain species, including *S. sessiforum* from Brazil and *S. oleraceum* from the West Indies and the Fiji Islands, were used as food.

A more familiar plant belonging to this genus is the Potato (*S. tuberosum*), which probably originated in the temperate regions of the Andes, where its tubers are believed to have been eaten as a food for over 2,000 years. This perennial herb, with rather weak branching stems 30–90cm/11–35in. high, and pinnate leaves with three or four pairs of ovate leaflets with smaller ones in between, bears white to purplish flowers with yellow anthers, followed by green or yellowish tomato-like fruits.

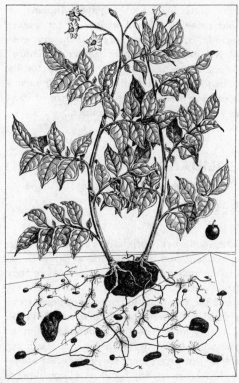

Solanum tuberosum

field crop. The cultivation of the plant also met with opposition in several other European countries.

As a medicinal herb the juice of the tuber was applied in fomentations, liniments and ointments 'for the pain of the gout, rheumatism and lumbago'. Even the carrying of a raw potato was regarded as a good 'preventative' for such complaints, while the mash of uncooked potatoes 'applied cold – cools burns and scalds'.

The Potato is used in the making of alcohol and liquors, such as schnapps, while its flour can be baked into cakes. However, the whole of the green plant, the leaves, berries and stalks are potentially poisonous, as are any tubers that have turned green on exposure to light.

The tuberous roots of several other species can be eaten as a food, including the Wild Potato (*S. fendleri*, syn. *S. tuberosum* 'Boreale') from the mountainous regions of northern Mexico and the south-western parts of the United States. Its small marble-sized tubers were much liked by the Navajo Indians, as were those of *Solanum jamesii*. Other species include *S. marginatum* from Ethiopia, employed in the tanning of leather; *S. indigoferum*, which is cultivated in Brazil for its indigo colour; while the fruits of *S. saponaceum* are used by the native women of Peru as a form of soap to whiten linen.

SOLIDAGO

Compositae, the Daisy family
Golden Rod

The Solidagos are primarily a North American genus, although several sorts are popular as ornamentals in much of Europe, where they have escaped and become naturalized. Of these the two most important species are the Canadian Golden Rod (*S. canadensis*) and the Early Golden Rod (*S. gigantea*), a similar plant also native to North America. Both are robust-growing perennials with erect stems and numerous tiny golden-yellow flowers borne in large pyramidal inflorescences. In

the past both were administered as vulneraries.

The principal species employed in European medicine was the Common Golden Rod (*S. virgaurea*), found in much of Europe, including the British Isles, growing in woods,

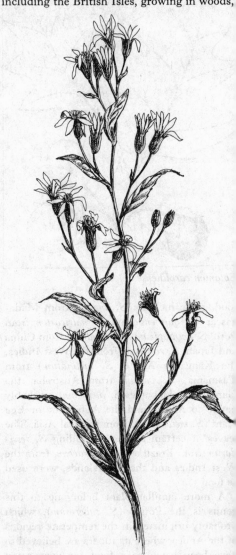

Solidago virgaurea

thickets, grassland and among rocks. A very variable, erect and hardy herbaceous perennial having several forms, the stems reach 10-75cm/4-30in. high, and bear in late summer plume-like clusters of tiny golden-yellow

lowers. Some of these forms or types are so
very distinct that in the past they were often
listed as different species. The word Solidago
is derived from the Latin *solidare*, to strengthen or join, referring to the 'principal
healing virtues' of the Common Golden Rod,
which was highly esteemed as 'a sovereign
wound herb, inferior to none, both for
inward and outward use'.

The young leaves, green or dried, were
most effectually prescribed, taken in a
'distillation' as 'a safe diuretic for removing
the gravel and stone of the reins or kidneys –
to ease the strangury – the bloody flux –
ulcers in the mouth and throat – ruptures –
and the spitting of blood'. As an external
application, decoctions were principally 'applied to green wounds, old ulcers and sores –
and as a lotion to wash the privy parts in
venereal cases'.

While the herb was thought to be a foreign
rarity, it was expensive and in great demand.
But when, in the mid-sixteenth century, it was
found growing wild near London, its reputation rapidly declined.

Culpeper prescribed this 'balsamic vulnery
herb' much as the apothecaries had before
him, but also to 'fasten the teeth that are
loose'.

Nowadays the Golden Rods are only
occasionally prescribed, although infusions or
liquid extracts taken frequently will promote
perspiration and help weak stomachs. Its
action is aromatic, carminative and stimulant.

The aromatic leaves of one of the smaller
American Solidagos, the slender, yellow-
flowering Sweet or Anise-Scented Golden
Rod (*S. odora*), which is native principally
from Maine and Vermont, south to Florida,
then west to Missouri and Texas, were
formerly used as a substitute for tea. This
beverage proved so good (in fact going under
the name of Blue Mountain Tea), that at one
time it was exported to China and is still
occasionally sold today.

An essence of it was employed as a diuretic
for infants and for relieving flatulence and
sickness. Infusions of its flowers are sometimes prescribed for their astringent aperient
and tonic principles, for removing gravel and
other urinary obstructions.

STACHYS
Labiatae, the Mint family
Marsh Woundwort, Hedge Woundwort

The Stachys genus consists of both hardy and
half-hardy mostly perennial flowering plants
(including one tuberous rooted vegetable).
They are native chiefly to the northern
temperate regions, through Europe to Asia.

Of these, the principal species used in
medieval medicine was the Marsh Woundwort (*S. palustris*), an erect, hairy and faintly
aromatic perennial reaching 1m/3ft high,
having lance-shaped toothed leaves, and
bearing whorls of dull pink or purplish
flowers from about June to September. It is
native to the marshy meadows, ditches and
watersides of most of Europe, except Iceland.

During the medieval period this particular
species was rated very highly as a 'vulnerary
herb' and was widely prescribed in the treatment 'of all fresh and green wounds – for
staunching blood flows – to dry up fluxes –
the humours of old and fretting ulcers – and
rotting or corroding cankers'. The juice of it,
in the form of a syrup, was regarded 'as
second to none' for 'bloody fluxes – inward
wounds – the breakings of the veins –
vomitings – the spittings of blood – and
ruptures'. For the latter, including 'the
ruptures of veins', an ointment or plaster of
the herb was also applied to the place. Gerard
gives an account of the herb's remarkable
efficacy in the treatment of an attempted
suicide. Within twenty days it had 'by God's
permission' perfectly cured 'a most mortall
wound in the throat [and] another deepe and
grievous wound in the breast'.

The tuberous roots of the species, often
listed as Woundwort, Marsh Stachys, Opop-
anewort, Panay, All Heal and Rusticum
Vulna Herba, were also boiled and eaten as a
nutritious food, as were the more tender, but
rather unpleasant-tasting, young shoots.

The herb is still prescribed for its antiseptic
and antispasmodic principles in the treatment
of cramp, vertigo, pains of the joints and
gouty infections, while the fresh juice in a
syrup will help stop bleeding and give some

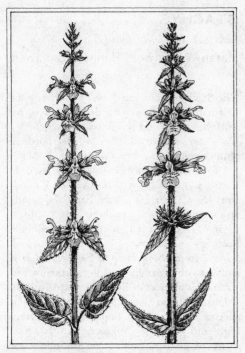

Stachys palustris (right), *Stachys sylvatica* (left)

relief in diarrhoea and dysentery. The bruised leaves applied direct to wounds will stop bleeding, as will the leaves of the Downy Woundwort (*S. germanica*). The latter is a whitish or silky haired erect growing biennial 30–80cm/11–31in. high, found in stony places and uncultivated soils in much of Europe, except the north.

The Hedge Woundwort (*S. sylvatica*), the most common of the European species, was sometimes substituted for the above. It is an erect hairy perennial 30–100cm/11–39in. tall, with creeping rhizomes, stalked, oval or heart-shaped, long, pointed toothed leaves, and from June to September bears whorls of claret-coloured flowers on slender leafless spikes. It is found in hedges, woods and similar shady places in most of Europe, except Iceland. Its leaves, which are very pungent when crushed, were applied direct 'to staunch flows of blood' or if pounded with vinegar were laid on 'wens – hard swellings – and inflammations', while 'a distillation of the flowers taken inwardly helps those that be melancholic'.

STRYCHNOS
Loganiaceae, the Logania family
Nux Vomica, Ignatius Bean

Most of the plants belonging to this genus of woody, climbing shrubs and trees are native to the tropical parts of both America and Asia. Several contain a virulent mixture of alkaloids, which, if taken orally, generally result in an agonizing death.

One or two of the more poisonous sorts however, for example such species as the Nux Vomica (*S. nux-vomica*), are also used in medicine. This medium-sized deciduous tree has opposite oval leaves smooth on both sides, and bears in the cold season clusters of small creamy-white unpleasant smelling flowers, followed by orange-like fruits filled with a white jelly-like pulp, containing three to five brownish-grey flattened disk-shaped seeds, each covered by a soft silky or woolly white substance. These are known as Strych-

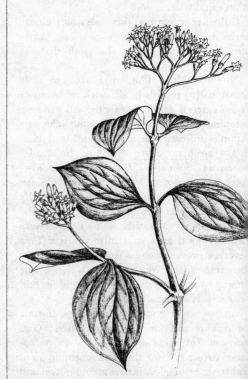

Strychnos nux-vomica

nine nuts and when ripe are collected, carefully cleaned and dried and exported, mainly from Madras, Cochin and other Indian ports. This area is the tree's natural habitat, although it is also found wild in Burma, Ceylon, the Malayan Archipelago and Australia.

From the dried seeds the alkaloids Strychnine and Brucine are extracted, together with a glycoside known as Loganin, a trace of copper and caffeo-tannic acid. As a medicinal herb in the nineteenth century, tinctures and fluids or liquid extracts of the powdered seed were prescribed in very small amounts and often mixed with other medicines for the tonic bitter and stimulant principles, as in 'atonic dyspepsia – neuralgia – debility – impotence – fatigue – chronic constipation – as a tonic in cardiac failure – pruritis – and for easing the pains and inflammations of the outer ear'. Professor O. Phelps Brown observes: 'It is a favourite medicine for paralysis and nervous debility generally. If a poisonous dose is given it will produce spasms like tetanus or lock-jaw. It is tonic, and increases the action of various excretory organs. Where want of nervous energy exists it is an admirable remedy.' Although known before the eighteenth century, the plant appears to have been left well alone in medicine. Both Parkinson and Joseph Miller write of it being used to poison cats, dogs, crows and even ravens.

The extracted alkaloids are still prescribed in official medicines for some of the illnesses mentioned above, and are generally mixed with other preparations, as in tinctures, extracts, tablets and pills. The alkaloid Brucine is similar to Strychnine in action but is regarded as slightly less powerful. The use of Strychnine in precisely measured amounts raises the blood pressure, improves the pulse, and is sometimes used as a tonic for the circulatory system in heart failure, or in cases of surgical shock. Larger doses will kill, causing a very high rise in blood pressure, leading to violent convulsions, with the hearing, vision, touch and smell all becoming very acute, and frequently accompanied by an intense fear. Death results from paralysis of the respiratory system. Strychnine is also used as an antidote for chloral or chloroform poisoning. In reverse, the violent convulsions caused by Strychnine can be controlled by dosing the victim or patient with chloral, chloroform or bromide.

Other names for the Nux Vomica include Quaker Buttons, Poison Nut and Semen strychnos.

The seed of the Ignatius Bean (*S. ignatii*, syn. *Faba ignatic* or *Ignatia amara*) is attributed with much the same properties as the

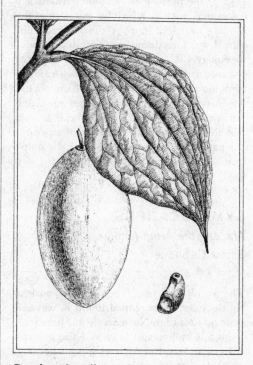

Strychnos ignatii

previous plant, and also contains the alkaloids Brucine and Strychnine. This species is a woody, climbing shrub, bearing large pear-shaped fruits, each containing 12 to 20 ovate, dull blackish-brown seeds or beans about 3cm/1in. long. Native to the Philippines, although now naturalized in parts of southeast Asia, it was administered there as a powerful stimulant and tonic.

At one time the bitter-tasting but odourless seed of this shrub was regarded as a 'useful remedy' against cholera, and was prescribed much like the previous species in the treatment of nervous disorders, debility, neuralgia and for certain types of heart trouble. The powdered seeds or tinctures of them – 'Tincture of Ignatia' – are still officially listed in several Pharmacopoeias.

An extract obtained from a South American species, *Strychnos toxifera*, was employed by certain Indian tribes there as an arrow poison under the name of Curare, Woorari or Urari. This deadly poison, which had been used for many years, was first studied scientifically in 1850 by the physiologist Claude Bernard. He discovered that it killed by paralysing the victim's muscles. In 1943 the alkaloid concerned was introduced successfully in anaesthesiology. A similar arrow poison was obtained from the juice of *Strychnos tieute*, a climbing shrub native to Java, which, should it penetrate the skin, soon causes agonizing convulsions and death from a heart attack. Not all the Strychnos species are of a poisonous nature: in Egypt and Senegal the pulpy fruits of *S. innocua* are sometimes eaten as a food.

SYMPLOCARPUS
Araceae, the Arum family
Skunk Cabbage

The Skunk Cabbage (*S. foetidus*) is a curious North American perennial found in wet and swampy soils from Nova Scotia to Minnesota, south to Carolina and Iowa and also in parts of Eastern Asia. In early spring it pushes up a purplish or purplish-brown, greenish-yellow mottled shell-like spathe enfolding a short oval, fleshy spadix, covered with tiny but numerous purplish flowers. In autumn these are followed by bright red pea-sized berries. The leaves which are large and fleshy appear after the spadix has formed, and often reach a height of 60cm/23in. and a width of 30cm/11in., while the tuber extends for some distance into the ground, by means of long fleshy fibres.

As a medicinal herb, the acrid-tasting seed and malodorous roots of the plant were the parts prescribed. Internally they were good as 'a stimulant, exerting expectorant, anti-

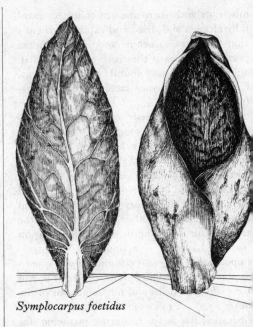

Symplocarpus foetidus

spasmodic, with slightly narcotic influences', in 'asthma, whooping cough, nervous irritability, hysteria, fits, epilepsy, convulsions, chronic catarrh, pulmonary and bronchial affections'. Externally applied in the form of an ointment 'it aids the reparative processes, discusses tumors . . . and eases pain . . .'

The root is still used, generally in the form of a liquid extract, for its antispasmodic, diaphoretic and expectorant principles, mostly for relieving asthma and other bronchial complaints. The powdered root is sometimes added as an ingredient to other compound mixtures and to herbal ointments for relieving pain.

The more tender leaves are quite edible. They can be boiled, changing the water two or three times to rid them of their smell.

In the past this plant has been botanically listed as *Spathyema foetida, Ictodes foetidus, Dracontium foetidum* and is commonly known today by several synonyms, such as Polecatweed, Skunk Weed and Meadow Cabbage.

TARAXACUM
Compositae, the Daisy family
Dandelion

About 10 species of Taraxacum are known in Europe: all contain a milky juice and have basal rosettes of sometimes downy leaves. The most familiar is the Dandelion (*T. officinale*, syn. *T. dens-leonis*, or *Leontodon taraxacum*), a stemless plant with a fleshy branching or simple tap-root and deeply serrated leaves. Its single bright yellow flowers, borne on solitary hollow stalks up to 50cm/20in. tall, appear at almost any time of the year, but mainly from April to November. Although native to Europe and Asia, the Dandelion is found in many other parts of the world, including Canada, the United States, Australia and New Zealand. It grows in meadows, pastures, gardens, along roads and in similar places.

The generic name of this very variable perennial, of which there are numerous micro-species and distinct forms, is believed to have been derived from the Greek *taraxis*, meaning disorder, and *akas*, a remedy, referring to its medicinal uses. It was known as Taraxacum to Avicenna, the great Arabian physician, who prescribed it in the early part of the eleventh century to evacuate bile, and as a medicine to gradually restore health.

The present name of Dandelion is derived from the French *dent de lion*, meaning tooth of the lion, the jagged leaves of the plant supposedly resembling the lion's teeth. The botanical name of Leontodon was allocated to the plant by Linnaeus and derives from the Greek *leon*, a lion, and *odous* or *odontos*, a tooth.

The principal part of the Dandelion prescribed in medicine was the root, which was regarded as 'most effectual for opening obstructions of liver, gall and spleen ... and such diseases that arise thereof', and 'therefore beneficial in rheumatisms, dropsy, gouts, the jaundice, and for removing torpor'. Matthiolus, in the sixteenth century, also prescribed the whole of the plant decocted for those afflicted with jaundice. Contemporaries

of his also applied the juice alone as a wash for scurvy, eczema or sores, and for other chronic diseases of the skin. Internally it was taken as a tonic to relieve indigestion and upset stomachs. The same would 'clear the bladder – remove uterine obstructions – relieve the heat of the ague – and is effectual in pestilential fevers.' The milky white sap from the flowering stems and leaves also 'withereth and removeth the worts'. Culpeper recommended it as it 'powerfully cleanseth imposthumes and inward ulcers in the urinary passages and by its drying and temperate quality doth afterwards heal them ...'

Parkinson, like Culpeper, referred to the herb as Piss-a-beds (or Bed) and writes it is 'very effectual for the obstructions of the

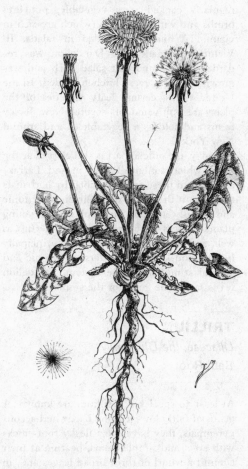

Taraxacum officinale

liver, gall and spleene, and the diseases that arise from them, as the jaundice and the hypochondriacall passion, it wonderfully openeth the uritorie parts, causing abundance of urine.' Other names for this species include Milk Gowan, Blow Ball, Swine's Snout and Priest's Crown.

The gipsies of Europe and Asia also made good use of this herb, adding it to their medicinal preparations and extracting from its roots a magenta-coloured dye.

As a rather weak substitute for coffee, the roots of the Dandelion can be gathered in the autumn, washed and dried, roasted until slightly brown then ground as ordinary coffee. They can also be blanched and eaten raw in winter salads. In France, where the plant is known as Pissenlit, the roots are regularly cooked as a vegetable, put into broths and with the leaves (which are rich in vitamin A and C) included in salads. In Victorian England, the Dandelion was regarded as an important salad herb and was grown in nearly every kitchen garden. In the United States certain leafy varieties of the plant are cultivated on several New Jersey farms and sold as a vegetable in and around New York.

Today, the official part is still classed as the roots, which contain Taraxacin and Tarraxasterol, and these are prescribed by herbalists throughout the world for their diuretic, tonic and slightly aperient principles. The young plants possess slightly narcotic properties as well, and as such are administered principally in liver and kidney disorders, as a tonic and general stimulant to the system. Dandelion tea is said to be good for the stomach.

TRILLIUM
Liliaceae, the Lily family
Beth Root

At least 30 species of Trillium are known. A genus of fairly low-growing hardy herbaceous perennials, they have short fleshy root-stocks with erect and simple stems, bearing at their summit a whorl of three broad leaves and, in early spring, a single three petalled flower the

colour of which varies in the different species from white to pink or purplish. About 20 species are found in North America (others in the Himalayan region and Japan) usually growing in woodland to the east of the Rocky Mountains, where they are collectively known under such names as Indian Shamrock, Wake Robin, Wood Lily, Ground Lily, Indian Balm, Nosebleed, Lamb's Quarters, Three Leaved Nightshade and Trinity Flower. The last two names refer to the triple arrangement of both the leaves and flowers, as does Trillium their generic name, a Latin word derived from *tri* or *trilex* meaning three.

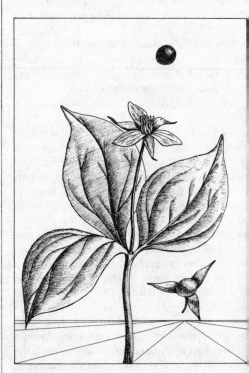

Trillium pendulum

Nearly all the species appear to have been used in medicine, although the plant most often resorted to was the Beth Root (*T. pendulum*), a familiar herb in the middle and western parts of the United States, where it is found in fairly rich soils, especially in damp shady woods, growing from 25–50cm/9–19in. tall and bearing its drooping solitary whitish flowers in May and June.

In medicine, the parts most used were the leaves and rhizomes. The latter have a faint turpentine odour and a peculiar aromatic, acrid taste, and when chewed greatly increases the flow of saliva. Both the roots and leaves were prescribed for their astringent, antiseptic and tonic effects, for 'bleedings from the lungs, kidneys and womb, excessive menstruation, and likewise in leucorrhoea or whites, and cough, asthma and difficult breathing . . . Boiled in milk, it is of eminent benefit in diarrhoea and dysentery.' Both the Indians and the early American settlers administered strong infusions of the powdered root to their womenfolk if they required help in childbirth; hence Birthroot, another common name. A poultice of rhizomes was considered 'very useful in tumors, indolent and offensive ulcers, stings of insects, and to restrain gangrene' while the leaves boiled in lard 'are a good application to ulcers, tumors . . .'

The powdered root is still prescribed for its astringent, pectoral, alterative and tonic principles for relieving pulmonary infections, internal bleeding, excessive menstruation and other women's complaints.

Other species of Trillium possessing similar medicinal properties include the Wake Robin (*T. grandiflorum*), a handsome plant 30–45cm/11–17in. tall, with three rich green leaves surmounted by a white flower turning pink as it ages; *T. nivale*, a similar but much smaller species, 8–10cm/3–4in. tall, with pure white flowers; *T. erythrocarpum* and *T. sessile*.

TUSSILAGO
Compositae, the Daisy family
Coltsfoot, Butterbur

Only one species of Tussilago is listed as indigenous to Europe – the Coltsfoot (*T. farfara*). This pretty little perennial plant bears bright yellow daisy-like flowers in early spring, on thick, erect, purplish coloured, scaly stems about 10–15cm/4–6in. tall, lengthening in fruit to 35cm/13in. Both flowers and fruit are produced before the stalked,

sea-green basal leaves appear. In the wild, this plant grows in waste places, on railway embankments, in quarries, on cliffs and in fields, favouring a damp, heavy or clayey soil. It is found throughout Europe, including the British Isles, Russian Asia, Siberia and Canada, and the north-eastern parts of the United States.

Its almost universal name of Coltsfoot refers to the hoof-like shape of the leaves. Other similar names include Foalfoot, Foolwort, Horsehoof, Bull's-Foot, Ass's-Foot and Hallfoot, while that of Son-before-Father (*Filius ante patrem*) refers to its habit of flowering before producing its leaves.

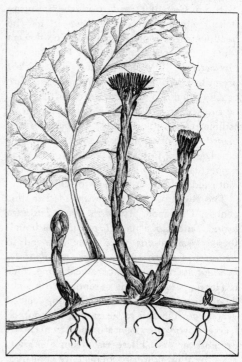

Tussilago farfara

The use of the Coltsfoot in medicine dates back to the time of the ancient Greeks and Romans, when it was prescribed in the treatment of various pulmonary complaints. This is referred to in its generic name of Tussilago, which evolved from the Latin *tussis* – a cough. The specific name *farfara* was taken from the Greek name for the White Poplar, whose leaves, like those of the Coltsfoot, have a downy covering on the underside, which at one time was used as a stuffing for pillows and beds.

Culpeper tells us 'the fresh leaves, or juice, or syrup thereof, is good for a hot, dry cough, or wheezing, and shortness of breath.' Besides this, the herb was prescribed, or rather 'the distilled water hereof . . . with elder-flowers and nightshade . . . as a singular remedy against all hot agues'. The leaves in a poultice 'helps those suffering from scrofulous tumours' while the powdered leaves 'form a good errhine for giddiness, headache and nasal obstructions'.

Several Pharmacopoeias formerly listed a 'Syrup of Coltsfoot' made from the flowering stalks, officially recommending it in the treatment of chronic bronchitis. The flowers contain the active constituents Faradial and Phytosterol. The leaves are still widely prescribed in herbal medicine, and are usually dried and used decocted (or they may be smoked as a tobacco) in the treatment of asthma, coughs and colds. All parts of the plant when dried have a somewhat bitter mucilaginous taste and will yield their properties to water or diluted alcohol. Coltsfoot candy is said to be good for coughs.

The Butterbur was once included in this genus, Culpeper listing it as *Tussilago hybrida*, and Linnaeus as *T. petasites*, although these classifications were later changed to *Petasites vulgaris* and again to *Petasites hybridus*, its present-day botanical name. This is a large, patch-forming perennial, with stout long creeping rhizomes, and long-stalked very large rounded to heart-shaped, toothed leaves, downy grey beneath and often 1m/3ft or more across. These rise from the roots after the stout flowering stems have appeared, the latter being covered by lance or strap-shaped scales, and bearing from March to May a large dense ovoid cluster of pale reddish to violet flowers, the males and females on different plants. It is found in much of Europe in wet meadows, marshes and by the riverside.

One of the principal uses of this plant was in the treatment of 'pestilence'. Lyte, in his 1578 *Herbal*, referred to it as a 'soveraigne

medicine against the plague' as did Gerard, who recommended the powdered root taken in wine 'because it provoketh sweat and driveth from the heart all venim and evill heate'. He says it also 'killeth worms' while the powder of the roots 'cureth all naughty filthy ulcers, if it be strewed therein'. Culpeper thought it 'a great strengthener of the heart and cheerer of the vital spirits . . . the decoction of the root, in wine, is singular good for those that wheeze much, or are short winded. It provoketh urine also, and women's courses, and killeth the flat and broad worms in the belly . . .'

Other names for this species include Plague Flower, Common Butterbur, Bogshorns, Butter-Dock, Cap-Dockin, Blatterdock, Flapperdock, Umbrella Plant, Langwort and Bog Rhubarb.

The bitter roots of the Butterbur are still given for their diuretic, stimulant and cardiac tonic principles, and are generally taken in warm infusions in the treatment of colds, fevers and asthma. Both the Butterbur and Coltsfoot are prescribed in the form of a tincture in homoeopathic medicine for relieving neuralgia.

ULMUS
Ulmaceae, the Elm family
Common Elm, Slippery Elm

The Ulmus genus consists of a group of deciduous trees and shrubs with alternate entire leaves. The various species range from bush height to very lofty timber-producing trees, native mainly to the northern temperate zone, including Europe, the British Isles, Asia, the Himalayas, China, North Africa and northern Mexico.

The use of at least one of the European species, probably the Common Elm (*U. procera*, syn. *U. campestris*), dates back to the time of Dioscorides, Pliny and Galen. All mention its astringent, demulcent and anti-inflammatory virtues, which led to its later use in the treatment of skin complaints. This tall, long-living tree with its numerous spreading branches is found in most of

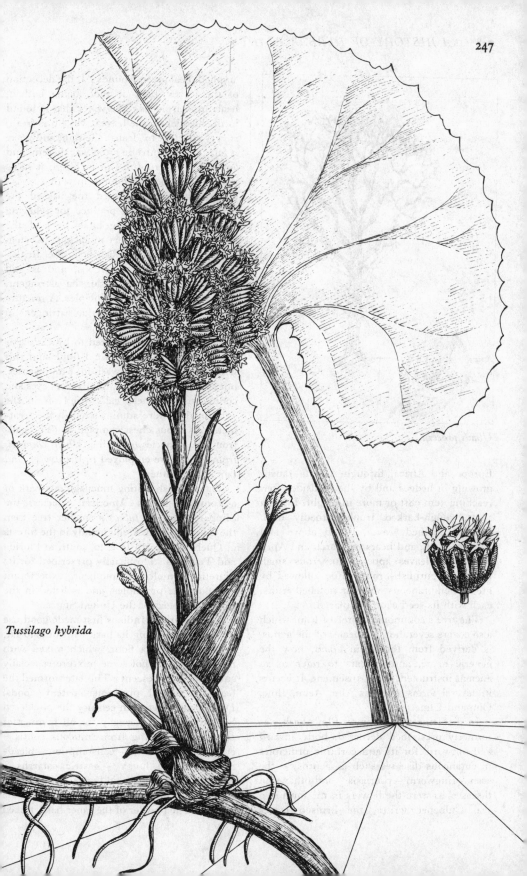

Tussilago hybrida

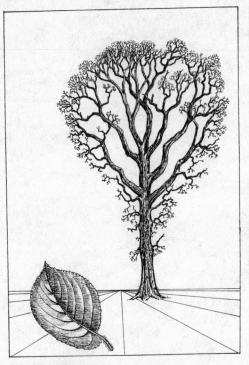

Ulmus procera

Europe and Africa, through Asia to Japan, growing in hedges and by the roadside often reaching 30m/98ft or more in height. It has a stout, rough-barked trunk, broadly oval, coarsely toothed leaves, rough above and hairy beneath, and bears in March and April before the leaves appear, numerous small flowers in purplish-brown tufts, followed by green membraneous obicular notched fruits, each with its seed centrally placed.

The tree's commonest name of Elm, which also covers several other species of the genus, is derived from the Latin *ulmus*, now the generic name, and appears to refer to an ancient instrument of chastisement. It occurs in several forms, such as Alm, Aelm, Ilme, Olm and Ulme.

In medicine the Common Elm's bark was formerly prescribed decocted, both 'inward and outward' for its antiscorbutic principles in cutaneous diseases such as 'leprosy – the scab – ringworm – psoriasis – and other skin diseases' as were the flowers in the form of a tea. Culpeper writes, the bruised leaves

'applied, heal green wounds . . . the decoction of the leaves, bark or root, being bathed, heals broken bones. The water that is found in the bladder on the leaves, while it is fresh, is very effectual to cleanse the skin, and make it fair; and if cloths be often wet therein, and applied to the ruptures of children, it heals them, if they be well bound up with a truss.'

Parkinson recommended the use of the bark in the form of a poultice for relieving gout. The bitter-tasting inner bark of the tree, which becomes very mucilaginous when wetted, was formerly listed in the British Pharmocopoeias of the 1860s, and is still prescribed by herbalists for its astringent, demulcent and diuretic principles. A tincture of the inner bark is used as an astringent in homoeopathic medicine.

The leaf bladders referred to by Culpeper contain a clear, sweet, viscid fluid, and this was used not only as a wash for skin diseases, but as an application to wounds, sore eyes and contusions. As these galls dried off in the autumn they were administered in the treatment of various chest complaints. (The galls from other species, including *Ulmus chinensis* from China, are employed in the dyeing and tanning of leather.)

The sweetish-tasting mucilaginous bark of a common North American species, the Slippery Elm (*U. fulva*) a smaller tree than the Common Elm, found mainly in the forests of Quebec to North Dakota, south to Florida and Texas, is still officially prescribed for its diuretic, demulcent, emollient, expectorant and nutritive principles, and is listed in the Pharmacopoeias of the United States.

The American Indians first made good use of this tree, cooking its bark with buffalo fat, grinding it into a flour, which mixed with milk formed a wholesome mixture especially suited for convalescents. This later formed the basis of several nutritious 'patent' foods. During the nineteenth century the powdered bark was taken internally for all manner of complaints, ranging from 'mucous colitis – enteritis – bronchitis – consumption – bleedings from the lungs – gastric catarrhs – racking coughs – typhoid fevers – affliction of the throat – pleurisy – diseases of the female organs'. The powder of the inner bark, mixed with hot water, and sometimes with other herbs, was applied to 'wounds of all kinds – swollen glands – inflammations – congestion – abscesses – and similar eruptions', and in gangrenous wounds 'equal parts of powdered Slippery Elm and fine charcoal, mixed either with an infusion of Wormwood or warm water', was applied direct, as an antiseptic poultice.

The bark was also prescribed for relieving intestinal and urinary ailments while the mucilage of the bark, mixed with the oil of the Male Fern (*Dryopteris filix-mas*, syn. *Aspidium filix-mas*) 'expels the tapeworm'.

The inner bark of the Slippery Elm is still prescribed for its demulcent, diuretic, emollient and pectoral principles. Finely powdered it makes a sustaining and nutritious food in cases of body weakness, bronchitis and inflammation of the stomach, having a soothing and healing effect on all the parts it comes in contact with. The coarse powder as a poultice helps to disperse inflammations and inflamed surfaces, speedily relieving various skin infections as well as burns, wounds and chilblains. It is also prescribed in lozenge form for irritation of the pharynx. Other names for this species include Red Elm, Moose Elm and Indian Elm.

The Slippery Elm above is not to be confused with the Californian Slippery Elm (*Fremontia californica*) a handsome, slightly tender deciduous shrub, bearing golden mallow-like flowers, the bark of which is said to possess similar medicinal properties.

URGINEA
Liliaceae, the Lily family
Squill

This small genus of bulbous plants is closely related to that of the Scilla and Ornithogalum, and is native mainly to southern Europe, the Mediterranean region and South Africa.

The species generally prescribed in the medicine of the ancient Greeks was the Squill (*U. maritima*, syn. *U. scilla* or *Scilla maritima*), also known as the Sea Onion or Sea Squill, a very variable perennial with

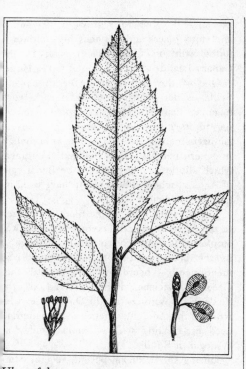

Ulmus fulva

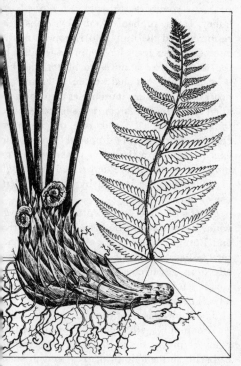

Dryopteris filix-mas

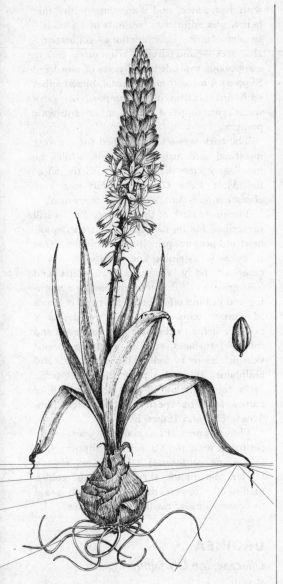

Urginea maritima

ranean region, where it grows in dry sandy and stony places and on rocky hills, although found wild in other places such as the Canary Islands and the Cape of Good Hope.

One of the Latin names for this plant, Scilla, is derived from an old Greek word meaning 'disturb' or 'excite', probably referring to its effect on the stomach if taken. Linnaeus named it *Scilla maritima*, although its generic name was later changed to Urginea, which alludes to the Arabic tribe Ben Urgin of Algeria, who are believed to have used its bulbs in medicine.

The medicinal use of the plant dates back to the classical period. Oxymel of Squill was employed as a cure for coughs by Pythagoras in the sixth century B.C., and was also mentioned by Theophrastus and several other Greek physicians. Pliny referred to the Scilla in his writings, as did Dioscorides who wrote of the different varieties and the method used for making what is known today as 'Vinegar of Squills'.

During the medieval period, several compounds and mixtures of Squill were used in Arabian countries, usually prescribed in honey. It was probably Arab physicians who re-introduced the bulb into European medicine. Culpeper records: 'The root is bitter to the taste, and so acrid as to blister the skin if it is much handled; taken internally in doses of a few grains, it promotes the expectoration and urine; in larger doses it vomits, and sometimes purges. It is one of the most certain diuretics in dropsical cases, and expectorants in asthmatical ones, where the lungs or stomach are oppressed by tough viscid phlegm, or injured by the imprudent use of opiates.'

During the nineteenth century the bulb was widely administered both in North America and Europe, much as above, and 'as a tonic for the heart – chronic bronchitis – catarrhal affections – as an emetic in croup or whooping cough' and was readily available commercially. The variety known as Red Squill was also laid down as a rat poison.

The bulb is still officially prescribed in many countries for its diuretic, expectorant, cathartic and emetic principles, and in small doses will relieve excessive secretions and

fibrous roots growing from large, often partly exposed bulbs up to 15cm/6in. across. In the autumn, on unbranched leafless stems 1–1½m/ 3–5ft tall, it bears numerous white flowers in a cylindrical cluster 30cm/11in. or more in length. Its large fleshy, broadly lance-shaped, shining dark green leaves appear after the flowers and persist until the following summer. It is native to much of the Mediter-

irritation of the mucous surfaces. As an expectorant it is administered for relieving catarrh, asthma, pneumonia, coughs and other bronchial complaints.

An Indian Squill (*U. indica*, syn. *Scilla indica*), which has a smaller bulb than the European sort, is used there and in other Eastern countries for very similar complaints. The bulb of a South African Squill (*U. altissima*, syn. *Ornithogalum altissimum*) possesses similar qualities. The bulb of a closely related plant, *Scilla peruviana*, which is native to such countries as Spain, Portugal, France and Italy, where it is found in damp, fertile soils, was sometimes substituted for that of the Squill.

Any of the above if over prescribed will cause sickness and vomiting, with abdominal pains and purging, accompanied by a fall in temperature, poor circulation, stupor, convulsions and sometimes death.

URTICA
Urticaceae, the Nettle family
Common Nettle

The various members of the Nettle family are indigenous to several parts of the world, including the tropical and temperate regions. Many of the species have stinging hairs on their leaves and stems, which is referred to in Urtica, their generic name, derived from the Latin *uro*, I burn. Several such species, especially those from the warmer countries, if carelessly handled can cause intense pain, including *Urtica heterophylla*, *U. crenulato* from India and *U. urentissima* from Java, the latter producing a painful inflammation that can last for several weeks. Fortunately the juice of the Nettle is also the antidote for its own sting, and when this is applied to the part affected it generally brings rapid relief.

The principal species with stinging hairs used in the medicine of medieval Europe was the Common Nettle (*U. dioica*), a stoloniferous and variable perennial, with many erect leafy stems up to 1½m/5ft high, bearing heart-shaped, long-pointed, stalked, saw-toothed, opposite leaves, and long tassel-like

usually one-sexed clusters of greenish yellow flowers. Found in waste places, woods, hedges, cultivated soils, on rubbish dumps and by habitation, throughout Europe, parts of temperate Asia, through to Japan, it is now widely naturalized elsewhere, for example, North and South America, Australia and New Zealand.

The commonest name of this plant, Nettle, is derived from the Anglo-Saxon *noedl*, meaning needle, referring either to its vicious sting, or to its use in the making of a thread, once used in western Europe in the weaving of different fabrics before the introduction of Flax and Hemp. The scanty remains of such a Nettle cloth have been discovered wrapping some cremated bones in a Danish burial dating back to the late Bronze Age. The plant's specific name *dioica* means two houses, an allusion to the one-sexed flowers that are found on separate plants.

Of its 'Vertues' Gerard wrote: 'Nicander affirmeth, that it is a remedie against the venomous qualitie of Hemlocke, Mushroms, and Quicksilver ... And Apollodorus saith that it is a counter-poison for Henbane, Serpents, and Scorpions.'

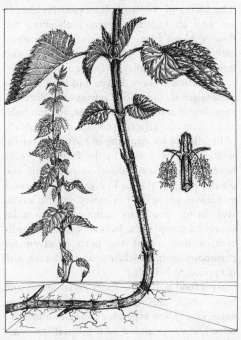

Urtica dioica

According to Culpeper: 'The juice of the leaves or the decoction of the root, is good to wash either old, rotten, or stinking sores or fistulas, and gangrenes ... manginess, and itch, in any part of the body – as also green wounds, by washing them therewith, or applying the green herb bruised thereto. It eases the pains, and dries or dissolves the defluctions. An ointment made of the juice, oil and a little wax, is good to rub cold and benumbed members. One handful of the leaves of green nettles, and another of Wall-wort, or Deanwort, bruised and applied simply themselves to the gout, sciatica, or joint aches in any part, hath been found an admirable help thereunto.'

In North America, the Stinging Nettle, or Great Nettle as it is sometimes called, has now naturalized itself from Newfoundland west to Minnesota, south to Carolina, Missouri and Colorado. During the nine-teenth century it was prescribed 'as an astringent, tonic and diuretic'. Decoctions of the root and leaves were regarded as 'valuable in diarrhoea, dysentery, and piles; also in haemorrhages, scorbutic and febrile affections, gravel, and other nephritic complaints ... The leaves of the fresh Common Nettle ... are also an excellent styptic, checking the flow of blood from surfaces almost immedi-ately upon their application. The seed and flowers are given in wine for agues.'

The dried flowers, leaves and seed are still administered for their astringent, diuretic, stimulating and tonic principles, for example, in infusions for relieving coughs and shortness of breath and for applying as a lotion to burns, while the fresh leaves in the form of Nettle beer or tea, makes a useful antiscorbutic and purifier of the blood. The juice of the roots and leaves prescribed in honey or with sugar, will bring relief in asthma and similar bronchial complaints. In homoeopathic medi-cine, a tincture of the herb is given for rheumatic-gout, chicken-pox, nettlerash and is applied to bruises.

As a food plant, the fresh green leaves and tops, which are rich in vitamin C, can be eaten as a spring vegetable (this has a laxative effect), may be added as a potherb to vege-table stews, or made into Nettle pudding.

Samuel Pepys, writing in his Diary in February 1661: 'We did eat some nettle porridge [which] was very good'.

The stem fibre of the plant was also spun coarse or fine and woven into rough or fine cloths, sailcloth, sacking and table linen, or was spun into rope or twine for fishing nets. A green colouring matter extracted from the leaves was once a popular wool dye, while the roots boiled with salt or alum yielded a beautiful yellow, for use on yarn. Nowadays Chlorophyll is extracted from the plant.

The dried herb, rich in minerals and protein, makes excellent fodder and will help increase egg and milk yields. Chopped up fresh it was at one time added to feed, to make the animals' coats and eyes shine. Other names for the Common Nettle include Ettle, Devil's Leaf, Devil's Plaything, Hoky Poky and Tanging Nettle.

The Small Nettle (*U. urens*) is a branching annual 10–60cm/4–23in. tall, with pale green, hairy, oval to heart shaped, stalked, saw-toothed leaves, and bears from May to October short clusters of greenish unisexual flowers. 'Possessing similar qualities', it was frequently substituted for the above species. This stinging plant is found in arable soils and waste ground throughout Europe and parts of Asia. Like the previous Nettle it is now extensively naturalized elsewhere, for example North America. Its other common names include Dwarf Nettle and Annual Nettle.

A North American species, the Stingless Nettle (*U. pamila*), also known as the Cool-Weed or Rich-Weed, was prescribed to give 'relief in inflammations, painful swellings, erysipelas and the topical poison of rhus'. The young leaves of the Slender Nettle (*U. gracilis*) are also known to have been eaten by the American Indians as a wholesome spring green, or were added as a potherb to their soups and stews.

The Roman Nettle (*U. pilulifera*) is an annual or biennial reaching 30–100cm/11–39in., native to the waste places and waysides of Mediterranean Europe although now naturalized elsewhere. According to the antiquary Camden in his *Britannica*, the Romans brought some Nettle seed with them and sowed it there for their use to rub and chafe their limbs, when through extreme cold they should be stiff or benumbed, having been told that the climate of Britain was so cold that it was not to be endured'. The general idea was to warm up the skin and to keep it smarting for the rest of the day, which probably developed into the practice of flogging those suffering from loss of muscular power or the pains of rheumatism with bunches of its stinging stems as a 'cure' – the hairs of this and other stinging species containing Formic Acid (HCO_2H).

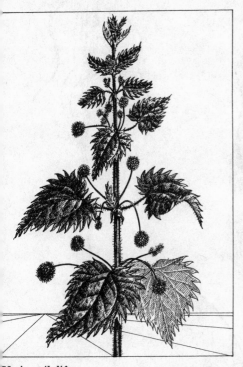

Urtica pilulifera

VERBASCUM
Scrophulariaceae, the Figwort family
Great Mullein, Dark Mullein

At least 250 species of Verbascum are known. A genus of coarse, erect, strong-growing hardy biennial or perennial herbs with alternate leaves and producing long terminal spikes of mostly yellow flowers, it is native to most of Europe, the Mediterranean region, temperate Asia and North America.

Of the species formerly used in medicine, the most important was the Great Mullein or Aaron's Rod (*V. thapsus*), a tall, robust biennial 30–200cm/11–78in. high, with greyish, downy or woolly basal leaves, and bearing from July to September club-shaped spikes of yellow flowers. It is found by roadside verges, on hillsides and sunny hedge banks, or in waste places throughout most of Europe and Asia to the Himalayas, although now widely naturalized elsewhere, as in North America.

The generic name of this plant, Verbascum, is believed to be a corruption of *barbascum*, from the Latin *barba*, meaning a beard, referring to the shaggy appearance of the genus, while *thapsis*, its specific name, may refer to the Greek island of that name, where the species originally thrived. Its commonest name of Mullein is derived from the Anglo-Saxon *molegn*, which evolved to the Middle English *moleyn*. These names are possibly derived from the Latin *malandria*, an ancient term used when referring to the blisters or pustules on the necks of cattle. In time the word *malandre* became applied to various cattle diseases, especially those of the lungs, and the Mullein, under the name of Cow's or Bullock's Lungwort, was used as a remedy for these. Both Gerard and William Coles recorded this as its principal use.

The Romans made good use of this resinous plant by stripping the leaves and flowers from the stems, and dipping them into tallow, to make simple torches or tapers. Parkinson in the seventeenth century writes: 'Verbascum is called of the Latines Candela regia, and Candelaria – because the elder age used the stalks dipped in suet to burne . . .' Later on, the whitish down of the plant, when thoroughly dried, was employed in the making of candle wicks, subsequently for those of oil lamps, and as a ready-made tinder when kindling with flint and steel.

The women of Rome also infused the flowers and mixed the resulting liquid with lye, using it as a wash to turn their hair golden yellow. This useful cosmetic remedy was repeated by Lyte in 1578. Poor people

Verbascum thapsus

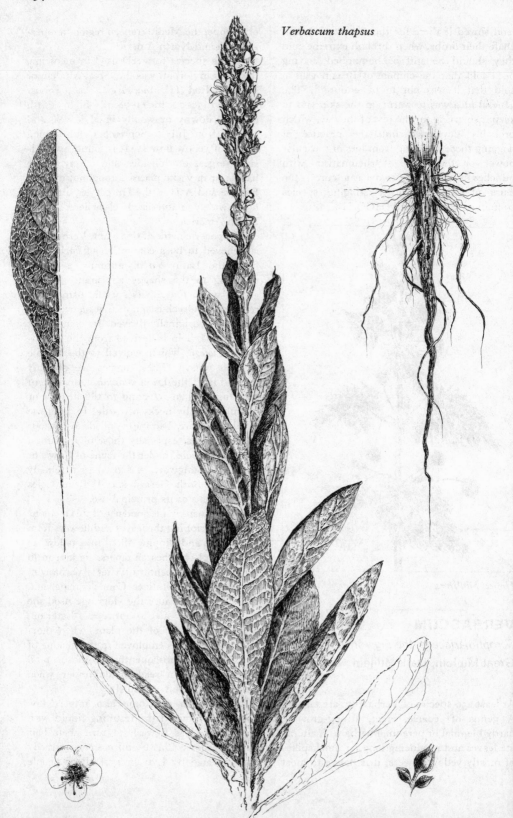

put the thicker, woollier leaves into their stockings as a means of keeping their feet warm, while the crushed seed, which is slightly narcotic, was fed into monastic fish ponds, or used by poachers, to make the fish sluggish, thereby enabling them to be more easily taken by hand. (Other species used in this way include *Verbascum sinuatum*, from the Mediterranean parts of Europe, which contains Saponin; and to a lesser degree *V. phlomoides* and *V. thapsiforme*, both common to southern and central parts of Europe.)

As a medicinal herb, the Great Mullein had many uses. Dioscorides administered the roots for diseases of the lungs, and Pliny gave its leaves to broken-winded horses. By the medieval period, the plant was widely prescribed throughout Europe. Decoctions of the roots, leaves and flowers were 'accounted pectoral' and 'good for wasting diseases – coughs – spitting of blood – consumption – and other afflictions of the breast', as 'profitable for those that are bursten inwardly' and of service in griping colic and likewise body pains, such as convulsions and cramps – and in laxes and fluxes against the body'. The decoction 'gargled, eases toothache – bleedings from the mouth and lungs – hoarseness – swellings of and sore throat' and 'the oil made by infusion of the flowers, is of good effect for the piles'. The decoction of the root in red wine or water 'is good for the ague' and boiled in milk 'especially helps all complaints of the bowels'. Hot fomentations of the leaves applied 'are excellent in tumours – burns – and in inflammations – will ease the swelling and pains of the piles' and if boiled in wine with the seed 'will speedily remove splinter and thorns from the skin – and ease the pains of the sinews or joints that be stiff'.

Its numerous names include Hedge Taper, High Taper, Hags Taper, Our Ladies Flannel, Old Man's Flannel, Our Lady's Candle, Adam's Flannel, Candlewick Plant, Blanket Herb, Begger's Stalk, Fluffwort, Fluffweed, Feltwort, Caddy's Lungs, Ag-Leaf, Clown's Lungwort, Jupiter's Staff, Peter's Staff, Shepherd's Club, Clot, Wild Ice Leaf, Mullein Dock, White Mullein, Velvet Plant, Velvet Dock and Lady's Foxglove.

In the United States during the nineteenth century the Great Mullein was prescribed for its demulcent, diuretic, anodyne and antispasmodic principles 'the infusion being useful in coughs, catarrhs, bleeding from the mouth or lungs, diarrhoea, dysentery and piles ... A fomentation of the leaves in hot vinegar and water forms an excellent local application for inflamed piles, ulcers and tumors, mumps, acute inflammation of the tonsils, malignant sore throat, etc. A handful of them may be also placed in an old teapot, with hot water, and the steam be inhaled through the spout, in the same complaints.'

The infused leaves and flowers, or liquid extracts of the Great Mullein, are nowadays given for their astringent, demulcent and pectoral principles, in the treatment of chest disorders, while the dried leaves are occasionally smoked for coughs.

Several other kinds of Mullein, although less common than the species mentioned above, were regarded as having similar medicinal properties. These include the Dark Mullein (*V. nigrum*) and the White Mullein (*V. lychnitis*), which were both cultivated in Elizabethan gardens; the Hoary Mullein (*V. pulverulentum*), also used to stupefy fish; the Large Flowered Mullein (*V. virgatum*); the Orange Mullein (*V. phlomoides*), formerly prescribed for expelling tapeworm; and the Moth Mullein (*V. blattaria*). Parkinson says the latter 'is so named because: Plinie saith that moths doe most frequently haunt where Blattaria either groweth or is laid'. The Purple Mullein (*V. phoeniceum*), which was introduced to Britain from central Europe sometime before 1597, was also cultivated as a medicinal herb.

The plants used for medicinal purposes are generally collected from the wild. In homoeopathic medicine, the dried leaves of several species are prescribed in the form of a tincture with spirits of wine, for relieving earache, continuous sick headache and migraine.

Verbascum nigrum

VINCA

Apocynaceae, the Dogbane family

Greater Periwinkle, Lesser Periwinkle, Madagascar Periwinkle

The Vincas make up a small group of trailing perennial herbs or sub-shrubs, usually with solitary bluish flowers. They are native mainly to the southern parts of Europe and the United States. Their generic name, Vinca, is derived from the Latin *vincio* meaning I bind, the long trailing pliable stems of some species having been used in the past for tying and binding, particularly in the making of wreaths and garlands.

The principal species used in medicine appears to have been the Greater Periwinkle (*V. major*), a robust perennial with trailing stems 1–2m/3–6ft long, rooting at the tips, oval or egg-shaped leaves of an evergreen nature, and large solitary lavender-blue flowers 4–5cm/1½–2in. across borne from about March to June. Probably native to the woods, hedges and similar shady places of the Mediterranean parts of Europe, it is now widely naturalized elsewhere as a result of its cultivation in gardens.

The use of this slightly acrid-tasting herb dates back to the time of the ancient Greeks. Little of its early history is recorded, although both Galen and Dioscorides are believed to have prescribed it in the treatment of 'fluxes'. By the time of Chaucer, who referred to it as 'Perwinke rich of hew', its use had become entwined in superstition and it was often used to help expel evil spirits from people. Apulieus, referring to the herb as *Vinca pervinca*, says that the plant was used to good advantage for many purposes, first against devil sickness, possession by demons and as a preventative against snakes, wild beasts, poisons, envy and terror. Variations of its name include 'Parwynke' from Macer's herbal and 'Penynke' as found in *The Boke of Secretes of Albartus Magnus of the Vertues of Herbs, Stones and Certaine Beastes*, which claimed: 'Perwynke when it is beate unto pouder with worms of ye earth wrapped about it and with an herbe called hous lyke, it

induceth love between man and wyfe if it be used in their meales . . .'

Other names for the Greater Periwinkle include Joy of the Ground, Flower of Death (from its use in the making of wreaths and garlands), Flower of Immortality, Cut Finger, Blue Finger, Blue Buttons and Pennywinkle.

Culpeper says of the herb: 'It is a great binder, and stays bleeding at the mouth and nose, if it be chewed. It is a good female medicine, and may be used with good advantage in hysteria and other fits. An infusion is good to stay the menses . . . It is

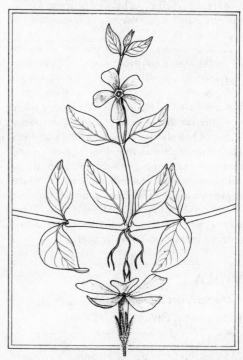

Vinca major (flower, below), *V. minor* (above)

good in nervous disorders.' He adds 'The young tops made into a conserve is good for the night-mare.' William Coles in 1657 observes that the 'branches' of this plant wrapped about the limbs is a remedy for relieving cramp. The bruised leaves in the form of an ointment with lard were also prescribed 'for all inflammatory conditions of the skin – and as an excellent remedy for the bleeding in piles', while 'periwinkle tea' was used as a general remedy for 'removing mucus in the intestines or lungs – for congestions – haemorrhages – various throat complaints, including inflammation of the tonsils.' The leaves of the herb are still administered for their astringent and tonic principles as in the treatment of menorrhagia and minor haemorrhages.

Culpeper recommended the small Periwinkle (*Vinca minor*) for similar complaints. This herb, now generally known as the Lesser Periwinkle, is a miniature version of the previous species, with evergreen leaves and solitary bluish-violet, or rarely white to pink flowers in spring. The fresh leaves in a tincture are still used in homoeopathic medicine.

A third species, the Madagascar Periwinkle (*V. rosea*, syn. *Lochnera rosea*, now *Catharanthus roseus*), a small sub-shrub up to 1m/3ft tall, bearing pinkish-white flowers, was formerly used in South Africa by the natives as a cure for diabetes. (The European species *V. major* had also been used for this purpose.) In the 1920s, it was found to contain several alkaloids, including two substances known as Vinblastine and Vincristine, both of which appear to inhibit the division of certain sorts of cancer-forming cells. Unfortunately the side effects of these substances were too severe for them to be really useful.

VIOLA

Violaceae, the Violet family
Heartsease, Sweet Violet

Most of this large genus is made up of hardy herbaceous perennials, although some are annuals, while a few are sub-shrubby plants, native to the tropical and temperate regions, including North and South America, Europe, the Mediterranean region, Asia, South Africa, Australia and New Zealand.

Of the medicinal species, one of the most familiar is the Heartsease or Field Pansy (*V. tricolor*). An erect or ascending branched annual, biennial or perennial up to 50cm/19in. tall, it has slightly downy, variable, heart to lance shaped leaves, and bears from March to November variable coloured flowers

of yellow, purple or white, or a mixture of all three. It grows in cultivated soils and grassy places throughout the whole of Europe, including the British Isles, North Africa and parts of Asia, Siberia and north-west India. In the wild the Heartsease also hybridizes with the Wild Pansy (*V. arvensis*) a variable, usually erect annual, generally with smaller flowers.

As a medicinal herb, the Heartsease was cultivated throughout Europe under the name of Herba Trinitatis or Trinity Herb which, with Three Faces in a Wood or Hood

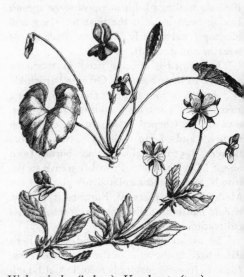

Viola tricolor (below), *V. odorata* (top)

and similar names, refers to the three colours in each flower. It was given 'for the heart – scald-head – pleurisy – skin diseases – convulsions – epilepsy and fits'. Gerard observes: 'It is good as the later physicians write for such as are sick of ague, especially children and infants – whose convulsions and fits of the falling sickness it is thought to cure.' Culpeper adds: 'A strong decoction or syrup of the herb and flower, is an excellent cure for the venereal disease.'

At one time the wild plant was listed in the Pharmacopoeias of the United States and is still prescribed there by herbalists, as it is in Europe, mainly for its diuretic and diaphoretic effects, in bronchitis, asthma and catarrh, especially in children, and as an

intment for treating various cutaneous
complaints such as eczema. A tincture made
from the whole plant with spirits of wine is
also used in homoeopathic medicine for skin
complaints and weakness of the heart.

Some of the Heartsease's other names
include Pansy (from the French Pensée),
Love-in-Idleness, Call (Cull)-me-to-you,
Bonewort, Biddy's Eyes, Trinity Violet,
Little-my-Fancy, Herb-Constancy, Kiss-me-
Love, Cuddle-Me, Jack-jump-up-and-kiss-
Me, Kiss-her-in-the-Buttry, Kit-run-in-the-
Fields, Pink-O-the-Eye, Godfathers, Pink-
eyed-John, Bird's Eye, Bullweed and Bane-
wort. Turner writes in his *Herbal*, the
Northern men 'call thys herbe banwurt
because it helpeth bones to knyt again . . .'

The use of the Sweet Violet (*V. odorata*) in
medicine dates back to the time of the ancient
Greeks. This low-growing, downy, creeping
perennial, has long rooting runners, with
rounded to heart-shaped leaves forming a
leafy rosette near the ground. It bears from
March to May sweetly scented deep violet or
white, occasionally lilac, pink or yellow
flowers, and is found in woods, hedges and
thickets throughout Europe and parts of Asia,
although now popular as an ornamental in
gardens and naturalized elsewhere. In the
wild the Sweet Violet often hybridizes with
the Hairy Violet (*V. hirta*) a similar European
species, but with narrower leaves with longer
hairs on the stalk, unscented flowers and no
runners.

In 300 B.C. Theophrastus recorded that
gardeners were so skilled in the cultivation of
the Sweet Violet, that plants with flowers on
were to be seen all the year round. Plutarch
later observed that the Romans planted it
among their garlic and onions. At about this
time the herb was bound to the head as a
preventer of headache, or giddiness, and as a
way of clearing hangovers. Its name frequently crops up in both the Greek and
Roman classics and it is mentioned by Homer
and Virgil. The herb was held in such high
regard in Athens that it became the city's
symbol, the Athenians using it to moderate
anger and bring about sleep. Pliny, on the
other hand, prescribed the root in vinegar as
a local application for relieving gout.

In ancient Britain the Celts are known to
have infused the flowers in goat's milk, their
womenfolk using it as a cosmetic, the Anglo-
Saxons in turn recommended the internal use
of the herb in the treatment of wounds, by
which time it was also regarded as an excellent
plant for dealing with wicked and evil spirits
or spells.

By the end of the sixteenth century several
different varieties of Sweet Violet were to be
found in English gardens. Gerard says of
their leaves, they 'are used in cooling plasters,
oyles and comfortable cataplasms or poultices,
and are of greater efficacies amongst other
herbs as Mercury, Mallowes, and such like
in clisters . . .' He also prescribed the herb
for inflammations, roughness of the throat, as
a comforter of the heart, as well as to
'assuageth the pains of the head' and to
'causeth sleep'. Tournefort writing about
syrup made from the flowers says it is 'a safe
and gentle Purger of young children'.
Besides this the plant was administered in
several forms for the 'ague in upgrown
people – falling sickness – fits – pleurisy –
jaundice – quinsies – diseases of the lungs –
hoarseness of the throat – the heat and
sharpness of the urine – and pains of the
bladder, back and reins.'

Towards the end of the nineteenth century,
fresh Violet leaves were externally applied in
hot compresses or fomentations and also
infused and taken internally for relieving the
pain of malignant tumours or cancers; several
reputed cures were reported. The fresh leaves
are still regarded as possessing certain antiseptic properties and can be applied as a local
compress, taken as a syrup or tea, or as a
liquid extract. As an expectorant the dried
flowers are prescribed in syrup or linctus for
the relief of coughs and colds.

The candied flowers of the Sweet Violet
were formerly taken as medicinal sweetmeats
and in Gerard's time were commonly known
as 'Violet Plates' and eaten not only for
pleasure, but as an expectorant for chest
complaints. Evelyn tells us the young leaves
could be fried and eaten with either orange
or lemon juice and sugar, and was of the
opinion they made a most 'agreeable har-
baceous dish'.

The flowers of the Spurred Violet (*V. calcarata*) were occasionally substituted for the above. Several other European species have been employed in medicine, including the Dog Violet or Heath Dog Violet (*V. canina*) a very variable plant with bright blue or pale blue flowers whose leaves and flowers were used in the treatment of skin disease. It also possesses strong cathartic and emetic principles. The Marsh or Bog Violet (*V. palustris*), which as its names suggest is found in bogs, marshes and wet heaths, was also used. A North American species known as Johnny-jump-Up or Early Blue Violet (*V. palmata*) was at one time used by the negroes to thicken soup, and this is generally found in mountain areas from Massachusetts to Minnesota and then south to Georgia.

The name of this genus, Viola, is derived from the Greek *ion*, violet-coloured, possibly referring to the flowers of many of the species.

VISCUM
Loranthaceae, the Mistletoe family
Mistletoe

Thirty or more species of Viscum are known to make up this genus of mostly parasitic plants, native chiefly to Europe, Asia, South Africa and Australia. Only one of these, the Common Mistletoe (*V. album*), was commonly used in medicine. This yellowish-green, semi-parasitic, mostly pendulous, branching evergreen shrub, attaches itself to several kinds of deciduous tree, usually on Apple trees, Poplars or Hawthorns. It bears thick leathery, elliptical stalkless leaves in pairs, and from February to April inconspicuous greenish-yellow flowers (the males and females on different plants) in stalkless clusters in the axils of the leaves. These are followed by round, white or occasionally yellow berry-like fruits. The species is found throughout most of Europe, central and northern Asia to Japan, south to North Africa.

The use of the Mistletoe dates back to the time of the ancient Druids, their High Priests crediting the plant with mystical powers. Pliny said the retreats of the Druids were in Oak groves, and whatever grew on an Oak tree was held in reverence by them, for it was regarded as a gift from heaven, especially the Mistletoe, probably because it was fairly rare. He goes on to say the Mistletoe was used as a cure for sterility and epilepsy, but to be effective it must never be allowed to touch the ground.

The generic name of this plant, Viscum, a very old Latin word, alludes to the viscous pulp of the berries, and is another name for birdlime. The specific *album*, simply means white, the usual colour of the berries. Its commonest name of Mistletoe is believed to

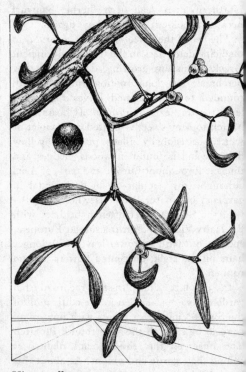

Viscum album

be derived from the Anglo-Saxon *misteltan*, where *tan* means twig, while *mistel* has possibly evolved either from *mist* in old Dutch meaning birdlime, hence Birdlime Twig, or *mistl*, meaning different, that is different from the tree it grows on. During the fourteenth century the name occurred as Mystyldene, which evolved in time to the present Mistletoe. According to another

Zingiber officinale (overleaf)

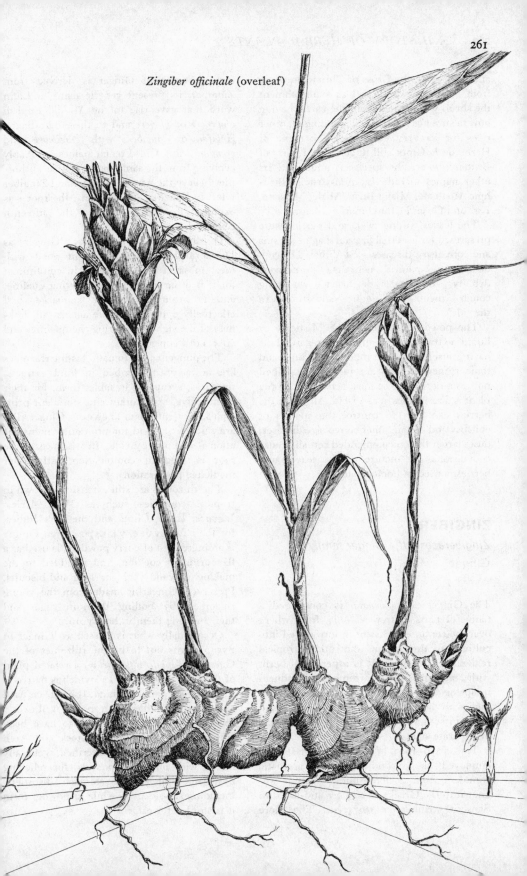

ancient legend, the Cross of Christ was made from Mistletoe wood, and as a punishment the shrub was banned from the earth, having now to suffer as a parasite depending on other trees for its very existence. The name of Herbe de la Croix still lingers on in parts of Brittany, where the species is abundant. Its other names include Lignum-Crucia, Bird-lime Mistletoe, Mislin Bush, Misle, Misselto, Kiss and Go and Churchman's Greeting.

The leaves, young twigs and berries were prescribed for 'internal haemorrhage – spasms and convulsive diseases – St Vitus's Dance – delirium – painful neuralgia – nervous debility – diseases of the heart – whooping cough – rheumatism – gout – and stitches in the side'.

The powdered leaves of the Mistletoe or liquid extracts of it, are still regarded as having useful antispasmodic, narcotic and tonic principles, but are mostly prescribed now as a nervine. The most active part of the plant is a resin known as Viscin. Although the berries can help to control the spasms of epilepsy and certain other convulsive diseases, doses larger than recommended actually cause convulsions. A tincture of the leaves and berries is used in homoeopathy.

ZINGIBER

Zingiberaceae, the Ginger family
Ginger

The Ginger (*Z. officinale*) is considered a native of parts of tropical Asia, from where over the centuries it has been introduced into cultivation throughout the other tropical regions of the world. It is a perennial herb, with a creeping jointed rhizome, that produces in spring a reed-like stalk about 60cm/23in. high with narrow green lanceolate leaves and bears in summer spikes of yellowish flowers on separate stems.

The dried root of this plant has been employed as a condiment and aromatic stimulant from ancient times, when it was known to the Greeks as *ziggiber* and listed in Sanscrit writings as *srngavera*. The more

familiar name of Ginger is derived from Zingiber, its present generic name, a Latin word that gave rise to the Middle English *gingivere* or *gingere* and to the Anglo-Saxon *gingifer* or *gingiber*, with *gingimbre* and *gimginre*, the Old French names, probably evolving from the same source. Other authorities believe the name of Ginger and Zingiber refer to Zanzibar from where the root was exported to Europe during the fifteenth century.

Of its uses Gerard says: 'Ginger as Dioscorides reporteth, is right good with meat in sauces, or otherwise in conditures; for it is of an heating and digesting qualitie, and is profitable for the stomacke, and effectually opposeth it selfe against all darkness of the sight; answering the qualities and effects of Pepper.'

The pungent and aromatic-tasting rhizomes are nowadays prescribed in fluid extracts, tinctures, syrups or in tablet form, for their carminative, expectorant and stimulant principles. Hot infusions known as Ginger Tea are said to be good for promoting menstruation if stopped by cold. In many cases the root is used in combination with other medicinal preparations.

The rhizomes are still extensively grown in tropical countries such as West Africa, Jamaica, India, China and the East Indies, for their food value, while powdered Ginger is an ingredient of curry powders, is used as a flavouring in cooking, and is added to the making of candy, ginger beer and biscuits. Preserved Ginger is made from the young rhizomes, by boiling them in sugar and then steeping them in hot syrup.

Occasionally what is classed as 'Ginger in Syrup' turns out to be the rhizomes of the Galanga (*Alpinia officinarum*) a related plant of the same Natural Order, which is native to the southern parts of China. It has been used as a spice in southern Europe for well over a thousand years and is known to have been employed in medicine by Greek and Arab physicians. It is still prescribed, generally mixed with other compounds, for relieving dyspepsia and similar stomach disorders, including sea-sickness, while in powder form it is snuffed for catarrh.

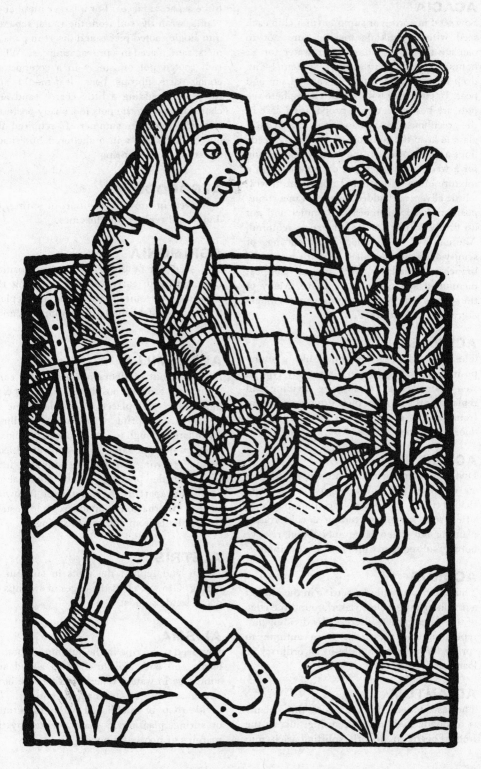

ACACIA

Sow seed in spring or summer (first chip each
seed with a penknife making sure not to
damage the 'eye' and soak in water for 24
hours), setting a little apart, 1–2cm/¼–¾in.
deep in well drained pots of sandy loam and
peat. In countries with a cool atmosphere the
pots are best placed in a propagating case in
the greenhouse, covering each with a sheet of
glass to keep the compost moist. As the seedlings appear, place on the greenhouse staging
for a week or so, then pot on separately in a
mixture of sandy loam and fibrous peat, with
a little silver sand added. Grow on in a sunny
position, keep soil moist in summer and pot
on firmly or plant out of doors as required.
Alternatively, in summer, insert cuttings of
semi-woody shoots pulled off with a piece of
branch attached, in pots of the compost
mentioned and grow on as above. Many of
the species require a minimum winter temperature of 4–7°C/40–45°F.

ACHILLEA

The two Achilleas mentioned like a sunny
position and will grow in almost any type of
well drained soil. Increase by dividing and
replanting the roots in their growing position,
from autumn to spring. Or sow seed out of
doors in spring.

ACONITUM

Divide roots in spring or autumn, planting in
an ordinary soil, in a sunny or partially
shaded position. Or sow seed in boxes of
sifted soil, spring, placed in a cold frame,
planting out when large enough on reserve
border, subsequently into growing position.

ACORUS

This plant is suitable for setting in the mud of
a marsh or the shallow water around the edge
of the water garden. Increase by dividing and
replanting the rootstocks from autumn to
spring. Will spread rapidly in an ordinary or
loamy soil.

ADIANTUM

The easiest method of increasing these plants
is to divide their roots in spring, just as the
fronds begin to uncurl, splitting each into

three separate pieces. For a larger number of
plants, wash the soil from the roots, separate
into single rooted pieces and insert in pans of
moist sand placed in a propagating case. When
well rooted pot on singly in a compost of
equal parts fibrous peat, leaf-mould and
turfy loam, adding a little coarse sand and
charcoal, placing the pots in a shady position,
watering freely in summer. If required for
out of doors plant in a sheltered but shady
moist position in spring.

AEGOPODIUM

Sow seed in growing position in spring, or
divide and replant the rhizomes.

AGRIMONIA

Sow seed out of doors in growing position
from spring to early summer, thinning the
seedlings as required. Or divide and replant
the roots of established plants from autumn to
early spring.

ALCHEMILLA

Sow seed out of doors in spring and early
summer in growing position. Or set in pots of
light sandy soil placed in a cold frame or
greenhouse in spring, transplanting seedlings
when large enough to 5cm/2in. apart, in boxes
of equal parts of sandy loam and rotted leafmould, growing on for the summer in a
partial shade, planting out of doors about
15cm/6in. apart in the autumn or following
spring. Alternatively, divide roots of established plants from autumn to spring.

ALETRIS

Divide and replant the roots in autumn or
spring. Grows well at the edges of swamps or
damp sandy woods.

ALISMA

Sow seed when ripe in the autumn, in pots of
loamy soil with a little charcoal added and
submerge in water. When seedlings are large
enough, plant in permanent position. Or
divide roots of established plants in autumn
or spring, planting in shallow water by the
margins of pools and ponds.

ALNUS
est raised from seed sown out of doors in
pring, in a bed of finely broken soil, or in
oxes of sandy soil placed in a greenhouse or
ame. When large enough plant seedlings out
5cm/6in. apart in lines in the nursery garden,
ansplanting every other year until required
r their permanent position. Will succeed in
wide range of wet and boggy soils, including
eavy clay. Alternatively, lift and replant the
uckers in winter.

ALTHAEA
ow seed out of doors in a sunny position,
te spring and summer, thinning seedlings to
5cm/6in. apart. On warmish soils transplant
flowering position in the autumn, other-
ise pot on and winter in frames, planting out
e following spring. Or sow seed in winter in
e greenhouse in boxes of sifted soil. When
rge enough plant seedlings in pots, harden
ff and plant out of doors in late spring,
referably in a deeply dug loamy soil, en-
iched with manure, watering well in dry
eather.

ANEMONE
Divide roots, or the rhizomes of the her-
aceous kinds, early spring or late autumn,
eplanting in growing position. Or insert root
uttings in boxes of sandy loam and leafmould
laced in a cold frame, setting out of doors the
ollowing spring. Alternatively, sow seed in
he autumn in pots of sandy soil placed in a
ame, although the seedlings tend to be slow
rowing.

ANETHUM
ow seed in spring, in shallow drills about
ocm/11in. apart, in a good garden soil, warm
unny position, thinning seedlings to 20cm/
in. apart. Gather stems as the lower fruits
pen, spread in an airy shed and thresh when
horoughly dry.

ANGELICA
ow seed in spring, preferably in a shady
osition, thinning seedlings when large
nough to 15cm/6in. apart. As they die after

flowering, renew by fresh ripe seed as necessary in late summer or early autumn. They
thrive particularly well near running water.

ANTHEMIS
Divide roots of established clumps, autumn
or spring, replanting a little apart. Or sow
seed in a well drained light to medium soil,
sunny position, from spring to early summer.

APOCYNUM
Divide roots and rhizomes of established
plants, autumn or spring, replanting a little
apart.

AQUILEGIA
The best method is to sow seed in a greenhouse in early spring, setting the seedlings
when large enough 7–8cm/2½–3in. apart in
trays of sandy loam and leafmould, growing
on in a cold frame. Plant out in early summer,
preferably in growing position to flower the
following year. Or sow seed out of doors,
early summer, thinning seedlings to 30cm/
11in. apart in autumn. Alternatively, divide
the roots of established plants in autumn or
spring, but as a rule these resent disturbance.
Will succeed best in an ordinary soil enriched
with leafmould, in a sunny or partially shaded
position.

ARISTOLOCHIA
Divide and replant the roots of the more
hardy herbaceous kinds in spring. Or insert
cuttings of ripe shoots in a sandy soil placed
in a cold frame, summer. Plant out of doors
the following year, when well rooted, early
spring or late autumn, in a good ordinary or
loamy soil. The climbing kinds are suitable
for growing over pergolas, walls and arches,
the herbaceous sorts are better set in the
herbaceous border. The more tender species
require a winter temperature of 12–15°C/
55–60°F and are often grown in the border of
the warm greenhouse in well drained pots or
tubs. The latter may be raised from seen
sown in spring, in a light rich soil, potting do
when large enough in a compost of two parts
fibrous loam, to one of leafmould and sharp
sand. Water freely in summer when growing.

ARTEMISIA

Divide and replant roots of the herbaceous kinds, autumn or spring. The more shrubby sorts are increased by cuttings inserted in a sandy compost, placed in a cold frame, late summer and early autumn, planting out when rooted the following spring, in an ordinary well drained soil, sunny position. Or sow seed out of doors in April.

. For a vigorous stock of Tarragon, remove cuttings of shoots from established plants in spring and insert in an ordinary soil under glass, planting outside when rooted. For a continuous supply of winter shoots, lift a few plants in the autumn, cutting back stems to 15cm/6in. and replant in boxes of ordinary garden soil, growing on in a greenhouse. In frost prone regions, the roots of plants out of doors are best protected with a layer of ashes during the colder months.

ARUM

Remove offsets or side pieces from established tubers during early autumn or spring. Replant in a partial shade, in an ordinary soil with leafmould added and protect with a layer of leaves in winter. Plant the more tender species at the foot of a protected wall or in the frost-proof greenhouse. If for pot cultivation, water freely when growing, drying off as the foliage dies.

ASARUM

Divide and replant the roots of established plants, autumn or spring. Sometimes used as an edging to the rock garden or shady border.

ASCLEPIAS

Sow seed in pots of sandy soil, placed in a cold frame, spring, planting out when large enough on reserve border. Or divide roots, autumn or spring, replanting in a peaty or leafy soil, sunny sheltered position. Some of the species, such as the Bastard Ipecacuanha require a minimum winter temperature of 15°C/60°F. Increase these in spring, by inserting cuttings of fresh young shoots in pots of sandy soil placed in a hothouse propagating frame. When rooted, pot on singly in a compost of equal parts peat, loam and leafmould.

ASPERULA

Divide and replant the roots of the perennia kinds in their growing position, autumn o spring. Or sow seed in spring in pots of sifted sandy soil placed in a shady cold frame planting out when rooted. Sow seed of annua kinds out of doors in a light rich soil in spring to flower during the summer months. A autumn sowing will produce flowers early th following year.

ATROPA

Sow seed in early spring in boxes of ordinar soil, with pieces of chalk or lime rubble adde for drainage, and place in a cool greenhous or frame. Plant out in early summer after th danger of frosts has passed and until estab lished water well, providing shade from th sun. Alternatively, sow seed out of doors spring or autumn, preferably in a light o gravelly soil with a chalky sub-soil, althoug germination is often patchy, sometimes takin several weeks. Cuttings of side branche removed from established plants in earl summer will also readily root.

BALLOTA

Divide and replant the roots of establishe plants, autumn or spring. Or sow ripe seed i growing position, thinning seedlings out a required.

BAPTISIA

Divide and replant the roots of establishe plants in autumn. Or sow seed in flowerin position in summer. They thrive in wel drained soil in a sunny position.

BELLIS

Lift and divide the roots as soon as th flowers have faded, spring or summer. Afte separating the pieces, replant about 8cm/3in apart on reserve border in a partial shad planting out in their permanent position i the autumn. This division of the plants best done annually, otherwise the flower deteriorate.

BERBERIS

Sow seed 2–3cm/½–1in. deep out of doors in a sheltered border in late autumn. Or set as soon as ripe (or early spring) in small trays placed in a cold frame. Compost 2 of loam, to 1 of leafmould and 1 of sand. When large enough plant singly in small pots, subsequently out of doors. Self sown seedlings are often to be found growing under the parent bushes, these can be dug up and replanted. Named varieties and hybrids that do not come true from seed are best increased by inserting cuttings of short ripened shoots 8–10cm/ 3–4in. long in a bed of sandy soil placed in a cold frame in late summer and early autumn, planting these out of doors the following year. Alternatively, layer the shoots in autumn or spring, or if they form detach and replant any suckers.

BETONICA

As for Stachys.

BIDENS

Sow seed of species mentioned in spring, in boxes of sandy soil placed in a greenhouse, planting seedlings out of doors in early summer, in a sunny position, ordinary soil. The Water Agrimony prefers a damp or wettish soil. Otherwise, divide and replant the roots of the perennial sort, autumn or spring.

BORAGO

Sow seed out of doors in spring, sunny position. When large enough thin seedlings to 30cm/11in. apart. Seed sown out of doors in autumn will flower the following year in early summer.

BRAYERA

Insert cuttings of firm ripened shoots in a very sandy soil in a greenhouse propagating case, late summer to early autumn. When large enough set singly in well drained pots of peat and loam with a little silver sand added. Requires a minimum temperature of 10°C/ 0°F.

BRUNFELSIA

Insert cuttings 5cm/2in. long in a greenhouse propagating case in summer, when rooted pot on singly in a compost of 2 parts fibrous loam to 1 part peat, 1 part leafmould and 1 part sand. Good drainage and firm potting is essential. Keep atmosphere moist by damping down floor and staging in summer, syringe foliage frequently and water freely when growing. Requires a minimum temperature of 10°C/50°F.

BRYONIA

Divide and replant roots in early spring. Or sow seed in growing position. Best positioned where there is something to ramble over, they thrive in almost any soil.

CALENDULA

Sow seed in an ordinary soil in spring to provide flowers in summer and early autumn, in September for blooms the following year. Thin seedlings or transplant as required.

CANNABIS

Sow seed thinly out of doors in growing position, spring. Lightly cover with soil, thinning seedlings to 45cm/17in. apart. Or sow seed in boxes of sandy soil placed in the greenhouse. When large enough prick out into other boxes, gradually harden off in a cold frame and plant outside in early summer.

CARUM

Sow ripe seed in a friable soil, late summer or the following spring, in drills 30cm/11in. apart, thinning the seedlings 15–20cm/6–7in. apart. The seed of the Parsley may take six weeks, or even longer to germinate. Water in dry weather.

CHELONE

Divide roots and replant in early spring, or in the autumn after the flowers have died. Or sow seed in pots of light soil placed in the greenhouse, spring. When large enough set seedlings 8cm/3in. apart in boxes. Compost, equal parts fibrous loam, leafmould and well rotted manure, adding a little sand. Grow on in a cold frame and plant out of doors the following year in early summer, sunny position.

CHENOPODIUM

All the species mentioned are easily raised from seed sown out of doors, preferably in deep, rich, fairly dry soil in spring, in a sunny place. For a succession of plants, sow seed of the various kinds at intervals throughout the summer, thinning to about 30cm/11in. apart when the seedlings are large enough. For use as a vegetable the young shoots are best harvested the following year, before the flowers develop.

CHIMAPHILA

Carefully divide and replant the roots in spring, taking care not to let them dry out. Set in a shady or semi-shady position, preferably in a sandy soil, well enriched with leafmould.

CHRYSANTHEMUM

Divide the roots of the herbaceous kinds, autumn or spring, replanting in growing position. Alternatively, both for these and the annual species, sow seed in flowering position in spring, thinning the seedlings out as required.

CICHORIUM

Sow seed of Chicory 1–2cm/½–¾in. deep in rows, late spring or early summer, preferably in a deeply-dug, well drained soil that was manured for the previous crop, thinning seedlings to about 20cm/7in. apart. During autumn lift the roots, cut the tops off and store in layers of sand or fine soil placed in boxes in a frost-proof shed. Alternatively, increase by root cuttings.

Endive is best raised from seed sown on a reserve bed, transplanting the seedlings when large enough to 30cm/11in. apart. If an autumn crop is required, sow seed in summer, in a well drained soil enriched with manure.

CICUTA

Divide and replant roots in a wet or very damp soil, autumn or spring.

CIMICIFUGA

Divide roots in autumn, replanting in a moist well cultivated soil, partially shaded position.

Or sow seed in a lightish soil placed in a cold frame, autumn, planting seedlings out of doors the following year.

CINCHONA

Insert cuttings of ripened wood in a mixture of loam and peat in a greenhouse propagator. When rooted pot on in a compost of equal parts of turfy loam and fibrous peat, with sand and a little charcoal added. Water freely when growing. Requires a minimum temperature of 12°C/55°F, but in the more temperate regions the species are sometimes grown in pots, tubs or the greenhouse.

COCHLEARIA

Sow seed of annual or biennial species in growing position, spring. The Horse Radish is readily increased by root cuttings inserted out of doors during the winter months. Good crops can be obtained by planting in a deeply dug, well manured soil.

COLCHICUM

Lift the corms as soon as the leaves die down, separate and replant immediately 5–8cm/2–3in. deep, about 15cm/6in. apart in a sandy or loamy soil enriched with leafmould. Do not disturb established plants unnecessarily. Alternatively, sow seed in summer or early autumn in pans or boxes of sandy loam and leafmould. Grow on in a frame and plant out of doors when twelve months old. Seedlings will take from 3 to 5 years to flower.

COLLINSONIA

Divide the roots or rhizomes, spring or autumn, replanting in a dampish soil, in partially shaded position.

CONIUM

Sow seed out of doors, spring, in growing position. (Some Pharmacopoeias recommend that only the leaves and young branches collected from plants in the wild should be employed in medicine.)

CONVALLARIA

Divide the roots of established clumps in autumn into crowns (each should have 2 or 3 buds), and replant about 8cm/3in. apart. Or sow seed in a reserve bed of light soil, March, when large enough plant out as above.

CORNUS

Besides layering the lower branches, or by removing the suckers from established shrubs, the majority of the species can be raised from seed which germinates freely. Sow as soon as ripe in a cold frame, or out of doors in spring. The roots of the herbaceous kind may be divided and replanted in spring. Alternatively, increase those with a shrubby nature by inserting cuttings of firm shoots in a sandy soil on a sheltered border in late autumn or winter.

CROTON

Insert cuttings of firm young shoots, singly in small pots of sandy soil, spring or summer, and place in a propagating case until rooted, potting on as required in a compost of 2 parts fibrous loam, to 1 of peat and sand. As most of the species require a minimum temperature of 12°C/55°F, they are generally raised in the temperate countries in the greenhouse, where they require a moist atmosphere and a position close to the glass. Water freely when growing.

CYCLAMEN

Sow seed of the more hardy kinds in well drained pans of light soil, spring, and place in a cool greenhouse or frame. As the first leaf develops transplant 2–3cm/¾–1in. apart in a light rich compost, and grow on in a cold frame allowing abundant air. Plant out in colonies, from summer to early autumn, in a rich friable loam with leafmould and a little brick or mortar rubble added. Position in a partial shade under trees or shrubs in the rock garden, or among hardy ferns. The more tender kinds are usually grown in the greenhouse from seed sown in late summer and autumn to provide blooms the following year. Simply press seeds into the compost and cover pans with a layer of moss until germination, which might take several weeks, keeping the soil fairly moist. When large enough, prick seedlings off into boxes, subsequently plant singly in pots in a compost of 2 parts loam, to 1 part leafmould with sand

added. Ventilate greenhouse in mild weather, but do not allow the temperature to fall below 7°C/45°F.

DAEMOMOROPS

Sow seed in pans of a sandy soil placed in a hothouse propagator, spring. When large enough, pot on in a compost of equal parts loam, peat, leafmould and sand. Although tropical plants requiring a minimum temperature of 15°C/60°F, they can be grown in a hothouse. Water freely when growing in summer, keep atmosphere moist and frequently syringe.

DAPHNE

Sow seed out of doors as soon as ripe in boxes of equal parts fibrous loam, peat and silver sand, covering with a layer of ashes. In early spring lift boxes and bring into a warm greenhouse, where the seed will usually germinate after several weeks. Alternatively, layer the shoots of the lower branches in autumn. When rooted plant in growing position, autumn or spring, preferably in a good light loam. Dryness at the roots should be avoided.

DATURA

The annual species including the common Thornapple are easily raised from seed sown out of doors, early summer. In cooler countries the seed is best sown in pots of light soil, placed in the greenhouse, spring, potting on singly, subsequently planting out of doors, early summer, in a light rich soil, sunny position. The shrubby sorts can be increaed either by seed or by inserting cuttings of shoots about 15cm/6in. long in pots of sandy soil placed in the greenhouse, spring or autumn. Cover with a bellglass until rooted, pot on as necessary, subsequently planting in spring into large well drained pots or tubs of equal parts loam and peat, with rotted manure and silver sand added. (These can be placed out of doors as ornamentals or dot plants in summer). Water freely when growing, very little from late autumn till spring. The majority of the shrubby species require a minimum winter temperature of 7°C/45°F.

DELPHINIUM

Sow seed of the annual species in their flowering position, spring, in a rich well drained ordinary soil. Or sow in boxes of light soil, placed in the greenhouse March. When large enough prick seedlings off into other boxes, harden off and plant out of doors, early summer, 15–20cm/6–7in. apart. Sow seed of the perennial species in the greenhouse, late winter; in a cold frame spring; or in the reserve border out of doors from spring to early summer, planting in flowering position, autumn or spring, into a deep well drained soil. Alternatively, insert cuttings of young basal shoots in small pots of sandy soil placed in a cold frame, spring. Keep frame closed and shade from the sun until rooted, then harden off and plant out of doors.

DIGITALIS

Sow seed in flowering position, spring or early summer, thinning seedlings if required to 15cm apart. They do best in a moist shady soil, and will seed themselves freely.

DRIMYS

Layer lower branches in spring. Or insert cuttings of ripened wood in a cold frame, autumn. Alternatively, sow seed in a warm greenhouse in spring. When large enough, plant seedlings out of doors in a sheltered border or grow against a warm wall, in a well drained loamy soil, with a little peat added. Will succeed in milder frost free regions only. Otherwise set in the border of a frost-proof greenhouse.

DROSERA

Divide the roots of the larger plants, spring, setting the individual crowns out of doors in the bog garden in live sphagnum moss. A more successful method is to cultivate these plants in the greenhouse, setting the roots in well drained pans of equal parts sphagnum moss and peat, with a little moss, sand, charcoal and crushed pot added, setting the pans in saucers of water. Alternatively, sow seed on the surface of a similar mixture at any time, but preferably spring, placing the pans in a saucer of water under a bellglass. Grow on in a sunny greenhouse or frame in a moist position.

DUBOISIA

Insert cuttings under a bellglass placed in the greenhouse, summer, potting on when rooted in a sandy loam. In the temperate regions these shrubs require the protection of a warm greenhouse.

EQUISETUM

Divide roots in spring, replanting in an ordinary soil in a moist shady position bog garden, or by the margins of pools and ponds.

ERIGERON

Sow seed out of doors in a light soil, sunny position, spring.

ERYNGIUM

Divide roots, spring or autumn, and replant in growing position, but do not disturb unnecessarily. Or sow seed in boxes of sandy soil placed in a cold frame, spring, setting out of doors the following autumn (or spring).

ERYTHRONIUM

Remove offsets from parent bulbs, early autumn, and replant 7–8cm/2–3in. deep, about 5cm/2in. apart, in a well drained but moist peaty or loamy soil, in a partial shade, sheltered position. If for the greenhouse set bulbs or offsets 2–3cm/¾–1in. deep, in pots of equal parts loam, peat and leafmould, summer, wintering pots in a cold frame, keeping soil fairly dry. Bring into the greenhouse in late winter and early spring to flower, watering moderately from this time.

ERYTHROPHLOEUM

Insert cuttings of half-ripened shoots with a heel attached, in a compost of equal parts sand and peat, placed in a propagating case, warm greenhouse. Or sow seed as soon as ripe under similar conditions. In temperate regions this tree requires the protection of a hothouse or stove.

EUCALYPTUS
In countries free from frost the various species, including the Blue Gum, can be raised from seed sown out of doors in a good soil and warm position. Otherwise sow in the greenhouse in pots of sandy soil, late winter and early spring. Alternatively, insert cuttings of side shoots in a similar soil, in a propagating case with a little bottom heat, early summer. When large enough, set singly in pots of 2 parts fibrous loam, to 1 part leafmould, sand and charcoal. Water freely in summer, moderately otherwise.

EUPHORBIA
Divide roots of the hardier kinds, spring or autumn, replanting in an ordinary or stony soil, on banks, dry borders and in sunny rockeries. Or sow seed in flowering position, late spring. Alternatively, insert cuttings in a sandy soil placed in a cold frame, summer. The more tender species usually succeed if raised in a sunny greenhouse. Increase by inserting cuttings 7–8cm/2–3in. long of young shoots, in well drained pans of sandy loam placed in a greenhouse propagator, late spring and summer. When large enough, pot on in a compost of equal parts fibrous loam and peat, with sand and some brick rubble added. Water freely when growing, carefully otherwise. Some of the latter group require a winter temperature of 10–12°C/50–55°F.

FOENICULUM
Sow seed in growing position, spring, thinning or transplanting the seedlings to 30cm/11in. apart. Or, at the same time, divide and replant the roots of established clumps. Both the Florence Fennel and the Carosella are readily raised from seed sown in drills, though the former requires rich, well-cultivated soil and plenty of water in dry periods.

FUMARIA
Sow seed, late spring in an ordinary soil, flowering position. If necessary train growth over a trellis.

GENTIAN
Most of the genus can be increased by seed, while the roots of some of the perennial kinds may be divided. To raise from seed it is best sown in the autumn in boxes, which are then exposed in the open to frost and snow. In spring, place the boxes in the shelter of a frame or greenhouse to encourage germination. The majority of the species are tolerant of a loamy soil.

GERANIUM
Sow seed of both annual and perennial kinds in a sunny growing position, spring. Or divide and replant roots of the perennials, autumn or spring. They thrive best in light, well-drained soils.

GEUM
Sow seed in boxes of ordinary soil placed in a cold frame, spring. When large enough set seedlings on the reserve border for the summer, replanting in their permanent places, autumn, where they will flower the following year.

GLECHOMA
Insert cuttings of flowerless shoots about 7–8cm/2–3in. long in a bed of sandy soil, shady position, in summer, covering with a cloche or handlight. Keep soil moist, but to avoid any damping off, remove moisture from the glass every morning. When well rooted, plant out in growing position.

GRATIOLA
Carefully divide and replant the roots or rhizomes in a dampish or wettish soil, autumn or spring.

HELLEBORUS
Divide and replant roots of well established plants in spring, leaving each individual piece at least four growth buds. Once established do not disturb for at least 5 or 6 years. They do best in moist, but well-drained soil, enriched with manure or leafmould.

HERNIARIA
Divide and replant roots in growing position, at any season.

HUMULUS

Divide and replant roots of the perennial sort, winter or spring. Or insert cuttings of young shoots 7–10cm/2–4in. long, singly in small pots placed in a warm frame, planting out of doors when rooted. Both the annual and perennial kinds can be raised from seed sown in the greenhouse, or outside in a warm sheltered position, spring. Will thrive in a soil enriched with manure and wood ash.

HYDROCOTYLE

Divide and replant the roots in spring, in a very damp or wet position.

HYOSCYAMUS

Sow seed thinly in early or late summer, growing position, preferably in a light fairly rich, well drained soil, thinning seedlings to 60cm/24in. apart. Germination is often patchy and in some cases the seed may remain dormant in the soil for several weeks.

HYPERICUM

Divide the roots of the herbaceous sorts, including the Common or Perforated St John's Wort, autumn or spring. Alternatively, insert short cuttings of soft shoots in a sandy soil placed in a warm frame, summer, planting the rooted cuttings out of doors from late autumn to early spring.

HYSSOPUS

Sow seed out of doors in a warm position, spring. Or insert cuttings in a shady border or cold frame, spring or towards the end of summer, planting out of doors when rooted about 30cm/11in. apart, watering until established.

ILEX

Sow seed, spring, out of doors, or in pots and boxes in the greenhouse, depending on whether hardy or not. Or insert cuttings of short shoots about 10cm/4in. long removed with a heel attached, in a sandy soil placed in a warm frame or greenhouse, where they will take several months to root. Some of the more tender species require protection from frost if grown in temperate countries, or they may be raised in the greenhouse. The seed of the Holly takes from 1 to 3 years to germinate although this is the usual method of increasing the species. The best method is to collect the berries, mix them in moist sand and place out of doors for a year, turning occasionally. Sow the seed after the second spring, keeping sand and seed together, and cover with a sandy or gritty soil. Transplant in autumn (not winter) when about 45cm/17in. high to growing position, making sure the roots are moist. It generally takes about 2 years for the Holly to recover after being transplanted, the trees may even lose their leaves, although these form again the following year.

INULA

Divide roots autumn or spring and replant in growing position. Or set pieces in boxes of sandy soil, placed in a cold frame, autumn planting out of doors the following spring. Alternatively, sow seed in reserve border spring, planting seedlings in growing position autumn.

IRIS

Divide and replant the rhizomes, bulbs and rootstocks of the various kinds in their growing positions as soon as the flowers are finished. Or sow seed when ripe in pans of light sandy soil placed in a cold frame, pricking the seedlings off into boxes subsequently planting out of doors. Germination of the seed is rather irregular and may take 15 months or more.

JUGLANS

Remove walnuts from the trees when ripe and stratify in sand for the winter to prevent them from drying out. Sow in spring preferably where they are to grow. Otherwise set on the reserve border and after the first year lift carefully, trim the roots and replant, transplanting annually until required for setting in permanent positions. Avoid frosty positions as spring frosts can damage the young growth of some species.

KRAMERIA

Insert cuttings in a sandy loam, greenhouse propagating frame, potting on when rooted in compost of sandy loam and fibrous peat. In temperate regions these plants will only grow in the hothouse.

LEONURUS

Sow seed in an ordinary soil, growing position, autumn or spring, transplanting when large enough to about 30cm/11in. apart.

LEVISTICUM

Sow seed as soon as ripe (otherwise in spring) in growing position, transplanting seedlings about 30cm/11in. apart. Alternatively, divide and replant roots in early spring. Prefers rich, moist, well-drained soil in a sunny position.

LIATRIS

Divide and replant the roots in growing position, spring. Or sow seed in a well prepared soil, summer, thinning seedlings out as required. Alternatively, sow seed in pots or boxes of sandy soil placed in a cold frame, spring. When large enough prick seedlings off into other boxes of light soil and grow on in a cold frame. When well established plant out of doors on reserve border and when large enough into their permanent quarters.

LIGUSTICUM

Sow seed out of doors, autumn or spring, in a rich moist, well drained soil, thinning seedlings to 30cm/11in. apart. Or divide and replant roots in spring.

LILIUM

Lift, separate and replant bulbs and bulblets in the autumn as the stems and leaves turn yellow. (An exception to this is the Madonna Lily, which produces a tuft of leaves in autumn and therefore should be divided earlier.) Or remove the looser scales from the bulbs, preferably spring, otherwise in the autumn, setting these in shallow pans of sandy soil, placed in a cold frame or greenhouse, and cover with a sheet of glass, later transplanting to the compost suitable for the species concerned. The majority of the species may also be raised from seed sown when ripe about 2cm/¾in. deep in drills, in a moist cool border out of doors, protected from the midday sun, the seedlings generally appearing by the following spring. When large enough set out in lines on the reserve border until large enough to plant in permanent positions. The rarer species are best sown in a sandy soil in an unheated greenhouse or frame. The Madonna Lily does best in a deep rich, lime containing soil, while the Tiger Lily and its varieties will thrive in an ordinary soil. The American Turk's Cap Lily, however, prefers a mixture of leafmould and sandy peat, or a lime-free sandy loam.

LINARIA

Divide and replant roots of the perennial kinds, autumn or spring, in growing position. Sow seed of annual species out of doors, or thinly in pans of light soil placed in a frame, spring. When large enough set seedlings some 5cm/2in. apart in boxes of similar soil and grow on until ready for planting out, preferably in a light well-drained soil. It is, however, apt to be invasive.

LUPINUS

Sow seed out of doors, late spring, thinning seedlings as required. Alternatively, sow sparingly in pots of sandy loam, placed in a greenhouse or frame, early spring, planting out of doors in growing position, early summer.

LYSIMACHIA

Divide and replant roots in growing position, autumn or spring. Or sow ripe seed out of doors from spring to early summer. Will grow well in sun or shade. Can also be increased by removing and planting the rooted runners.

MALVA

Divide and replant roots of perennial kinds in an ordinary soil, autumn. Or sow seed outside on reserve border, late spring, transplanting the seedlings when large enough to growing positions. Sow seed of annual kinds as soon as ripe, or in spring.

MANDRAGORA

Sow seed when ripe, or in spring, out of doors or in a frame, transplanting seedlings towards the end of summer into a lightish rich well-drained soil. Otherwise, divide and replant roots in spring.

MARRUBIUM

Divide and replant roots in spring. Or insert cuttings, spring, in a sandy soil placed in a cold frame, keeping frame closed until roots have formed. Alternatively, sow seed thinly out of doors, early summer, transplanting seedlings to 15cm/6in. apart on reserve border, and to their final positions the following year.

MARSDENIA

Insert cuttings of shoots in a warm close frame, summer, planting when rooted in an ordinary soil, sheltered position. In cooler or frost prone regions, set in the greenhouse border, training growth up a wall.

MELIA

Insert cuttings of well ripened side shoots, removed with a heel of old wood attached, in pots of sandy soil, placed under a handlight or glass out of doors in summer, airing for a few minutes daily to prevent excessive dampening. When rooted, pot on singly in a mixture of 3 parts loam to 1 part sand. In milder regions plant out of doors in a sandy loam, sunny sheltered position, keeping roots moist in summer. Otherwise grow on in large pots or tubs in the greenhouse. Requires a winter temperature of 4°C/40°F.

MENISPERMUM

Lift, divide and replant the suckers or underground stems in the autumn. Or sow seed out of doors, growing position, early summer. The Levant Nut if grown in cooler countries requires the shelter of the hothouse and can be increased by inserting root cuttings in an ordinary soil. The Pareira vine needs similar treatment and is best increased by inserting cuttings of shoots in pots of fibrous loam, summer, although it will take up a lot of room.

MENTHA

Divide and replant roots in a moist growing position, spring, each piece having a joint should grow. Or insert cuttings of young shoots in a shady border, summer. Alternatively, insert cuttings in a moist closed frame, planting out when rooted.

MITCHELLA

Divide roots, early spring, replanting in a light moist soil enriched with leafmould. Or sow seed in a light soil, frame or greenhouse, spring. Does well in rock gardens if in a semi-shaded position.

MUCUNA

Sow seed in pots of lightish soil, spring, placed in a greenhouse propagating frame, potting on singly when rooted. Usually grown in the temperate countries as a hothouse ornamental.

MYRISTICA

Insert cuttings of ripe shoots in pots of sand placed in hothouse propagating case. Or if obtainable sow fresh seed under similar conditions, taking care not to damage the tap root. When large enough, pot on cuttings or seedlings in a sandy loam and fibrous peat. In cooler countries the Nutmeg can only be grown in a hothouse.

NEPETA

Divide and replant roots in growing position, spring. Or insert cuttings of flowerless side shoots in pots or boxes of sandy soil, placed in a closed, shaded cold frame, summer, moistening occasionally. As the roots form gradually ventilate, water more freely, and when ready plant outside on reserve border or permanent site.

NICOTIANA

Sow seed in pots or pans of light soil placed in a warm greenhouse, late winter or early spring, providing shading until seedlings appear. When large enough, prick seedlings off into boxes, about 5cm/2in. apart, in a compost of loam and leafmould, subsequently setting singly in pots. In early summer harden off in a frame and plant out of doors, growing position, in a good well-drained sandy soil. The leaves for smoking are generally harvested in twos or threes in early autumn as they begin to mottle, a second picking being made a week or so later. These however, should be properly dried and 'cured' before using.

OCIMUM
Sow seed out of doors, early summer, or in pans or boxes of equal parts loam and leaf-mould, placed in a warm greenhouse, early spring. When large enough, prick seedlings off into boxes of a similar compost, planting outside, early summer, in a well-drained soil, sunny sheltered position.

OPHIOGLOSSUM
Divide the roots, autumn or spring, replanting in growing position, lightly covering the rhizomes with soil. Prefers fairly moist loamy soil with leafmould added, in a partially shaded place.

ORIGANUM
Divide and replant the roots of the perennial kinds, autumn or spring. As some of the species are only half-hardy and likely to damage by frost, they are sometimes grown as annuals, and raised from seed sown out of doors in late spring, or a little earlier in boxes of sandy soil placed in a heated greenhouse. When large enough prick off seedlings 7–8cm/2½–3in. apart in boxes of light soil, keeping shaded and fairly well watered until established, before hardening off and planting out of doors, early summer, in a well-drained soil enriched with manure. Alternatively, increase the more shrubby kinds in spring, by inserting cuttings of side shoots in small pots of sandy soil, placed in a warm greenhouse, potting on as the roots form. Some of the more tender species are best grown in the greenhouse with a winter temperature of not less than 7°C/45°F.

OROBANCHE
These plants will only grow if in contact with a suitable host. Therefore sow seed near the roots of the appropriate plant. The perennial sorts often live on the roots of their hosts for several years before sending up their flowering stems.

OSMUNDA
Divide and replant roots in growing position, spring or autumn. Alternatively, sow ripe spore in pans of well-drained finely sifted compost sprinkling a little charcoal on the surface. (Do not cover the spore.) Set container in a saucer of water, cover with a sheet of glass and place in a cold frame. As the fronds begin to develop, this may take several weeks, prick off 2–3cm/¾–1in. apart into pans of a similar compost, keeping the plants shaded for a time, subsequently potting on for use in the greenhouse or setting out of doors. The Royal Fern thrives best in a deep moist situation, especially if planted by the edge of a pond or stream. The Moonwort is much more tolerant of a drier soil.

PAPAVER
Sow seed thinly out of doors, sunny position, spring or late summer, in an ordinary but friable, well raked soil, preferably one that was manured for the previous crop, thinning the seedlings as required.

PARIS
Divide and replant roots in their growing position, autumn or spring. Does best in a shady position in light, moist soil.

PHYSOSTIGMA
Sow seed in hothouse propagating frame, summer, potting on when rooted, subsequently planting in large tubs or hothouse border. In temperate regions the Calabar Bean will only grow in the hothouse, where it requires plenty of room.

PHYTOLACCA
Divide and replant roots in their growing position, autumn or spring. Alternatively, sow seed in a sheltered position, spring.

PLANTAGO
Sow seed of both annual and perennial species out of doors, spring, in growing position. Or divide and replant roots of the perennial kinds, autumn or spring.

POLYGONATUM

Divide and replant roots in their growing position, autumn or spring. Or sow seed in autumn, which will germinate in early spring. Can also be grown in the unheated greenhouse to provide early flowers, by potting up pieces of root in the autumn in a loamy soil, watering through winter as the soil dries.

PRIMULA

Sow seed as soon as ripe in a shady position, transplanting seedlings when large enough to permanent quarters. Or sow in pans of sifted loam and leafmould with a little silver sand added. Water well after sowing, cover containers with a sheet of glass and a piece of paper and place in a cold frame, pricking seedlings off into boxes, subsequently planting in growing position out of doors. Alternatively, divide and replant the roots of the perennial kinds such as the Cowslip and Primrose in autumn.

PSYCHOTRIA

Divide and replant the roots in a moist soil, shady position, autumn. Only rarely grown in the temperate countries, where it requires the shelter of a warm greenhouse.

PULMONARIA

Divide and replant the roots in growing position, preferably slightly shaded, in autumn or spring.

RHUS

Sow seed in a well-drained light loamy soil, placed in a cold frame, spring, planting seedlings out of doors the following year. Species with strong shoots and long leaves, i.e. the Staghorn Sumach, can be increased by cutting up pencil thick pieces of root into lengths about 20cm/7in. long, setting these in boxes of leafmould or very leafy soil, in the greenhouse, or out of doors, spring. Alternatively, increase those with thin shoots, by inserting cuttings of half-ripe shoots about 10cm/4in. long in a propagating case in summer.

ROSMARINUS

Insert cuttings of firm side shoots out of doors, or in a cold frame, late summer or early autumn. Transplant the following autumn to about 30cm/11in. apart on reserve border, subsequently into their permanent positions. For a bushy habit pinch out tips. Alternatively, layer the lower branches, severing when rooted and replant in growing position. It does best in a light, well-drained soil in a sunny position.

RUTA

Sow seed out of doors, spring, thinning seedlings to 15cm/6in. apart, transplanting when large enough to their growing positions. Or insert cuttings of side shoots in a similar soil, late summer and early autumn, planting out when well rooted. Does best in a light, well-drained soil, in a partially sheltered position. At one time the plant was used as a low dividing hedge between beds in kitchen gardens.

SALVIA

Divide and replant roots of the perennial sorts, autumn, although plants increased this way generally take time to recover. Or insert cuttings of shoots 7–8cm/2½–3in. long in a sandy soil in a close frame or greenhouse, planting out of doors when rooted. Alternatively, sow seed in a greenhouse or frame, spring, covering containers with glass, keeping moist and shaded until germination. When seedlings reach about 5cm/2in. high, set out of doors on reserve border or growing position. Otherwise sow seed of annual kinds out of doors, spring and early summer, flowering position, thinning seedlings to 15cm/6in. apart. Most of the species will thrive in a well-drained loamy soil in a sunny position.

SAMBUCUS

Sow seed as soon as ripe out of doors, or in boxes of loamy soil placed in a frame or greenhouse. When large enough, set seedlings on reserve border subsequently into permanent position. Or insert cuttings of firm shoots out of doors, autumn. Otherwise, divide roots of the herbaceous kind at about the same time.

SANICULA

Divide and replant the roots in their growing position, preferably in autumn (otherwise through to spring), setting the pieces about 20cm/7in. apart. Prefers a rich, moist soil, in a shady position.

SAPONARIA

Divide and replant the rhizomes in growing position, from autumn to spring. Or sow seed in a cold frame, from spring to early summer, planting out when large enough.

SASSAFRAS

Remove and replant suckers in a loamy, well-drained soil, autumn or spring. Or sow seed in a sunny sheltered position, or in the greenhouse if district liable to frosts, planting out of doors when large enough.

SCABIOSA

Divide and replant roots in growing position, spring. Or sow seed out of doors, autumn or spring. When transplanting set in groups, making sure to firm soil around roots.

SCOPOLIA

Sow seed out of doors, autumn or spring, in growing position, thinning seedlings as required.

SENECIO

Sow seed of the annual and biennial kinds out of doors in permanent position, spring and early summer. Divide and replant the roots of the herbaceous sorts, autumn or spring. Alternatively, sow seed of the latter group out of doors, early summer, transplanting seedlings to reserve border, and when large enough to their permanent site. The more shrubby ones may be increased by inserting cuttings of well ripened shoots in pots of sandy soil placed in a cold frame, autumn, planting out of doors when rooted.

SIEGESBECKIA

Sow seed out of doors in permanent position, early summer. Or treat as a half-hardy annual, by sowing in a warm greenhouse, spring, planting seedlings out of doors, early summer, in an ordinary soil.

SIMABA

Insert cuttings of ripe wood in sand, placed in a hothouse propagating frame, or sow imported seed. When rooted or large enough, pot on in a compost of well-drained turfy loam. In temperate regions the Cedron requires the shelter of a hothouse.

SOLANUM

Sow seed of the hardier species out of doors in a well-drained soil, spring, thinning seedlings as required. Or as with the perennial kinds insert cuttings of young wood in pots of sandy soil placed in a greenhouse with a little bottom heat. Or sow seed early spring, in well-drained pans of sandy soil placed in the greenhouse, potting on for use as greenhouse ornamentals, or harden off and plant out of doors. Alternatively, in spring, divide and replant the roots of the tuberous kinds, i.e. the Potato and Horsenettle. Some of the species are rather tender and require a night temperature of $7°C/45°F$, and are therefore best grown in a greenhouse.

SOLIDAGO

Divide and replant the roots of the more vigorous plants from autumn to early spring. Will succeed in a sunny or partially shaded position.

STACHYS

Divide and replant the roots and rhizomes in their growing position, autumn or spring.

STRYCHNOS

The species of this genus are rarely cultivated. In temperate countries they are occasionally seen as climbers in the hothouse, and can be increased by sowing seed in a hothouse propagating frame in summer.

SYMPLOCARPUS

Divide roots, autumn, replanting in a wet or very moist soil, well enriched with decaying leaves.

TARRAXACUM

Sow seed thinly out of doors in permanent quarters, spring or autumn, thinning seedlings as required.

TRILLIUM

In spring divide and replant roots in required site, preferably a cool and partly shaded one. Or sow seed as soon as ripe (otherwise in spring) in a cold frame, in pans of loam and leafmould with a little silver sand added.

TUSSILAGO

Divide and replant the roots or rhizomes in their growing positions, autumn.

ULMUS

Sow ripe seed thinly out of doors on reserve border, growing on there until large enough to plant in permanent positions. Otherwise detach and replant the suckers, autumn. (The Male Fern mentioned can be increased in early spring, by division of its rootstock or rhizomes, and is best planted in a compost of equal parts loam and peat. Set out of doors in open woodland or shady position, or in the greenhouse).

URGINEA

Remove and replant the offsets from the parent bulbs in spring. In countries susceptible to frost these are best pot grown in a light airy greenhouse. If grown this way, half bury the bulbs in a compost of equal parts loam and leafmould with sand freely added, watering sparingly until growth commences, freely as the roots form, reducing in the autumn.

URTICA

Divide and replant the roots of the perennial species in their growing position, spring and early summer. Alternatively, sow seed, as with the perennial sorts, in spring.

VERBASCUM

Sow seed as soon as ripe, or in early summer, on reserve border, transplanting seedlings to 15cm/6in. apart, subsequently setting in their growing positions, autumn.

VINCA

Divide and replant the roots in their growing position, autumn or spring. In cooler regions the Madagascar Periwinkle requires the protection of a greenhouse.

VIOLA

Sow seed out of doors in early summer, thinning seedlings as required. Or sow in spring, in pans of loam, leafmould and silver sand placed in a frame, pricking off when large enough into boxes of a similar compost, planting out of doors in summer. Alternatively, divide the roots of the perennial sorts, or remove and replant the rooting runners when flowering is over.

VISCUM

If for cultivation the Mistletoe can be established on a host plant in spring by rubbing the seed fresh from the berries into the crevices of the tree, or in the clefts between the branches, leaving enough of the sticky fruit to hold the seed in place. As the male and female flowers form on different plants to ensure a good crop of berries, it is necessary to establish plants of both sexes. The two most suitable hosts are the Hawthorn and the Apple, and others include the Maple, Poplar, Willow, Cedar, Larch, Oak, Mountain Ash and similar trees with a softish bark. A second species, *Viscum cruciatum* from south-west Spain, with red berries was sometimes substituted for the above.

ZINGIBER

Divide the roots into small pieces and replant on ridges of well worked soil, early spring. In temperate regions the Ginger will only grow in a hothouse.

Glossary of Medicinal Terms

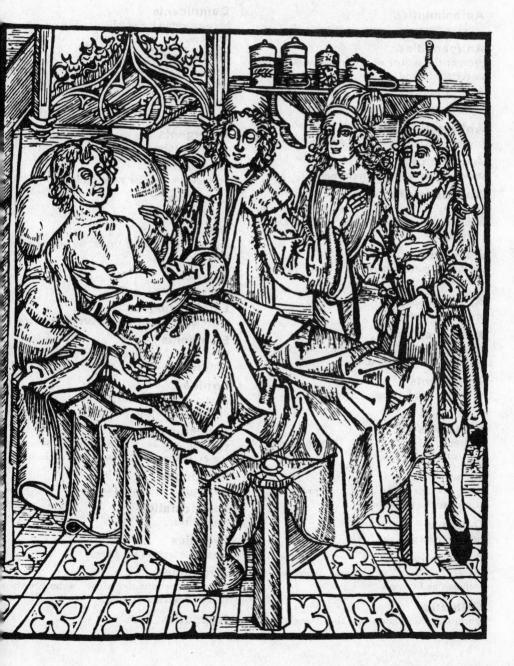

Absorbents or Antacids
counteract acidity of the stomach and bowels.

Alteratives
gradually restore the normal functions of the body.

Anodynes
relieve pain.

Anthelmintics
expel or cause the death of worms in the body.

Antiperiodics
prevent the return of periodic diseases, such as certain fevers.

Antiscorbutic
to be used against scurvy.

Antiscrofulous
prevent or cure scrofulous diseases.

Antiseptics
prevent infection or putrefaction.

Antispasmodics
relieve or cure spasms, or irregular and painful action of the muscles, as in St Vitus' Dance, epilepsy, etc.

Aperients
produce a natural movement of the bowels – a laxative.

Aphrodisiacs
excite sexual desire.

Aromatics
have a fragrant smell, generally with an agreeable, pungent taste.

Astringents
shrink or bind, causing a contraction of the tissues.

Balsamics
soothing medicines of a smooth and oily consistency.

Bitters
sharp acrid or biting medicines, prescribed to stimulate the appetite.

Cardiacs
have an effect on the heart.

Carminatives
dispel flatulency or griping pains of the stomach and bowels.

Cathartics
stimulate the action of the bowels – a purgative.

Cholagogues
produce or evacuate bile.

Correctives
improve or restore to a healthy state.

Decoction
essence of plant extracted by boiling the plan down.

Demulcents
have a soothing or emollient effect on inflame surfaces.

Deobstruents
remove obstructions, can clear or open th natural passages and ducts of the body.

Depuratives
cleanse or purify.

Detergents
cleansing substances.

Diaphoretics
promote or increase perspiration.

Digestives
aid the digestion.

Diuretics
increase the flow of urine, by acting on th kidneys.

Emetics
cause vomiting.

Emmenagogues
assist and promote the menstrual discharge.

Emollients
have a soothing and softening effect on th body tissues.

Errhines
generally snuffed into the nose to increase th discharge of mucous fluid and cause sneezing

Expectorants
cause an increase in expectoration, promotin the excretion of mucous from the chest.

Febrifuges
help reduce or control fevers.

Haemostatics
control bleeding.

Hepatics
have an effect on the liver.

Hydrogues
remove accumulations of water, causin watery evacuations.

Hypnotics
cause sleep.

nsecticides
ill insects.

rritants
ause irritation.

Laxatives
oosen the bowels and relieve constipation.

Mydriatics
ilate the pupils of the eyes.

Myotics
ontract the pupils of the eyes.

Narcotics
iminish the action of the nervous and
ascular systems, causing drowsiness,
ethargy, stupor and insensibility.

Nephritics
ave an effect on the kidneys.

Nervines
ooth and calm the nerves, restoring them to
natural state.

Nutritives
ourish the body, promoting growth or
ealth.

Parasiticides
estroy parasites.

Parturients
nduce labour and help in childbirth.

Pectoral medicines
elp to relieve affections of the lungs.

Purgatives
vacuate the bowels, but more forcefully than
n aperient or laxative.

Refrigerants
educe fevers, relieve thirst and bring a feeling
f coolness.

Resolvents
elp to relieve and reduce swellings or
flammations.

Rubefacients
pplied as counter irritants to the skin, causing
edness and blistering.

Sedatives
ssen nervous excitement, irritation and pain.

Sternutatories
ritate the mucous membrane and cause
eezing.

Stimulants
roduce energy.

Stomachics
digestive tonics.

Styptics
help to control bleeding by contracting the
tissues or blood vessels.

Sudorifics
cause or increase copious perspiration.

Taenicides
expel tapeworms from the body.

Tonics
invigorate or stimulate, producing a feeling of
well-being or strength.

Vermifuges
expel worms and other parasites from the
body.

Vulneraries
used in the healing of wounds.

Bibliography

General Books of References, Sources and Further Reading

The following list is by no means a complete one, but is a general account of the works referred to in the course of research. The dates given are not necessarily the dates of the original printing.

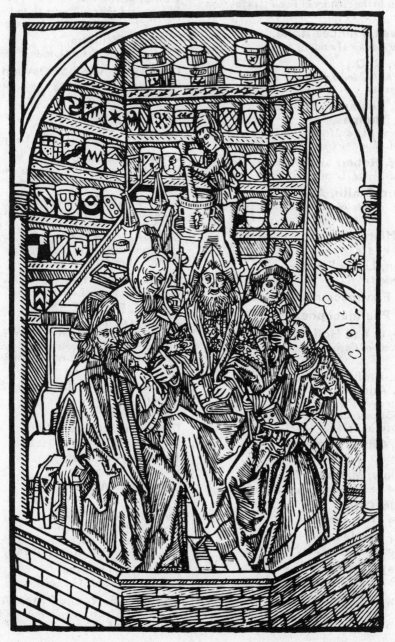

Amherst, Alicia,
A History of Gardening in England (London)
1897

Andrews, Edward Deeming,
Shaker Herbs and Herbalists (Stockbridge,
Massachusetts) 1959

Arber, Agnes,
Herbals Their Origin and Evolution
A Chapter in the History of Botany 1470–1670
(Cambridge) 1953

Bardswell, Frances Anne,
The Herb Garden (London) 1911

Barlow, R. O.,
The Complete Modern Garden Herbal (Pennsylvania) 1945

**Barton, Benjamin, H. and
Castle, Thomas,**
*The British Flora Medica; or History of the
Medicinal Plants of Great Britain* 1845

Bentley, Robert and Trimen, Henry,
Medicinal Plants (London) 1880

Bernhard-Smith, A.,
Poisonous Plants of All Countries (London)
1923

Bock, Hieronymus,
His Herbal 1552

Bowden, Lorna Frances,
Wild Flowers of Europe (London) 1969

British Pharmaceutical Codex

British Pharmacopoeia

Britten, J. and Holland, R.,
A Dictionary of English Plant Names (London)
1886

**Britton, Nathaniel and
Brown, Addison,**
*An Illustrated Flora of the Northern United
States, Canada and the British Possessions*
(New York) 1913

Brown, Oliver Phelps,
The Complete Herbalist (London) 1871

Brownlow, Margaret Eileen,
Herbs and the Fragrant Garden (London) 1957

Brunfels, Otto,
Herbarum Vivae Eicones 1532

Bryant, Charles,
Flora Diætetica (London) 1783

Bulkeley, Robert,
His Book 1641

Bullein, William,
*Bulleins Bulwarke of Defense Againste all
Sicknes, Sorhes and Woundes* (London) 1562

Chaucer, Geoffrey,
(1340?–1400) *The works of, various editions*

Chittenden, Frederick James,
Dictionary of Gardening (Oxford) 1971

Clendening, Logan,
Source Book of Medical History (London/New
York) 1942

Coats, Alice M.,
Flowers and their Histories (London) 1968
The Book of Flowers (London) 1973

Cobbett, William,
The English Gardener (London) 1833

Cockayne, Thomas Oswald,
*Leechdoms, Wortcunning and Starcraft of
Early England* (London) 1864

Coles, William,
Adam in Eden (London) 1657
The Art of Simpling (London) 1656

Cooper, Samuel,
*A Dissertation on the Properties and Effects of
the Datura Stramonium* (Philadelphia) *c.*1797

Culpeper, Nicholas,
A Physicall Directory (London) 1649
The English Physician etc. (London) 1652
Culpeper's Herbal or the English Physician etc.
1652; published by Dr George Alexander
Gordon (London) 1802

Curtis, William,
Flora Londinensis (London) 1835

Deakin, Richard,
*The Flora of the Colosseum of Rome or, Illus-
trations and Descriptions of Four Hundred and
Twenty Plants Growing Spontaneously upon
the Ruins of the Colosseum of Rome* (London)
1855

**Dispensatory of the United States of
America**
(Philadelphia)

Dodoens, Rembert,
Cruÿde boeck (Antwerp) 1554

Drayton, Michael,
Poly-olbion (London) 1622

Emboden, William,
Narcotic Plants (London) 1972

Evelyn, John,
Acetaria (London) 1699
A Discourse of Forest Trees (London) 1776
Kalendarium Hortense (1664) 1679

Fairchild, Thomas,
The City Gardener (London) 1722

Fitter, R. S. R. and Fitter, A.,
*The Wild Flowers of Britain and Northern
Europe* (London) 1974

Foster, Gertrude,
Herbs for Every Garden (New York) 1966

Fraser, Sir Thomas,
On the Characters, Actions and Therapeutic Uses of the Ordeal Bean of Calabar (Edinburgh) 1863

Fuchs, Leonhard,
De Historia Stirpium (Basel) 1542

Gardener, Richard,
Kitchen Gardening 1599

Gerard, John,
A Catalogue of Plants (1596–99); edited by B. D. Jackson (London) 1876
The Herball or Generall Historie of Plants 1597

Gerard's Herbal
Enlarged by Thomas Johnson 1636

Gilmour, John Scott and Walters, Stuart Max,
Wild Flowers (London) 1969

Gorkom, K. W. van,
A Handbook of Cinchona Culture (Amsterdam and London) 1883

Gray, Asa,
A Manual of the Botany of the Northern United States etc. (New York and Chicago) 1867

Grieve, Maude,
Culinary Herbs and Condiments (London) 1933
A Modern Herbal (London) 1974

Grete Herbal
1526

Grew, Nehemiah,
Anatomy of Plants (London) 1682

Grigson, Geoffrey,
A Herball of all Sorts (London) 1959
The Englishman's Flora (London) 1955

Guthrie, D.,
History of Medicine (London) 1947

Hanmer, Sir Thomas,
The Garden Book; Edited by Ivy Elstob 1933

Harley, John,
The Old Vegetable Neurotics: Hemlock, Opium, Belladonna and Henbane etc. (London) 1869

Hatfield, Audrey Wynne,
How to Enjoy Your Weeds (London) 1969
Pleasures of Wild Plants (London) 1966
The Magic of Herbs (London) 1970

Hedrick, U. P.,
A History of Horticulture in America till 1860 (London and New York) 1950

Hill, John,
(calling himself Sir John Hill)
A General Natural History, etc. (London) 1751
The British Herbal (London) 1756
The Family Herbal (Bungay) 1820

Hvass, Else,
Plants That Serve Us (London) 1960

Hyll, Thomas,
The Proffitable Arte of Gardening (London) 1568

Inglis, B. D.,
Wild Flowers of Britain (London) 1969

Johnson, G. W.,
History of English Gardening 1829

Johns, Rev. C. A.,
Flowers of the Field (London) 1882

Josselyn, John,
New England Rarities Discovered (London) 1672

Kelly, Stan,
Eucalypts (London and Sydney) 1970

Kent, Elizabeth,
Flora Domestica (London) 1823

Kingsbury, John M.,
Deadly Harvest (London) 1967
Poisonous Plants of the United States and Canada (Englewood Cliffs, New Jersey) 1964

Langham, William,
The Garden of Health (London) 1579

Law, Donald,
Herb Growing for Health (London) 1969

Lawson, William,
The Countrie Housewife's Garden (London) 1617

L'Ecluse, Charles de,
Rariorum Plantarum Historia (Antwerp) 1601

Lindley, John,
Flora Medica (London) 1838

Lloyd, J. U.,
Origin and History of all the Pharmacopoeial Vegetable Drugs (Cincinnati) 1929

Loudon, John Claudius,
An Encyclopaedia of Plants (London) 1829
An Encyclopaedia of Gardening (London) 1860

Lupton, Thomas,
A Thousand Notable Things (1660 edn) (London) 1579

Lyte, Henry,
A Niewe Herball (1619 edn) 1578

Macleod, Dawn,
A Book of Herbs (London) 1968

Markham, C. R.,
Peruvian Bark (London) 1880

Markham, Gervase,
The Country Housewife's Garden (London) 1613
The English Husbandman (London) 1613
The English HusWife (London) 1615

Masefield, G. B., Wallis, M., Harrison, S. G. and Nicholson, B. E.,
The Oxford Book of Food Plants (London) 1969

Matthiolus,
Commentarii 1560

Mawe, Thomas and Abercrombie, John,
Every Man His Own Gardener (17th edn) (London) 1776

McClintock, D. and Fitter, R. S. R.,
The Pocket Guide to Wild Flowers (London) 1956

McIntyre, A. R.,
Curare – Its History, Nature and Clinical Use (Chicago) 1947

Mead, William Edward,
The English Medieval Feast (London) 1931

Medsger, Oliver Perry,
Edible Wild Plants (New York) 1966

Miller, Joseph,
Botanicum Officinale, or a Compendious Herbal (London) 1722

Miller, Philip,
The Gardener's and Florist's Dictionary (London) 1724
Catalogus Plantarum (London) 1730

Monardes, Nicolas,
Joyfull Newes Out of the Newe Founde World (1569) Translated into English by John Frampton in 1577

Moulton, C. W.,
A Biographical Encyclopaedia of Medical History (New York) 1905

Muenscher, W. C. and Rice, M. A.,
Garden Spice and Wild Pot-herbs (New York) 1955

Nelson, A.,
Medical Botany (Edinburgh) 1951

Newton, James,
A Complete Herbal (London) 1805

North, Pamela,
Poisonous Plants and Fungi in Colour (London) 1967

Osol, A. and Farrar, G. E.,
The Dispensatory of the United States of America (Philadelphia) 1960

Palladin,
On Husbandry (*c.*1420) A late undated copy

Parkinson, John,
Paradisi in Sole, Paradisus Terrestris 1st edn 1629 2nd edition, much enlarged and corrected, 1656
Theatrum Botanicum (London) 1640

Passe, Crispin de,
Hortus Floridus etc. 1614

Pechey, J.,
Compleat Herbal of Physical Plants (London) 1707

Pitton de Tournefort, Joseph,
The Compleat Herbal 1719

Phillips, Henry,
Flora Historica (London) 1824
History of Cultivated Vegetables, etc. (London) 1822

Platt, Sir Hugh,
The Garden of Eden (London) 1594

Polunin, Oleg,
Flowers of Europe (London) 1969

Polunin, Oleg and Huxley, Anthony,
Flowers of the Mediterranean (London) 1972

Polunin, Oleg and Smythies, B. E.,
Flowers of South-West Europe (London) 1973

Prior, R. C. A.,
Popular Names of British Plants (London) 1863

Ray, John,
A Collection of Curious Travels and Voyages in Two Volumes (London) 1697
Historia Plantarum etc. Vol. I 1686; Vol. II 1688; Vol. III (London) 1704
Synopsis Methodica Stirpium Britannicarum etc. 1694

Rea, John,
Flora, Ceres and Pomona (London) 1665
Flora; Seu, De Flora Cultura (London) 1676

Rhind, William,
A History of the Vegetable Kingdom 1887

Robinson, W.,
The English Flower Garden (London) 1883

Rohde, Eleanour S.,
The Story of the Garden (London) 1932
The Old English Gardening Books (London) 1972

Salmon, William,
Botanologia. The English Herbal: or History of Plants etc. (London) 1710

Sanders' Encyclopaedia of Gardening
Revised by A. G. L. Hellyer (London) 1971

Scott, J.,
The Mandrake Root (London) 1946

Sheldrake, Timothy,
Botanicum medicinale, A Herbal of Medicinal Plants etc. (London) 1759

Slavik, Bohumil,
Wild Flowers, Ferns and Grasses (London) 1974

Step, Edward,
Wayside and Woodland Trees (London and New York) 1904

Stevenson, Rev. Henry,
The Gentleman Gardener's Director (London) 1769

Stoerck, A.,
An Essay on the Internal Use of Thornapple, Henbane and Monkshood 1763

Stuart, G. A.,
Chinese Materia Medica (Shanghai) 1911

Sydenham, Thomas,
A Treatise on the Gout (London) 1660

Taylor, G. M.,
British Herbs and Vegetables (London) 1947

Taylor, Joseph,
Nature the Best Physician: or A Complete Domestic Herbal 1818

Taylor, Norman,
Plant Drugs that Changed the World (London) 1966

Theophrastus,
His Enquiry into Plants translated by Sir Arthur Hort, 1916

Thomas, H. H.,
The Book of Hardy Flowers (London) 1920

Thomas, H. H. and Forsyth, Gordon,
The Popular Encyclopaedia of Gardening (3 vols.)

Thornton, Robert John,
A Family Herbal (London) 1810

Tradescant, John,
Musaeum Tradescantianum (London) 1656

Trease, George Edward,
A Textbook of Pharmacognosy (London) 1961

Turner, William,
Libellus de Re Herbaria novus etc. (London) 1538
A New Herball (in 3 parts) 1551–68

Tusser, Thomas,
Five Hundred Pointes of Good Husbandrie (1810 edn) (London) 1573
July's Husbandry (London) 1577

Withering, William,
An Account of the Foxglove and Some of its Medicinal uses etc. (Birmingham) 1785

Woodville, William,
Medical Botany 1794

Wren, R. C.,
Potter's New Cyclopaedia of Botanical Drugs and Preparations (London) 1956

Indexes of Botanical and Vernacular Names

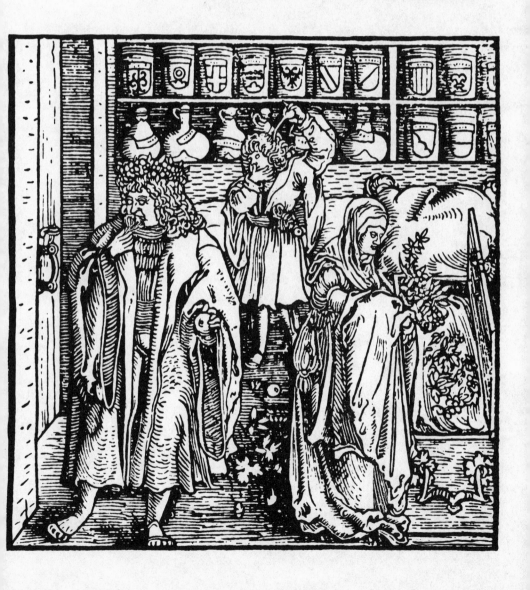

Index of Botanical and Vernacular Names

BOTANICAL INDEX

Figures in brackets refer to the pages on which illustrations appear

VERNACULAR NAME INDEX

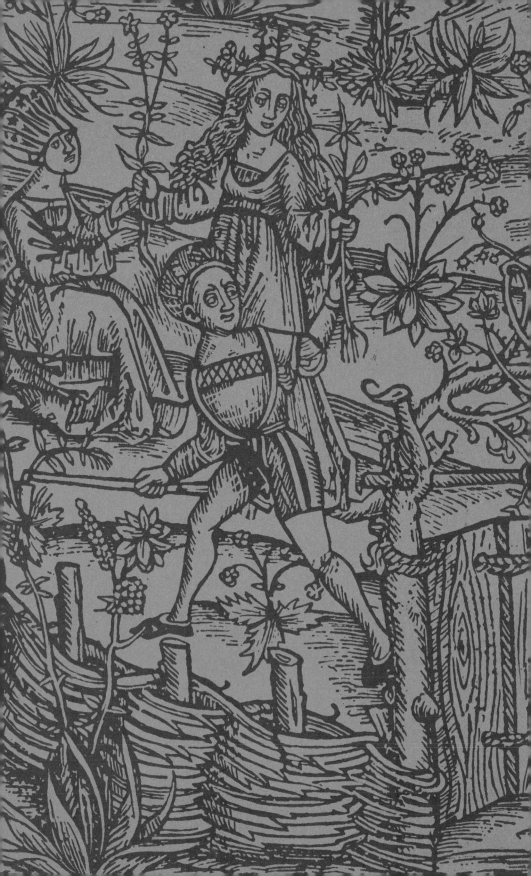